Trivedi's Gynaecology

Dr Amarendra Nath Trivedi, MBBS (Honours)

Diploma in Obstetrics, MRNZCOG, FRANZCOG, DDU, AFRACMA

Obstetrician, Gynaecologist, and Ultrasonologist

Associate Professor, Monash University Melbourne

Former Director, Women's, Children's, and Adolescent Health,
Peninsula Health, Melbourne, Australia

Examiner for Monash University and RANZCOG

Former Examiner for New Zealand Registration Examination

Assessor RANZCOG for Specialist International Medical Graduates

Dr Ashish Pandey, MBBS (Honours)

Austin Hospital, Melbourne

First edition August 2017

ISBN: 0648085503
ISBN 13: 9780648085508

The authors can be contacted at
reception@drtrivedi.com.au

Dedication

The book is dedicated to my teachers, especially Dr. Norman E. MacLean, and my family—Alka, Ayush, Ayesha, and Akash—for standing by me through thick and thin and making me what I am today.

—Amarendra Nath Trivedi

I would like to heartily thank my whole family, my close friends, and especially my inspiring coauthor, who continue to guide, nurture, and support me.

—Ashish Pandey

Table of Contents

Dedication iii

Table of Contents v

Foreword viii

Preface ix

How to Use This Book x

Chapter 1. How to Answer Short Answer Questions 1

Chapter 2. Menstruation and Its Disorders 5

2.1. Clinical Physiology of Menstruation 5

2.2. Dysmenorrhoea 6

2.3. Premenstrual Syndrome (PMS) and Premenstrual Dysphoric Disorder (PMDD) 8

2.4. Dysfunctional Uterine Bleeding 17

2.5. Heavy Menstrual Bleeding 22

2.6. Primary Amenorrhoea 29

2.7. Secondary Amenorrhoea 45

Chapter 3. Disorders of Puberty 53

3.1. Delayed Puberty 53

3.2. Precocious Puberty 58

Chapter 4. Early Pregnancy Complications 67

4.1. Miscarriage 68

4.2. Recurrent Miscarriage 85

4.3. Ectopic Pregnancy 96

    4.3.1. Tubal Pregnancy 98

    4.3.2. Cornual Pregnancy 104

    4.3.3. Ovarian Pregnancy 105

    4.3.4. Abdominal Pregnancy 105

    4.3.5. Cervical Pregnancy 106

4.4. Gestational Trophoblastic Disease 117

Chapter 5. Gynaecological Infections 133

5.1. Sexually Transmitted Infections (STIs) 133

5.2. Vaginal Discharge 142

Chapter 6. Pain 151

6.1. Pelvic Inflammatory Disease 151

6.2. Chronic Pelvic Pain 158

6.3. Dyspareunia 165

6.4. Endometriosis 169

Chapter 7. Disorders of Fertility 179

7.1. Polycystic Ovarian Syndrome 179

7.2. Infertility 192

    7.2.1. Infertility 193

7.2.2. Ovarian Hyperstimulation Syndrome (OHSS)..................................204

7.2.3. Assisted Reproductive Technology 206

7.2.4. Hyperprolactinaemia..206

7.2.5. Unexplained Infertility..211

7.2.6. Male Infertility..211

7.2.7. Surrogacy 213

Chapter 8. Contraception..231

8.1. Combined Oral Contraceptive Pill..231

8.2. Oestrogen-Only Contraception 233

8.3. Progestin-Only Contraception..236

8.4. Intrauterine Contraceptive Devices 239

8.5. Emergency Contraception..242

Chapter 9. Menopause...253

9.1. Menopause 253

9.2. Premature Menopause (Premature Ovarian Failure) 260

9.3. Benefits and Risks of HRT...261

9.4. Postmenopausal Bleeding (PMB)..263

Chapter 10. Urogynaecology 275

10.1. Pelvic Organ Prolapse...275

10.1.1. Anterior Vaginal Wall Prolapse (Urethrocoele and Cystocoele) 282

10.1.2. Posterior Vaginal Wall Prolapse (Rectocoele and Enterocoele).....284

10.1.3. Uterine Prolapse..285

10.1.4. Vaginal Apical Prolapse 286

10.1.5. Summary of History and Examination..288

10.1.6. Summary of Management 289

10.2. Urinary Incontinence 300

10.2.1. Incontinence..301

10.2.2. Urinary Tract Infection...303

10.2.3. Urethral Syndrome (Urethral Pain Syndrome) 305

10.2.4. Painful Bladder Syndrome (Interstitial Cystitis) 305

10.2.5. Stress Incontinence 307

10.2.6. Urge Incontinence..310

10.2.7. Mixed Incontinence..313

10.2.8. Overflow Incontinence 313

Chapter 11. Benign Diseases of the Uterus 329

11.1. Fibroids 329

11.2. Adenomyosis...345

11.3. Endometrial Polyp 348

11.4. Uterine Perforation during Hysteroscopy/Curettage 350

Chapter 12. Benign Diseases of the Cervix 355

12.1. Clinical Physiology of the Cervix..355

12.2. Cervical Intraepithelial Neoplasia 356

12.3. Cervical Polyps 364

12.4. Nabothian Follicle (Cyst)...364

12.5. Ectropion..364

Chapter 13. Benign Diseases of the Ovary **377**

13.1. Ovarian Cysts and Benign Neoplasms...377

13.2. Ovarian Cysts in Pregnancy 385

Chapter 14. Benign Diseases of the Vulva **399**

14.1. Lichen Sclerosus 401

14.2. Lichen Planus..402

14.3. Lichen Simplex 403

14.4. Psoriasis Vulvitis 404

14.5. Candida Vulvovaginitis...405

14.6. Vulvodynia..406

14.7. Vulvar Intraepithelial Neoplasia..407

Chapter 15. Malignant Diseases of the Uterus **417**

15.1. Endometrial Cancer 417

15.2. Uterine Sarcoma 424

Chapter 16. Malignant Diseases of the Cervix **439**

16.1. Cervical Cancer...439

Chapter 17. Malignant Diseases of the Ovary **453**

17.1. Ovarian Cancer 453

17.2. Borderline Malignant Ovarian Tumours 459

Chapter 18. Malignant Diseases of the Vulva **473**

18.1. Vulvar Cancer..473

Chapter 19. Drugs Used in Gynaecological Surgery **481**

19.1. Antibiotics in Gynaecological Surgery 481

19.2. Thromboprophylaxis in Gynaecological Surgery.............................482

Foreword

It is with pleasure and great honour that I write this foreword for Trivedi's Gynaecology.

Amarendra (Amar) Trivedi has been a colleague and a friend for more than 10 years. I have had the privilege to visit his unit at Peninsula Health numerous times and to see how he has transformed it into an excellent teaching and training unit.

For a nobody to write a Foreword is challenging but I was amazed at Amar's persistence.

As an academic it is very clear to me that our speciality is obstetrics 'heavy'. Therefore, it is wonderful to have a book such as Trivedi's Gynaecology to highlight the importance of gynaecology in the management of women's health.

The two goals in the preface clearly state why the book was written and the preamble on MCQs and SAQs is a must read for all students – undergraduate and post graduate.

The chapters cover all of Gynaecology in a succinct way and each chapter is capped with some priceless resource of SAQs and MCQs. The language is easy to understand the sub headings have a clear link all throughout.

To put up to date references and show levels of evidence for each chapter means this body of work will need to continue year after year!

I thoroughly recommend this book to all undergraduate and post graduates of all levels.

Congratulations Amar – work for a life time begins.

Best wishes,

Professor Ajay Rane OAM
MBBS MSc MD FRCOG FRCS FRANZCOG CU FICOG (Hon) PhD FRCPI (Hon)
Mater Pelvic Health Education & Research Unit
Townsville-Cairns, Australia

Preface

The medical profession is a lifelong journey of learning. We learn by reading books and journals, by talking to other colleagues, by our own experiences, and—last but not least—by our mistakes, both intended or unintended, and our near misses.

We have been and will remain part of this journey for the rest of our careers. As part of this journey, Dr Trivedi has been fortunate to be involved with the enjoyable responsibility of imparting knowledge, mentoring, assessing, writing questions and setting standards at all levels of examinations in multiple countries. We have been students, examinees, and examiners at all levels.

Experiences gained while perfecting our skills for this craft have enabled us to give a shape to this book. Our endeavour has been to provide to our readers a comprehensive, contemporary, and evidence-based concept of disease processes. The style of expression builds from basics to advanced facets of the principles and practices of gynaecology. The multiple-choice and short-answer questions with their model answers also reflect the same pattern. Students (undergraduate, diploma, and fellowship) can absorb and assimilate depending upon their level, requirements, and aptitude.

Dr Pandey has been the Dux of King's College, Auckland, New Zealand, and excelled in the MBBS examination of Monash University, Melbourne. This was not just by chance. In fact, nothing was left to chance. This was possible because of his ability to understand the processes mentioned above, to introspect, and to reflect. We have endeavoured to dissect and then disseminate this information to the doctors of tomorrow. The doctors of today will find this book fruitful, functional, and factual.

We would like to express our immense gratitude to our students, registrars, and colleagues for their constructive feedback and encouragement. Without that, the contents of the book would not have been as useful to the different levels of readers.

This book is an unparalleled collection containing a description of diseases with levels of supporting evidences, ultrasound appearance of lesions, and over 450 multiple-choice and 170 short-answer questions with their model answers. We are confident that this book will not disappoint those in pursuit of excellence in clinical practice as well as in preparation for examinations.

—Amarendra Nath Trivedi and Ashish Pandey

How to Use This Book

A very unique feature of this book that has intimately shaped how it has been written is the partnership between an experienced clinician with extensive knowledge on the topic and examination setting and a recently graduated doctor who excelled in his medical degree. This has resulted in a book that is relevant for all levels of readers and is appropriate for both examination revision and as a point of reference.

This book has been written with two goals:

- To help different levels of students and examinees (undergraduate, diploma students, and postgraduates) in enriching their knowledge base and to enable them to excel in the examinations.
- To act as an easy resource to doctors practicing gynaecology.

Let us discuss the first goal. The book has a chapter on almost every gynaecological condition. The text is up-to-date with all of the scientific information and level of evidence, where available. Most chapters have short-answer and multiple-choice questions. The text provides a detailed concept of the disease, whereas the questions extend the boundaries of the reader's knowledge even further.

To prevent repetition, the answers to the questions are mostly not in the text. So, to get a wide knowledge of the topic, the reader is encouraged to read both the main text and the questions at the end. The questions have different degrees of difficulty and complexity. Undergraduate students may choose to confine themselves to simple questions such as history, differential diagnosis, management of a condition, or equipment needed to examine a woman with uterovaginal prolapse. For postgraduate students, there are more complex questions, such as whether hysterectomy should be part of all vaginal-prolapse surgery, the current state of use of mesh in gynaecological surgery, whether CIN III should be treated by a hysterectomy, and so on. A large number of questions are based on past examinations of different levels in Australasia, the United Kingdom, and the Indian subcontinent. There is also a section on how to answer short-answer questions; it is largely based on our experience and observations, and it will be very useful to examinees.

This book has over 450 multiple-choice questions and over 170 short-answer questions with model answers, in addition to the main text. This will provide an unparalleled resource to readers, all in one place.

We are confident that this book has all the information required to excel in an examination.

With regard to the second goal of this book, there are plenty of flowcharts and treatment options, with their pros and cons. Doctors practicing in gynaecology will find the book an easy resource and reference.

The evidence classification has been taken from the Royal College of Obstetricians and Gynaecologists. Following are the criteria for different levels of evidence:

- IA: Evidence obtained from meta-analysis of randomised controlled trials
- IB: Evidence obtained from at least one randomised controlled trial
- IIA: Evidence obtained from at least one well-designed controlled study without randomisation
- IIB: Evidence obtained from at least one other type of well-designed quasi-experimental study
- III: Evidence obtained from well-designed nonexperimental descriptive studies, such as comparative studies, correlation studies, and case studies
- IV: Evidence obtained from expert committee reports on opinions and/or clinical experience of respected authorities

How to Answer Short Answer Questions

A very important part of succeeding in medical school examinations—or any specialty examinations—beyond having an in-depth knowledge of the content, is to be able to apply knowledge to answer multiple-choice questions (MCQs) and short-answer questions (SAQs) to get the full marks.

There is no single way to prepare for examinations. People have different methods of learning and understanding, and so it is not possible to prescribe an exact way to study. However, there are some general rules that are applicable to everyone, regardless of whether you study better alone or in a group, whether you listen to music or draw pictures, or whether you transcribe textbooks to your own notebook in perfectly neat handwriting.

First, you should have a clear plan of what you need to study and by when you would like to have each topic completed. Second, when you sit down to study, you must ensure that all distractions are removed and that your full focus is dedicated to your studies, to ensure that the time you spend reaps the greatest reward. Third, as you go through the year and steadily amass your knowledge and understanding, continually reflect on your strong and weak areas. An excellent way to do this is with practice questions, which can help you quickly identify areas in which you may not be as competent as you might have thought. This also means that you can go back to the weaker areas and study them again, because it is well known that repetition is a highly effective habit to consolidate knowledge.

Many colleges and universities provide model answers to the examiners to remove subjectivity and enhance reproducibility as far as humanly possible during marking. A marking schedule is also provided for the same reason. The candidate is awarded marks only when his or her answers carry the same meaning as the model answer or have the same words as in the model answer. The candidate does not get any mark or gets very few marks if that answer, even though correct, is not in the model answer.

Short-answer questions are open-ended questions that ask the candidate to display a firm understanding of the topic as well as the ability to adapt content to a variety of patient vignettes. It is crucial, therefore, that you can answer questions in the most direct and concise way (to save time) possible to ensure you attain all available marks. Because these examinations are often time-pressured, the technique of answering short-answer questions as briefly in words as possible, is very important. At the same time, your answer should be as broad as possible, so that it includes all the areas mentioned in the model answer. Single words, such as "bilateral" (instead of "the tumour is bilateral") and "Incidence = 60%" (instead of "the incidence of this tumour is 60% in the general population") will also fetch the full marks. Identifying the key words in a question that will advise the level of detail and type of answer that is required to get the marks cannot be overemphasised. Some of these words are shown in the table in this chapter.

Time permitting, answer the question in an easy-to-read prose style with good grammar and correct spelling. But often the questions are so many and the time so little that this will not be achievable. Incorrect spelling gives a poor impression to the examiner, which may reflect in marking, where the examiner has some discretion.

Where the answers to multiple-choice questions (MCQs) are limited to only a handful of possible selections, the possible answers to short-answer questions (SAQs) are wide-ranging; however, the examiner will only give marks based on one set of correct answers or answers that are in the model answer. To assist a candidate to provide the necessary information in the answer without surplus, examiners use specific words in the question as a guide to the length of answer.

For example, consider the following question: "Compare the levonorgestrel-containing IUCD with endometrial ablation in the treatment of heavy menstrual bleeding." The key "question word" in this question is *compare*, which means the examiner wants the candidate to discuss the similarities and differences between two or more things. An example of how to answer this would be to create a table in which the two items being compared, *levonorgestrel-containing IUCD* and *endometrial ablation*, would form the two column headings. Each row would then be a different characteristic of treatment of heavy menstrual bleeding—for example, *mode of action*—and then the similarities and differences could be entered in the corresponding parts of the table.

The following is a list of question words that are used in SAQs, with the kind of information that you should provide:

List	Just name the answers; there is no description or explanation needed.
Define	A statement of the exact meaning of the word, without description. Putting only synonyms will not be sufficient.
Outline	A general description or plan showing the essential features of the topic, without the details.
Discuss	Write in detail (within the stipulated time) and cover issues like advantages and disadvantages, with supporting evidence.
Evaluate	Judge the quality, importance, and value of a given treatment or investigation. You must provide the level of evidence if available.
Compare (and contrast)	Write the differences and similarities in a tabular form.
Analyse/critically analyse	Similar to "evaluate." Examine the topic in detail, mentioning its suitability, relevance, pros and cons, merits and demerits, etc.
Assess	Same as "evaluate" and "analyse"
Explain	Write in detail (within the stipulated time), revealing all facts and controversies about the topic.
Identify	To recognise or correctly name what is being asked.
Justify investigation or treatment	Outline the merits and demerits of the given investigation/treatment with supporting level of evidence, showing that the advantages outweigh the disadvantages.
Summarise	A brief restatement showing the main features.

Table 1.1. Terms used in short-answer questions

It is also crucial for the candidate to read the entire question, as sometimes a question about management will ask for treatment options only for postmenopausal women—or only the surgical treatment options. Paying close attention while reading the question can save a great deal of time and help to focus your thinking to provide the most suitable answer.

SAQs may be split into separate parts, and each part may be worth a different number of marks. Identifying the number of marks for a given question also gives an indication of how much information that examiner is seeking for it. It should also guide you to allocate a proportional amount of time to a question, based on how many marks it is worth relative to all of the other questions.

For example, in a sixty-minute SAQ paper that is worth forty marks, you should aim to allocate one minute and thirty seconds for each mark. This means that you should complete an eight-mark question within twelve minutes.

Once you have decided how long to spend on a given question, apportioning that time effectively will ensure that you complete a well-rounded answer. The first thing to do for a couple of minutes initially is to plan your answer, jotting down the key points and structure of the answer. This prevents you from forgetting any important information or remembering something once you have started the answer and so needing to include it in the wrong section of the answer. Occasionally, you will need to leave an answer unfinished during an exam to return to it later (if heavily time-constrained); a plan guarantees that you can immediately pick up where you left off.

An important part unique to SAQs is the requirement for candidates to corroborate their statements with a level of evidence from the literature. A level of evidence corresponds to how well supported a claim is in the medical literature, hence providing an indication of how strong a recommendation one can make based on the claim. Examiners want to assess a candidate's ability to critically analyse the information he or she has learned and to show that the candidate keeps up to date with the latest research and changes to best practices within his or her country of practice. To assist readers in preparing for this part of the examination, this book provides levels of evidence where available so that candidates can use this information directly in their examinations.

Chapter 2
Menstruation and Its Disorders

Chapter 2.1. Clinical Physiology of Menstruation

Definition

Menstruation is the physiological, cyclical shedding of the functional layer of the endometrium between menarche and menopause. The age of menarche in the developed world is between 12 and 13 years. Over the next 3 to 4 years after menarche, the menstrual cycle becomes ovulatory and hence regularised.

Characteristics of a Normal Menstrual Cycle

Length of bleeding:

- Usually 3–4 days and < 7 days.
- Expressed as numerator (see below).

Length of cycle: (number of days between the start of one period to the start of the next)

- Usually 21–35 days.
- Some variation is normal. The major determinant is quality and rate of follicular development.
- Expressed as denominator. For example, if a woman menstruates for 5 days and her cycle length is 30 days, her menstrual cycle will be shown as $\frac{5}{30}$.

Amount of blood loss:

- Around 30 mL per cycle.
- > 80 mL is abnormal.
- In routine clinical practice, it is assessed subjectively, but in research settings, it is assessed more accurately by pictorial diagrams.

Different Phases of the Menstrual Cycle

A normal menstrual cycle has two phases—proliferative (follicular) and secretory (luteal)—separated by ovulation.

Proliferative Phase

This is the phase in which a sequence of chemical changes promotes the development of the primordial follicle (50 μm) to a preovulatory follicle (20 mm diameter). It usually lasts 10–14 days. The endometrium has a characteristic 3-layered appearance on a transvaginal ultrasound and hence can be easily diagnosed.

The proliferative phase starts with the beginning of menstruation and ends with ovulation.

Secretory Phase

This is the phase in which the granulosa cells of the ruptured follicle luteinise to form the corpus luteum. The corpus luteum secretes progestogens that make the endometrial glands tortuous, dilated, and rich in glycogen and mucus. This prepares the endometrium for the implantation of a fertilised egg, in case a pregnancy eventuates. The duration of this phase is always constant, around 14 days. Hence, the timing of ovulation can always be back-calculated. For example, if the menstrual cycle length is 35 days, ovulation would have occurred on day 21 (35 minus 14). A midluteal progesterone level greater than 25 nmol/L suggests ovulation.

On transvaginal ultrasound scan, a secretory phase endometrium appears hyperechoic and up to 12–14 mm thick. The 3-layered appearance seen in the proliferative phase is not seen. The corpus luteum appears as a complex adnexal mass with increased peripheral vascularity ("ring of fire" seen on ultrasound scan in 30% of cases).

Chapter 2.2. Dysmenorrhoea

Dysmenorrhoea is the cyclical lower abdominal pain/exacerbation of pain that may start 1–2 days before menses and ends before the menses ends. The pain is midline, crampy, and may radiate to the lower back and upper thighs. Bowel symptoms, such as nausea and vomiting, may coexist. An estimated 20–90% of women in between menarche and menopause suffer from dysmenorrhoea in different degrees. Psychosocial factors, lifestyle and emotional stress all contribute to dysmenorrhoea. Women with family members suffering from dysmenorrhoea have a higher incidence.

Types:

i. Primary
ii. Secondary

Primary Dysmenorrhoea

Primary dysmenorrhoea is defined as pain with menses for which there is no known physical cause to explain the symptoms. It usually starts in adolescence.

Pathogenesis

Arachidonic acid, the precursor of prostaglandin $F_{2\alpha}$, E_2, and leukotrienes, is found in a higher concentration in the uterus. These prostaglandins cause uterine hypercontractility, ischaemia and sensitisation of pain fibres. All these changes cause painful menses. In addition, the prostaglandins $F_{2\alpha}$ and E_2 also affect the bowel and cause GIT symptoms.

Diagnosis

The history of relevant symptoms and their cyclical nature will strongly indicate the diagnosis. Any other pelvic pathology should be excluded by a thorough gynaecological examination, including cervical and vaginal swabs to exclude infection. A transvaginal ultrasound scan will help in excluding any uterine pathology such as an endometrial polyp or a leiomyoma, adenomyosis, endometrioma, or any ovarian neoplasm (evidence level III). A hysteroscopy or a laparoscopy may be needed if the transvaginal ultrasound scan shows any pathology.

Management

A minor degree of dysmenorrhoea may not require any pharmacological treatment. A low-fat and vegetarian diet, relaxation exercises, and removal of stress at home and work may help. Pharmacological treatment will depend on contraceptive needs. If contraception is needed, the combined oral contraceptive pill is the starting treatment. It reduces the prevalence and severity of dysmenorrhoea. The low-dose pill (20 µg ethinyl oestradiol) is equally effective. The combined pill acts by suppressing ovulation, endometrial proliferation, and prostaglandin synthesis. Women not requiring contraception should be started on nonsteroidal anti-inflammatory drugs (NSAIDs) before the commencement of the symptoms. Women with known hypersensitivity to NSAIDs, peptic ulcers, nasal polyps, angioedema, or asthma should not be prescribed this drug. NSAIDs act by inhibiting prostaglandin synthesis and reducing intrauterine pressure. Mefenamic acid, which is an aryl carboxylic acid, has a higher concentration in the uterus and hence is more effective in reducing myometrial contractility. Other types of NSAIDs—such as aryl propionic acid (ibuprofen, naproxen, and ketoprofen), indoleacetic acid (indomethacin), and selective cyclooxygenase (COX–2) inhibitors (celecoxib)—are also very effective in treating the symptoms. Any other analgesic (narcotic/nonnarcotic) could also be used as add-on treatment. When the family is complete, endometrial resection or ablation may also help. Levonorgestrel-containing intrauterine devices have also been used to treat this condition. Zinc sulphate, 50 mg daily, reduces the duration and severity of dysmenorrhoea by affecting the metabolism of prostaglandins (Zekavat OR et al., 2015). Transcutaneous nerve stimulations and heat fomentation are more effective than placebos. Laparoscopic uterine nerve stimulation and presacral neurectomy are not supported by current evidence to treat this condition (2005 Cochrane meta-analysis, Evidence IA). Vaginal childbirth also helps in reducing the severity of primary dysmenorrhoea, possibly by interfering with the pain conduction mechanisms.

Secondary Dysmenorrhoea

Secondary dysmenorrhoea results when one or more pelvic pathologies are present to account for the painful menses. This usually starts later in the reproductive life.

Pathologies that could cause secondary dysmenorrhoea are the following:

1. Endometriosis
2. Adenomyosis
3. Pelvic infection
4. Cervical stenosis
5. Endometrial polyps/leiomyoma
6. Ovarian neoplasms
7. Müllerian abnormalities
8. Life stressors
9. Pelvic congestion

Endometriosis

Pain increases during menstruation. Infertility and dyspareunia may be present. There may be clues during a clinical examination, such as uterosacral nodularity and tender adnexa. A transvaginal ultrasound scan may show an endometrioma. Endometriosis is dealt with in another chapter.

Adenomyosis

A clinical examination may show an enlarged, nodular, and tender uterus. A transvaginal ultrasound scan has the characteristic appearance of adenomyosis.

Pelvic Infections

Chlamydia, gonorrhoea infections, infections arising from intrauterine devices, or appendicitis may cause painful menses. Pain is aggravated by oedema, the inflammatory response, and later on, scarring and adhesions.

Cervical Stenosis

Pain usually lasts throughout the menstrual bleeding, and bleeding is scant. It usually results from stenosis at the internal os level, which may be congenital or acquired. Acquired cervical stenosis commonly results at the external os level from cervical surgery or hypoestrogenism. This condition is suspected on the basis of a suggestive history, a scarred or very narrow external cervical os, and maybe the presence of a hematometra on a transvaginal ultrasound scan.

Other

Other conditions, such as uterine or ovarian neoplasms and Müllerian abnormalities, could be diagnosed by a transvaginal ultrasound scan with or without a hysteroscopy/laparoscopy. Treatment of secondary dysmenorrhoea will be individualised. Each condition should be treated appropriately.

There is controversy about whether "pelvic congestion syndrome" really exists or contributes to secondary dysmenorrhoea. There is no defined treatment for this condition.

The psychosocial aspects and life stressors should also be addressed by a change in lifestyle, behavioural treatment, relaxation exercises, and, very rarely, by low-dose antidepressants/anxiolytics.

Chapter 2.3. Premenstrual Syndrome (PMS) and Premenstrual Dysphoric Disorder (PMDD)

PMS is defined as a group of cyclical, mild-to-moderate physical (headache, breast tenderness, swelling), emotional (fatigue, depression/anxiety, anorexia) and behavioural (aggression, loss of concentration) symptoms that happen in the secretory phase of the menstrual cycle. There is always a symptom-free interval of 1–2 weeks.

PMDD is a more severe form of PMS in which emotional and behavioural symptoms predominate, and there is severe inability to function normally. Although PMS is quite widely prevalent in all cultures, nearly 40% of women with PMDD are incapacitated by this condition.

Risk Factors

- Family history of emotional problems
- Preexisting psychiatric conditions
- Postpartum depression
- Alcohol or substance abuse
- Smoking
- Early menarche
- Obesity

Causes

PMS/PMDD is a multifactorial psychoendocrine disorder. Changes in ovarian hormonal secretions due to ovulation lead to changes in neurotransmitters in the brain, which in turn cause reduction of the serotonergic function in the second half of the menstrual cycle.

Diagnosis

PMS is diagnosed by the presence of the relevant symptoms in the second half of the menstrual cycle in a cyclic fashion. Other organic causes of the symptoms must be excluded. Patients are required to maintain a diary of symptoms over successive cycles. The severity of symptoms should be such that it affects quality of life.

PMDD is diagnosed by the presence of at least 5 symptoms of PMS, including at least 1 affective symptom. Examples of affective symptoms are: mood lability, anxiety, feelings of sadness, hopelessness, helplessness, and constant anger and aggression.

Management

- Ovarian suppression: This is achieved by the monophasic combined oral contraceptive pill (COC), especially pills having drospirenone (evidence level IB). These pills could be given with or without sugar pills. Progesterone alone has no effect (Evidence Level IA). In severe cases, GnRH analogues may be used.
- Selective serotonin reuptake inhibitors (e.g., venlafaxine): These drugs are very effective in PMS and are the main treatment for PMDD. They improve the physical and behavioural symptoms (evidence level IA) within 1–2 days. These drugs could be administered either cyclically in the luteal phase or continuously. Side effects include GIT, CNS and sleep disturbance, and sexual dysfunction.
- Diet and exercise: These include aerobic exercises, rest and relaxation, stress management, behavioural therapy, vegetarian diet, and calcium and vitamin B6 supplementation.
- Bromocriptine and evening primrose oil: These are cyclically used for mastalgia.
- Bilateral oophorectomy: If none of the above treatments have worked and there is cessation of symptoms with GnRH analogues, then bilateral oophorectomy could be considered, with or without a hysterectomy.

Short-Answer Questions

Question 1

Why do prepubertal girls not menstruate?

Answer:

During prepubertal years, the hypothalamic-pituitary-ovarian axis remains suppressed, and hence menstruation does not occur. The gonadotropin-releasing hormone–producing cells (GnRH-producing cells) in the hypothalamus remain supressed. The mechanism of this is uncertain. A gene in the GnRH-producing cell, which is controlled by leptin produced by the adipocyte, may be responsible for this. By about 9–10 years, the GnRH is secreted by the hypothalamic cells. This leads to the production of FSH—initially at night in spikes but after a few years during the daytime as well. The FSH stimulates the development of follicles in the ovaries and hence the hypothalamic-pituitary-ovarian axis becomes activated, leading to the menstrual cycle.

Question 2

Why are menstrual cycles following menarche anovulatory?

Answer:

Menarche (age of first menstruation) occurs after the peak of pubertal growth spurt has been reached. The menses remain anovulatory until the oestrogen starts to exert its positive feedback on the hypothalamus and pituitary. This feedback promotes the midcycle surge of LH, which is essential for ovulation.

Question 3

Briefly discuss the mechanism of the onset of menses.

Answer:

In the absence of a pregnancy, the corpus luteum undergoes luteolysis around 9–11 days after ovulation. The mechanism of luteolysis is unclear. Prostaglandin $F_{2\alpha}$ from the ovary and oestradiol released from the corpus luteum itself play a part in the luteolysis. The luteolysis of the corpus luteum results in the fall of oestrogen, progesterone and inhibin A levels. The fall in progesterone levels leads to endometrial spiral arteriolar constriction and subsequent endometrial ischaemia and shedding of the functional endometrium (stratum compactum and spongiosum) and bleeding. The above mechanism is very similar to the withdrawal bleed from the cessation of a combined oral contraceptive pill.

Question 4

Why is menstrual bleeding self-limiting?

Answer:

Menstrual bleeding is self-limiting due to these reasons:

   i. The beginning and end of menses are due to a definite sequence of events and affect the entire endometrium simultaneously.

ii. The endometrial shedding is orderly, progressive, and is due to progressively increasing duration of constriction of spiral arterioles. Hence, random breakdown of endometrium is prevented.

iii. Bleeding vessels are sealed by clotting factors, and oestrogen-mediated regeneration of the endometrium starts. Destruction of the endometrium and regeneration follow simultaneously.

iv. Myometrial contraction contributes very little to the cessation of menstrual bleeding.

Question 5

Why does ovulation occur?

Answer:

The level of LH rises steadily in the second half of the follicular phase of the cycle, as a result of the stimulation from the follicular oestrogen. The LH causes luteinisation of the granulosa cells, which start to secrete an increasing amount of progesterone. This progesterone, through its action on the pituitary, causes marked increase in LH levels, a phenomenon called LH surge. The LH surge stimulates meiosis of the oocyte and synthesis of progesterone and prostaglandins in the developing follicle. Progesterone stimulates the proteolytic enzymes, which cause rupture of the follicular wall. Ovulation occurs nearly 10–12 hours after the peak of the LH surge. Prostaglandin synthetase–inhibiting drugs such as aspirin and ibuprofen will inhibit ovulation by inhibiting the synthesis of prostaglandin.

Question 6

Ovulation occurs more frequently from the right ovary. Discuss.

Answer:

This statement is true. The right ovary is the dominant ovary for most of the reproductive life. Due to the differences in the venous return of the two ovaries, the left ovarian venous return is slower than the right ovary. Because of this, the left-sided corpus luteum takes longer to disappear, which reduces the chance of ovulation from the left ovary in the following month. Nothing of that sort happens on the right side; hence the right ovary ovulates more commonly. As a result of all that, 64% of pregnancies originate from eggs released by the right ovary.

Question 7

How does conception prevent the onset of menses?

Answer:

Just before implantation, the zona pellucida disintegrates, and the developing blastocyst (hatched) starts to adhere to the decidua. At this stage, the blastocyst also produces hCG, which acts on the corpus luteum to maintain the production of progesterone and oestradiol. This prevents the onset of menstruation and allows the early pregnancy to continue.

Question 8

An 18-year-old year-12 student has severe dysmenorrhoea and is concerned about its adverse effects on her final end-of-year examination preparation. How would you manage this situation?

Answer:

History:

- Age at menarche
- Menstrual cycles: frequency; duration of bleeding; heaviness of bleeding; severity, onset, and duration of any associated pain
- Presence or absence of nausea, vomiting, diarrhoea, dizziness, or headache during menstruation
- Impact of symptoms on daily activities such as school attendance, sports participation, and other social activities
- Medication use: type, dose, timing in relation to the onset of cramps/pain, and perceived effectiveness in terms of relief and ability to engage in all daily activities
- Sexual history: current sexual activity, type of contraception, history of sexually transmitted diseases, and history of pelvic inflammatory disease
- Associated stress factors
- Sexual abuse

Examination:

- Vaginal
  - Only limited to external genital inspection if virgin
  - Bivalve speculum examination: normal anatomy, discharge, bleeding, microbiological swabs, cervical cytology
- Bimanual examination: size, shape, axis, mobility of uterus, nodules in the POD, cervical excitation, any abnormal adnexal mass
- Transvaginal ultrasound scan (translabial or abdominal if virgin)

The above tests will not pick up endometriosis. An ultrasound scan, however, will be able to pick up endometrioma.

Treatment options:

If all the above tests are normal, the diagnosis is primary dysmenorrhoea.

- NSAIDS, paracetamol: start before pain
- Combined oral contraceptive pill with periodic skipping of sugar pills to avoid menses
- Progestins: e.g., norethisterone or medroxyprogesterone acetate cyclic for 2 weeks or continuous
- Etonogestrel (Implanon®), depot medroxyprogesterone acetate injection 150 mg IM every 3 months
- If abnormal scan or if refractory symptoms after 3 months, consider laparoscopy to exclude endometriosis or PID

Multiple-Choice Questions

Q1. Which of the following is the last event in the process of ovulation?

A. LH surge

B. Release of oestrogens from the granulosa cells

C. Luteinisation of the granulosa cells

D. Release of proteolytic enzymes in response to increased progesterone secretion

Answer: D

Q2. Which is the most common cause of regular menses in a 9-year-old with a history of thelarche and adrenarche?

A. Hypothyroidism

B. Gonadal tumours

C. Brain tumours

D. Idiopathic

Answer: D

Q3. In a regular 35-day cycle, when will the serum progesterone level reach its maximum?

A. Day 14

B. Day 17

C. Day 21

D. Day 25

Answer: C

Q4. Subnucleolar vacuolation in the endometrial cells is a sign of which of the following?

A. Menstrual phase endometrium

B. Proliferative phase endometrium

C. Ovulation

D. Decidualisation

Answer: C

Q5. Which of the following statements is true for decidua?

A. Decidual cells are derived from endometrial stromal cells under the influence of progesterone.

B. Decidual cells are derived from endometrial stromal cells under the influence of LH.

C. Decidual cells are derived from endometrial stromal cells under the influence of oestradiol.

D. Decidual cells do not secrete prolactin.

Answer: A

Q6. Which of the following statements is **not** true for the menstrual cycle?

    A. Its length is determined by the rate and quality of follicular growth.

    B. It is normal for the cycle to vary in individual women.

    C. Most anovulatory cycles occur between 20 to 40 years of age.

    D. Nearly half of women have a perfect 28-day cycle.

Answer: C

Q7. Which of the following statements is most true for intermenstrual bleeding?

    A. Small intermenstrual bleeding can easily be ignored.

    B. Intermenstrual bleeding is pathological and should be investigated.

    C. Only large, regular intermenstrual bleeding should be investigated.

    D. Intermenstrual bleeding indicates a hyper-oestrogenic state of the endometrium.

Answer: B

Q8. Which of the following statements is **not** true for the management of intermenstrual bleeding?

    A. STI screen should be done in the management of IMB.

    B. Cervical smear should be repeated if the last cervical smear was > 3 months ago.

    C. Hysterectomy is the best treatment option.

    D. Hysteroscopy and curette have a role.

Answer: C

Q9. Which of the following leads to the resolution of corpus luteum?

    A. Increased oestradiol

    B. Increased progesterone

    C. Decreased LH

    D. Decreased FSH

Answer: C

Q10. Which is the most common cause of secondary dysmenorrhoea?

    A. Pelvic congestion

    B. Ovarian neoplasm

    C. Leiomyoma

    D. Endometriosis

Answer: D

Q11. Which of the following statements about oestrogen is **not** correct?

    A. Oestrogen administration caused vasodilatation.

    B. Oestriol synthesis in pregnancy is enhanced by aromatisation in the fetal adrenal gland.

    C. Oestrogen increases the effect of nitric oxide on vascular smooth muscle.

    D. Oestrogen is a positive inotrope.

Answer: B

Q12. Which of the following drugs is most useful for the treatment of PMS?

A. Progesterone

B. Anxiolytics

C. Vitamin B6

D. Selective serotonin reuptake inhibitors

Answer: D

Q13. Anorexia nervosa:

A. Is associated with anovulation with normal oestrogen level

B. Is associated with increased FSH and LH

C. Can cause severe osteoporosis if prolonged

D. Is not associated with skin collagen changes or wrinkling

Answer: C

Q14. Which one of the following has autosomal recessive inheritance?

A. Marfan's syndrome

B. Huntington's disease

C. Cystic fibrosis

D. Adult onset polycystic kidney disease

Answer: C

Q15. Which of the following is the main factor that causes the onset of menstruation?

A. Progesterone withdrawal

B. Estrogen withdrawal

C. LH withdrawal

D. FSH withdrawal

Answer: A

Q16. An established clinical indication for antiprogestogens is:

A. Routine contraception

B. Postcoital contraception

C. Endometriosis

D. Premenstrual syndrome

Answer: B

Q17. Which of the following is **not** needed for the diagnosis of PMS?

A. A symptom complex consistent with the diagnosis

B. A luteal-phase pattern

C. Severity sufficient to disrupt life

D. Objective physical findings

Answer: D

Q18. Which of the following would **not** enhance contraction of a myometrial cell?

A. Binding of intracellular calcium to calmodulin to activate calcium-dependent myosin light-chain kinase

B. Voltage-operated calcium-channel activation

C. Receptor-operated calcium-channel activation

D. Sarcoplasmic reticulum calcium uptake

Answer: D

Q19. Which of the following statements regarding anticoagulation with warfarin is correct?

A. The effect of warfarin is most rapidly reversed by administering fresh frozen plasma.

B. Paracetamol in normal dosage may cause a drug interaction.

C. Treatment should be monitored by measuring the partial thromboplastin time.

D. Breastfeeding is contraindicated.

Answer: A

Q20. Which of the following is **not** correct?

A. Iron requirement in a menstruating, nonpregnant female is approximately 2 mg/day.

B. Iron requirement in a pregnant female is approximately 9 mg/day.

C. Iron absorption in the nonpregnant adult is approximately 5% of daily intake.

D. Cord-blood serum ferritin is greater than maternal serum ferritin.

Answer: B

Q21. What is the incidence of severe PMS?

A. 1%

B. 5%

C. 10%

D. 15%

Answer: B

Q22. A 25-year-old suffers from emotional lability and depression for 10 days prior to her periods. She has a history of premenstrual fatigue, bloating, and breast tenderness. Her symptoms improve with the start of her periods. Contraceptive pills have helped her partly. Which of the following will best treat her?

A. Spironolactone

B. Evening primrose oil

C. Fluoxetine

D. Vitamin B6

Answer: C

Q23. A 20-year-old has severe pain, nausea, and headache during her periods since menarche. The rest of the history and pelvic examination are normal. What will be her initial treatment?

A. Antiprostaglandins

B. Danazol

C. GnRH analogues

D. Ergot derivatives

Answer: A

Chapter 2.4. Dysfunctional Uterine Bleeding

Definition

Dysfunctional uterine bleeding (DUB) is defined as irregular vaginal bleeding with no demonstrable genital or extragenital organic cause. It is a diagnosis of exclusion.

Clinical Physiology

There are two types of DUB:

- Anovulatory (80% incidence)
- Ovulatory (20% incidence)

Anovulatory DUB

This is a disease of adolescent and premenopausal (> 41 years old) age groups. In both age groups, the pathogenesis revolves around anovulation from any cause in the presence of oestrogen and a lack of progesterone causing decreased $PGF_{2\alpha}$ and other prostaglandins. The bleeding is mostly painless.

Because of insufficient oestrogen, the LH surge, and consequently ovulation, does not occur. In the absence of ovulation, the corpus luteum does not form, and progesterone secretion does not start. However, due to the presence of developing follicles, a prolonged supply of oestrogen is maintained, which leads to endometrial proliferation and hyperplasia. Such an endometrium lacks a stromal support matrix and so becomes fragile and undergoes superficial breakage and bleeding. This leads to endometrial shedding in patches. Due to the lack of progesterone, $PGF_{2\alpha}$ is in short supply, and hence the vasoconstrictive action is missing. This leads to continuation of bleeding.

Ovulatory DUB

This is a disease of 21–40-year-olds. The pathogenesis revolves around an increased synthesis of vasodilatory prostaglandins rather than vasoconstrictive prostaglandins, despite ovulation and a normal level of progesterone. Due to an excess of vasodilatory prostaglandins, bleeding is heavy, and due to the presence of $PGF_{2\alpha}$, the bleeding is painful (dysmenorrhoea). Histologically, the endometrium is secretory.

History

A detailed history should be obtained, which should include the following:

- Duration and severity of bleeding
- Pattern of bleeding, whether regular or irregular
- Associated pain, postcoital bleeding
- Age of menarche
- Gravida and parity
- Last cervical smear
- Use of contraception
- Any associated medical and surgical history
- Any regular drug use

Examination

- Vital signs
- Pallor
- Thyroid examination for goitre
- Abdominal examination, looking for masses or peritonism
- Vaginal examination with a bivalve speculum
  - Confirm presence of a normal vagina and cervix
  - Look for signs of infection
  - Take high vaginal swabs
- Bimanual examination
  - Uterine size
  - Adnexal masses

Investigations

- FBE, TSH, iron studies.
- Transvaginal (translabial if virgin) ultrasound, including saline sonohysterography. The ultrasound scan should ideally be performed in the proliferative phase of the menstrual cycle.
- Coagulation profile (BT, PT, APTT):
  - 20% of teenagers with this problem will have a coagulation defect.
- Hysteroscopy and endometrial biopsy, if ultrasound is suggestive of endometrial pathology or failed medical treatment.

With the above history, examination, and investigations, any organic cause of genital or extragenital bleeding can be excluded.

Exact quantification of the blood loss is not essential in clinical practice, beyond the information obtained during clinical assessment. The correlation between the woman's perception of the heaviness of bleeding and the actual blood loss is poor. A woman should be treated if she desires to be treated, on account of her perception of heavy bleeding, or if the bleeding is abnormal based on the clinical assessment.

Management

The treatment of DUB is mostly medical and rarely surgical. Apart from replacing iron or transfusing packed red blood cells, the principles of medical treatment are as follows:

Nonhormonal

Antifibrinolytic Agents

Example: tranexamic acid

This acts by reducing fibrin degradation in the spiral arterioles and their branches. It achieves a 50% reduction in blood loss. In women with ovulatory DUB, increased fibrinolytic activity has been shown in the spiral arterioles and their branches. Hence, this drug is especially useful for this condition.

Dose: 1 g, TDS

Side effects: GIT disturbance, headache, DVT, disturbance to colour vision

Contraindication: active intravascular clotting

Prostaglandin Synthetase Inhibitors

Examples: mefenamic acid, ibuprofen

These drugs inhibit conversion of arachidonic acid to various prostaglandins and also block prostaglandin receptors in the endometrium. They reduce blood loss by 25%. They also relieve menstrual pain.

Dose (mefenamic acid): 500 mg TDS, with food, for the first 3 days of menses

Side effect: gastric irritation

Contraindication: asthma, allergy, peptic ulcer disease

Hormonal

High-Dose Oestrogen

This is only used in an emergency where quick control of bleeding is needed. A dose of 25 mg of conjugated equine oestrogen is administered intravenously every 4 hours until the bleeding is controlled. Oestrogen promotes rapid regeneration of the endometrium, sealing the denuded surface. This treatment controls blood loss in 72% of women. All oestrogen must be followed by progestin coverage and withdrawal bleeding.

Combined Oral Contraceptive Pill

This is the most commonly used drug in the treatment of anovulatory DUB. Bleeding is reduced by 50%. It causes orderly regression of excessive endometrial thickness to normal. It should be discontinued after 3 months to allow the unopposed endogenous oestrogen to reactivate the endometrium.

Side effects: nausea, DVT

Progestogens

Examples: norethisterone, medroxyprogesterone acetate, norethynodrel

These are the drugs of choice for anovulatory DUB. Progestins help in the conversion of oestradiol to oestrone sulphate, which is rapidly excreted. Progestins also diminish oestrogen effect on target cells by inhibiting oestrogen receptors, and they suppress oestrogen-mediated transcription of oncogenes. These actions lead to the antimitotic, antigrowth impact on the endometrium, which causes reversal of hyperplasia and limitation of growth postovulation.

Menstrual blood loss is reduced by 30%. It can be used cyclically orally or with an intrauterine device, where it reduces blood loss by 90%. A levonorgestrel-containing IUCD is as effective as endometrial ablation, more effective than cyclical norethisterone, and is the most effective medical treatment for DUB. It is cheap and well tolerated, it does not usually interfere with coitus, and it prevents a hysterectomy in at least 60% of such women.

GnRH Analogues

GnRH analogues cause amenorrhoea by inhibiting pituitary production of gonadotropins. They are expensive, and they cause severe menopausal symptoms and osteoporosis. This group of drugs is primarily used prior to myomectomy for reducing the size of myomas, making surgery easier with less blood loss. It is also used to thin the endometrium prior to endometrial resection/ablation.

Multiple-Choice Questions

Q1. What is the cause of a midcycle bleeding in a 30-year-old?

    A. Decrease in oestrogen level immediately before ovulation

    B. Increase in oestrogen level immediately before ovulation

    C. Decrease in progesterone level immediately before ovulation

    D. Increase in progesterone level immediately before ovulation

Answer: A

Q2. Which of the following statements is correct with reference to intermenstrual bleeding (IMB)?

    A. A small amount of infrequent IMB could be ignored.

    B. IMB is often due to pathology.

    C. It is seldom due to chlamydia infection.

    D. It is often due to low oestrogen levels.

Answer: B

Q3. Which of the following is **not** a cause of anovulatory DUB?

    A. PCOS

    B. Obesity

    C. Immaturity of HPO axis in postpubertal girls

    D. Submucous fibroid

Answer: D

Q4. A 30-year-old who has been on the combined oral contraceptive pill for many years starts to get irregular uterine bleeding with scant or absent periods. Her pregnancy test is negative. How will you treat her?

    A. Exclude uterine fibroids

    B. Prescribe additional norethisterone for 7 days

    C. Prescribe additional oestradiol for 7 days

    D. Replace pill with a levonorgestrel IUCD

Answer: C

Q5. A woman on depot medroxyprogesterone acetate injection every 3 months consults you with irregular spotting. How will you treat her?

    A. By prescribing additional oral progestin

    B. By prescribing additional oral oestrogen

    C. By prescribing mefenamic acid

    D. By prescribing antifibrinolytic agent

Answer: B

Q6. Which of the following is not important for the control of menstrual bleeding?

    A. Thrombin generation at the basal endometrium

    B. Deposition of fibrin at the basal endometrium

    C. Platelet aggregation at the bleeding site

    D. Myometrial contraction

Answer: D

Q7. During a laparoscopic hysterectomy for DUB, a 2x3-cm hole is seen at the dome of the urinary bladder. Which of the following will you do?

    A. Repair the hole in 2 layers with ethibond and insert a suprapubic catheter for 5 days

    B. Repair the hole in 2 layers with polyglactin suture and insert a urethral catheter for 7 days

    C. Repair the hole in 2 layers with PDS, insert urethral catheter for 48 hours, and perform a cystogram prior to removal

    D. Repair the hole in 2 layers with PDS and omental patch and insert a urethral catheter for 10 days

Answer: B

Chapter 2.5.   Heavy Menstrual Bleeding

This was previously known as menorrhagia.

Definition

Heavy menstrual bleeding (HMB) is bleeding lasting more than seven days during menstruation or a quantity of blood loss exceeding 80 mL during menstruation.

Bleeding may be very heavy and of sudden onset, requiring emergency hospitalisation. Chronic, heavy periods may cause iron deficiency anaemia in 60% of women. 20% of teenaged and 15% of adult women will have coagulation defects, mainly von Willebrand's disease (13%) and factor XI deficiency (4%). The risk of endometrial cancer in women > 40 years of age with HMB is 1%.

Types

- Idiopathic, synonymous with ovulatory DUB.
- Secondary to organic disease, such as:
  - Pelvic pathology: submucous fibroids, endometrial polyps, adenomyosis
    - Intracavitary lesions cause increased bleeding due to increased endometrial and vascular fragility and abnormal prostaglandin levels.
    - Intramural fibroids cause increased bleeding due to topographic endometrial abnormalities, endometrial glandular atrophy overlying the fibroid, venous congestion, and alteration in prostaglandin levels.
  - Coagulation disorders: von Willebrand's disease, idiopathic/thrombotic thrombocytopaenic purpura.
  - Endocrine disorders: hypothyroidism, Cushing's syndrome.

History

The history as described in the chapter on DUB should be applied to HMB also.

The aim of the history should be to ascertain the heaviness of bleeding and presence of any organic diseases. Questions regarding the following points will help in this:

- Number and frequency of sanitary pad/tampon use and change
- Whether tampons and pads are used together
- Presence of large clots
- Soiling of clothes
- Any restriction to activities, such as time off work/school or limitation of movement
- Tiredness, exhaustion

The following symptoms and conditions will indicate the presence of an organic cause:

- IMB/PCB: endometrial or cervical polyps, ectropion, cervical intraepithelial neoplasia (CIN), cervical cancer

- Dyspareunia/dysmenorrhoea: endometriosis, adenomyosis
- Easy bruising, excessive bleeding on dental extraction: bleeding disorder
- Tiredness, listlessness, oedema: hypothyroidism

Examination

The examination will be the same as described in the chapter on DUB.

Investigations

The investigations will partly depend on the information obtained from history and clinical examination. The investigations could be as follows:

- FBE and iron studies to check for anaemia
- TSH, to screen for hypothyroidism.
- Clotting studies (BT, PT, APTT), for von Willebrand's disease (vWF antigen, ristocetin cofactor assay) and platelet count for thrombocytopaenia.
- Transvaginal ultrasound scan in the proliferative phase (ideally between days 5 to 10) of the menstrual cycle to look at:
  - Endometrial thickness.
  - Regularity of endometrium.
  - Endometrial polyps.
  - Submucous or intramural fibroid.
  - Myometrium for features of adenomyosis.
  - Ovaries for neoplasms such as granulosa cell neoplasm.
  - The secretory endometrium may falsely look like endometrial polyp on ultrasound scan. Hence, it is recommended that the scans should be done in the proliferative phase of the menstrual cycle.
- MRI is seldom necessary.
- Hysteroscopy and endometrial biopsy, if ultrasound is inconclusive or suggests pathology, such as endometrial polyps, hyperplasia, or submucous fibroids.

Management

The management should be individualised depending on the woman's situation, symptoms, and needs. For example, treatment would differ if the woman desired contraception or if she was experiencing concurrent dysmenorrhoea.

Medical

This is the first-line treatment option, unless there is a pelvic organ pathology present. Medical treatment is described in DUB.

Surgical

- Dilatation and curettage:
  - This is primarily done for its diagnostic value, but it can also be therapeutic for a variable length of time.
- Endometrial ablation or resection:
  - Available techniques include diathermy, thermal balloon, microwave, and laser.
  - The entire full-thickness endometrium should be resected/ablated; otherwise the endometrium will regenerate.
  - The following are contraindications for this procedure:
    - Pregnancy
    - Possible or confirmed endometrial hyperplasia or cancer
    - Woman wishing to conceive in the future
    - Active pelvic infection
    - Intrauterine contraceptive device (IUCD) in situ
    - Uterine scar, other than LUSCS scar
    - Congenital uterine anomaly such as bicornuate uterus (only for bipolar and thermal ablation)
- Myomectomy/resection of submucous myoma in women desiring to keep the uterus to maintain fertility. The type of surgery depends upon:
  - The number, size, and location of the fibroids
  - The gynaecologist's skills
- Hysterectomy can be performed when all other treatments have failed and the woman does not desire fertility. The risk of:
  - Damage to the bowel or bladder: 1%
  - Blood transfusion: 6%
  - Death: 1 in 10,000 cases

Short-Answer Questions

Question 1

What is the difference between dysfunctional uterine bleeding (DUB) and heavy menstrual bleeding (HMB), also known as menorrhagia?

Answer:

DUB is irregular bleeding from the genital tract in the absence of an organic cause, largely due to anovulation. It is usually painless.

In contrast, HMB is regular bleeding from the genital tract, with or without an organic cause. It is mostly ovulatory and often painful.

The drug of choice for DUB is either cyclical progestogen or the COC, whereas the levonorgestrel-containing IUCD is the drug of choice for HMB.

Question 2

Compare and contrast with evidence the different techniques for endometrial ablation: bipolar radiofrequency, thermal balloon, and rollerball ablation.

Answer:

The indication for endometrial ablation is the treatment of ovulatory menorrhagia in premenopausal women.

Type of ablation	Bipolar radiofrequency	Thermal balloon	Rollerball diathermy
Method	Hysteroscopy should be performed prior to ablation to rule out malignant conditions and focal pathology that may be causing DUB.		
	An electrode array, protected by a sheath, uses bipolar radiofrequency impedance technology to ablate the uterus. The cavity must be assessed for integrity (with CO_2) prior to commencing the procedure, to ensure there is no perforation.	Latex or silicone balloon is placed in the uterine cavity and a preheated liquid (e.g., 5% dextrose in water) is circulated for a set time.	Electrosurgical current passes through an electrode to destroy the basalis layer of the endometrium under hysteroscopic vision. It requires pretreatment with GnRH agonists, danazol to thin the endometrium.
Advantages	Fast procedure. Higher initial rates of amenorrhoea (46–58%) than other procedures (Evidence Level IA). Fewer minor complications than rollerball ablation. Can be performed by less experienced surgeons. Easier to learn the technique.	Can be performed by less experienced surgeons. Fewer minor complications than rollerball ablation. Easier to learn the technique.	Cheaper to perform. Relatively longer learning curve.
Disadvantages	Expensive. Higher risk of equipment failure, postoperative nausea/vomiting, and uterine cramping (Evidence Level IA).	Expensive. Higher risk of equipment failure, postoperative nausea/vomiting, and uterine cramping (Evidence Level IA).	Higher rates of complications, such as irrigation fluid overload, cervical laceration, and haematometra (Evidence Level IA). Must be performed in an operating theatre. Longer operation time. Greater need for general anaesthesia.
Outcome	Comparable outcomes over long term—as measured by amenorrhoea, patient satisfaction, and subsequent surgery—between all methods of ablation (Evidence Level IA). Same incidence of severe complications, such as uterine perforation, haemorrhage, and endometritis (Evidence Level IA).		

Table 2.1. Comparison of different techniques for endometrial ablation

Question 3

Compare the levonorgestrel-containing IUCD with endometrial ablation in the treatment of HMB.

Answer:

	Levonorgestrel-containing IUCD	Endometrial ablation
Mode of action	Reduces endometrial proliferation Inhibits ovulation	Ablates endometrium via a variety of methods
Outpatient procedure?	Yes	No
Need for anaesthetic?	Mostly not	Yes
Success rate	90% reduction in blood loss May cause amenorrhoea	90% reduction: Of those, 40% amenorrhoea, 40% reduced bleeding, 40% need another surgery in 5 years
Patient satisfaction rate	70%	70%
Duration of treatment	5 years	Hopefully lifelong
Fertility	Acts as a long-term reversible contraceptive	Does not provide contraception Should not get pregnant after this surgery
Important contraindications	PID Nulliparity	3 or more caesarean sections Large uterus Large myoma
Complications	Irregular bleeding for first 3–4 months	Uterine perforation Electrolyte imbalance if glycine used

Table 2.2. Comparison between levonorgestrel-containing IUCD and endometrial ablation in the treatment of HMB

Question 4

List the differential diagnoses for HMB in a 15-year-old girl.

Answer:

- Uterine abnormality: uterine didelphys; endometrial or cervical polyps and fibroids very uncommon in this age group
- Ovarian neoplasms: granulosa cell tumour
- Bleeding disorder: von Willebrand's disease, idiopathic thrombocytopaenic purpura
- Endocrine disorders: hypothyroidism, Cushing's syndrome, immaturity of HPO axis
- Systemic disorders: chronic liver disease, chronic kidney disease

Question 5

A 24-year-old woman presents to you with HMB, and you diagnose the cause to be von Willebrand's disease. Describe the disorder.

Answer:

Von Willebrand's disease is the most common inherited heterogenous group of bleeding disorders, affecting 1% of the population. In woman with HMB, the prevalence goes up to 13–20%.

Inheritance:

- Autosomal dominant—type I (most common), type II
- Autosomal recessive—type III (most severe)
- Acquired—when antibodies to vWF are developed, such as in SLE

Physiology: The function of vWF is to promote the formation of the platelet plug at the site of vessel trauma. It does so by transporting factor VIII, thus reducing its excretion by 20 times.

Pathology: The disease results from defects in the synthesis or function of vWF, causing disordered platelet aggregation. Physiologic fluctuations in the level of vWF do occur.

Symptoms: Easy bruising, epistaxis, haemorrhage from even minor surgical procedures, HMB

Diagnosis: Suggestive history, vWF antigen, ristocetin cofactor assay; repeated testing may be required due to the physiologic variation.

Treatment:

1. Desmopressin nasal spray
2. Plasma-derived concentrates rich in the high-molecular-weight multimers of von Willebrand's factors

Question 6

Evaluate the nonmedical treatment options in a 34-year-old nulliparous woman with HMB.

Answer:

The following factors will impact the nonmedical treatment options in this woman:

- Desire to maintain fertility
- Causes of heavy menstrual bleeding, such as fibroids or adenomyosis

The following nonmedical treatment options will be considered in a woman desirous of maintaining her fertility:

- Hysteroscopy and curettage:
  - The value of this surgery is mainly diagnostic, but it also results in a therapeutic benefit, the duration of which varies.
  - It is a short and easy surgery, with rapid return to work.
  - The risks, such as bleeding, infection, and uterine perforation, are very uncommon in this age group.

- Myomectomy (or hysteroscopic resection of a submucous fibroid, if present):
  - Myomectomy could be done laparoscopically or by a laparotomy.
  - Hysteroscopic resection of the fibroid could be done as a day case with return to work in 2–3 days. More than one attempt at resection may be needed if the fibroid is large.
  - If myomectomy is done by a laparotomy, it will require 4–6 weeks of convalescence.
  - Risks of bleeding, infection, and unintended damage to viscera are very low.
  - In some cases, not all fibroids are able to be removed, and so symptoms may recur.

The following nonmedical treatment options could be considered if the woman does not desire future fertility:

- Endometrial ablation by a second-generation device (microwave or thermal balloon):
  - They are mostly performed under general anaesthetic.
  - The operative time is very short, and the postoperative recovery is quick; hence the risk of VTE is not increased.
  - Endometrial priming with danazol is also not needed with the second-generation devices.
  - Patient satisfaction rates are about 70–80%.
  - Recurrence of bleeding is more common in women with adenomyosis.

- Hysterectomy, either laparoscopic, abdominal, or vaginal:
  - This is the definitive treatment of HMB in women not desirous of future fertility.
  - In the short term, it is expensive, with a recovery time of approximately 6 weeks.
  - Complications are similar to other surgical methods.

The following radiological procedures could be considered if the woman wanted to preserve her uterus and all other treatments had failed or were not wanted by the woman:

- Uterine artery embolisation (UAE):
  - This technique, performed by an interventional radiologist, reduces uterine arteriolar blood flow, causing ischaemic necrosis and shrinkage of the uterine fibroids, while allowing the surrounding myometrium to recover.
  - HMB resolves in 85–95% of women.
  - It should only be done once any sarcomatous change in the fibroid has been excluded.
  - UAE is controversial in women desirous of maintaining fertility, but it may have a limited role because of surgical risk, failed previous surgery, or the woman's choice.
  - Because of a lack of good-quality evidence, its routine use in the younger age group is not advocated.
  - The effects of UAE on fertility and pregnancy are uncertain.
  - Advantages of UAE compared with other surgical methods:
    - No significant difference in patient satisfaction and quality of life
    - No difference in short- or long-term complications
    - Significantly reduced length of stay and recovery time
    - No difference in the rate of premature menopause
  - Complications of UAE:
    - Vaginal discharge and fever (4%)
    - Failed procedure (4%)

- VTE (0.3%)
- Groin haematoma
- Allergy to contrast
- Artery dissection

  o Two randomised control trials (REST and EMMY) have shown reintervention rates between 28.4–32% at 5 years for UAE, compared with 2–10.7% for the surgical methods.

- Magnetic resonance–guided focused ultrasound surgery (MRgFUS):
  o This is a noninvasive technique for large fibroids and is not commonly available.
  o It employs an MRI thermal-imaging system to continuously measure temperature changes inside the uterus.
  o A high-intensity ultrasound beam is focused in the different areas of the fibroid, where it raises the temperature, causing necrosis.
  o Its effect on future pregnancies is not yet established. However, it does result in symptomatic improvement in HMB that is caused by large fibroids.

Chapter 2.6.   Primary Amenorrhoea

Definition

Primary amenorrhoea is defined as the lack of onset of menstruation at the age of 16 years in the presence of secondary sexual characteristics or at the age of 14 years in the absence of secondary sexual characteristics.

Secondary sexual characteristics imply breasts (mainly) and pubic and axillary hair development.

Cryptomenorrhoea implies obstruction to the outflow of the menstrual blood in the genital tract, either due to a septum or imperforate hymen.

Oligomenorrhoea implies menstruation at more than 35 days' interval.

Incidence

0.3% of girls experience primary amenorrhoea.

Clinical Physiology

Primary amenorrhoea is a symptom, not a disease. The menstrual flow is an end result of the complex and synchronised interaction of the different components of the hypothalamic-pituitary-ovarian-uterine axis. Once the CNS-hypothalamic axis becomes less inhibited by oestrogen, the hypothalamus develops the pulsatility for GnRH secretion, which is modulated by neurotransmitters. The GnRH promotes secretion of FSH and LH from the anterior pituitary gland, which leads to ovarian follicular development and eventually ovulation.

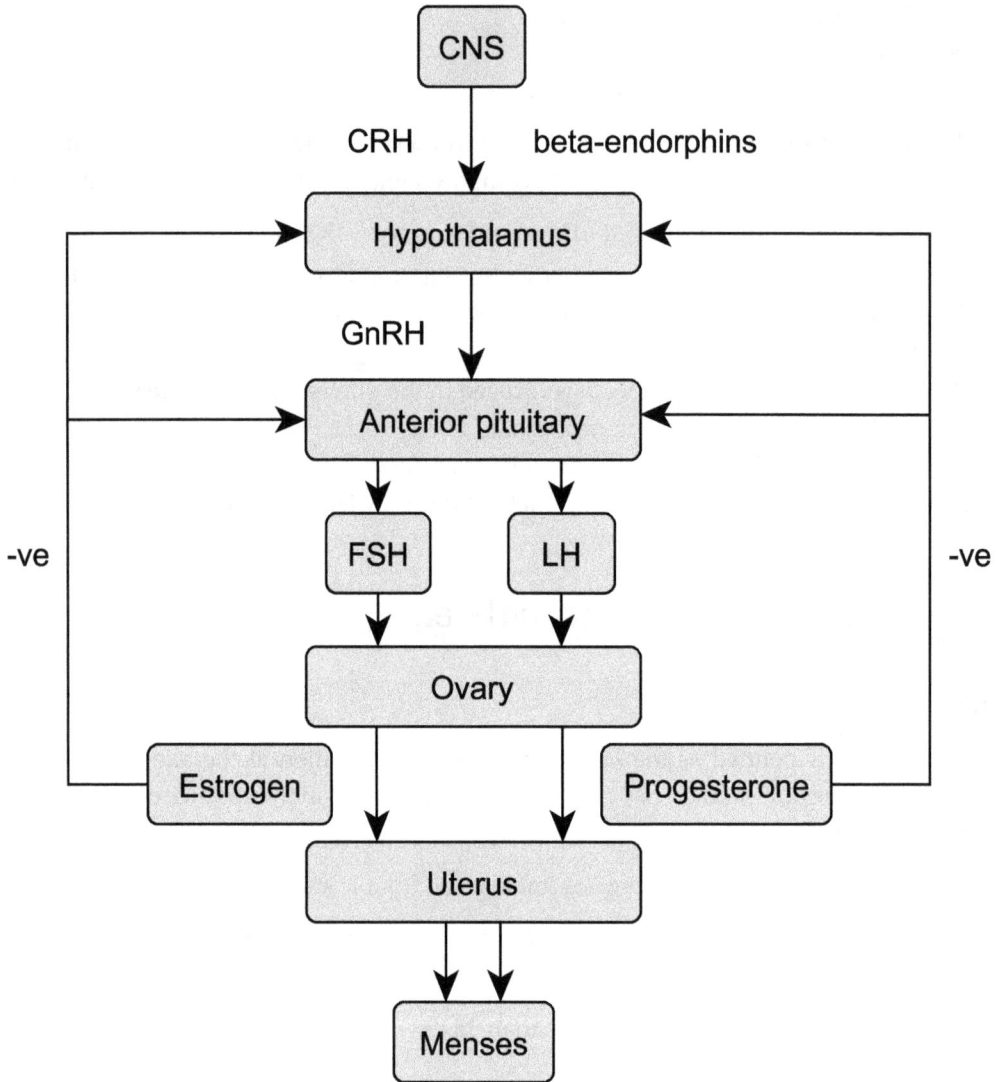

Figure 2.1. Flow diagram showing CNS-hypothalamic-pituitary-ovarian-uterine axis

After ovulation, the follicle converts into the corpus luteum, which starts to secrete progesterone, in addition to oestrogen. In the absence of a pregnancy and hCG, the corpus luteum withers, and the secretion of oestrogen and progesterone decreases, resulting in a withdrawal bleed.

Problems at any stage of this axis will result in amenorrhoea. The problems could be structural, genetic, or endocrinological. The structural causes are not many and can mostly be discerned with a focused history and thorough clinical examination. The diagnostic pillars to distinguish between hypogonadotropic and hypergonadotropic hypogonadism are the presence of a uterus and breast development and, secondly, the level of FSH.

Causes

On the basis of the presence or absence of breasts and a uterus, primary amenorrhoea can be classified into 4 groups:

1. Breasts absent, uterus present—most common
2. Both breasts and uterus present—second most common
3. Breasts present but uterus absent
4. Both breasts and uterus absent

It is important to make an exact diagnosis because there are different diseases that manifest into primary amenorrhoea and the prognosis for fertility varies.

Breasts Absent, Uterus Present

Women in this group have no ovarian oestrogen, either due to ovarian (gonadal), pituitary, or hypothalamic disorders.

Ovarian disorders include the following:

- 45X (Turner's)
- 46X, abnormal X (e.g., short- or long-arm deletion)
- Mosaicism
- Pure gonadal dysgenesis
- 17-α-hydroxylase deficiency

Gonadal failure is the most common cause of primary amenorrhoea and is mostly due to the deletion of all or part of the X chromosome. Deletion of the whole X chromosome or its short arm results in short stature; however, deletion of only the long arm does not result in short stature. These chromosomal disorders are due to random events and are not inherited.

Pituitary failure, which causes low gonadotropin levels, can be due to the following:

- Thalassaemia major
- Retinitis pigmentosa
- Chromophobe adenomas

The structural and/or endocrinological problems of the hypothalamus results in decreased gonadotropin secretion, which then leads to low oestrogen levels. Hypothalamic failure (hypogonadotropic hypogonadism) disorders include the following:

- Kallmann syndrome—anosmia, increased arm-span-to-height ratio
- Craniopharyngioma

Both Breasts and Uterus Present

Approximately 25% of these cases are caused by a prolactinoma. The remaining women have amenorrhoea that is caused by the same aetiologies that cause secondary amenorrhoea. Refer to the chapter on secondary amenorrhoea for more information regarding this.

Breast Present but Uterus Absent

There are two diseases in this group:

- Androgen resistance (testicular feminisation):
    - This disease is genetically transmitted, either by a X-linked recessive or autosomal dominant mode of inheritance.
    - The affected individuals have XY karyotype but suffer from a lack of testosterone receptors in the target organs and hence exhibit a lack of differentiation of male external and internal genitalia.
    - The external genitalia remain female, with a short or absent vagina.
    - Pubic and axillary hairs are absent because of a lack of testosterone receptors.
    - There are no male or female internal reproductive organs.
    - The oestrogen level is low but still able to cause breast development in the absence of the opposing action of testosterone. Testes, if present, should be removed before 20 years of age because of the risk of gonadoblastoma formation (20%).

- Congenital absence of uterus (Mayer-Rokitansky-Küster-Hauser syndrome or MRKH, or Müllerian agenesis):
    - These disorders are developmental accidents and are rarely inherited. Affected individuals have XX karyotype.
    - There is normal breast development and normal pubic and axillary hair but an absent vagina and uterus.
    - There could be concomitant renal (33%), skeletal (12%), and cardiac abnormalities.

Both Breasts and Uterus Absent

This is a rare group of disorders, characterised by insufficient oestrogen for breast development. The karyotype is XY with increased gonadotropins but low testosterone levels.

History

The history in a case of primary amenorrhea should cover the following areas:

- Recent weight changes
- Exercise regimen
- Life stressors
- Eating disorders
- Chronic illnesses: thyroid, prolactinoma
- Development of breasts, and pubic and axillary hair
- Any cyclical pelvic pain
- Breast discharge
- Family history of similar problems

Examination

There should be a thorough examination of all systems, with special reference to the following:

- The development of breasts, and pubic and axillary hair
- External genitalia
- Weight, height, and arm span
- Vaginal examination, if possible, checking for haematocolpos
- Any dysmorphic features

Investigations

- FBE, UEC, LFT, β-hCG, autoimmune antibodies
- FSH, LH, oestradiol, prolactin, TSH, testosterone
- MRI brain if prolactin level very high
- Pelvic ultrasound scan
- Karyotype
- X-ray of left wrist for bone age

Management

If the uterus is present, follow the algorithm outlined in Figure 2.2. If the uterus is absent, follow the algorithm outlined in Figure 2.3.

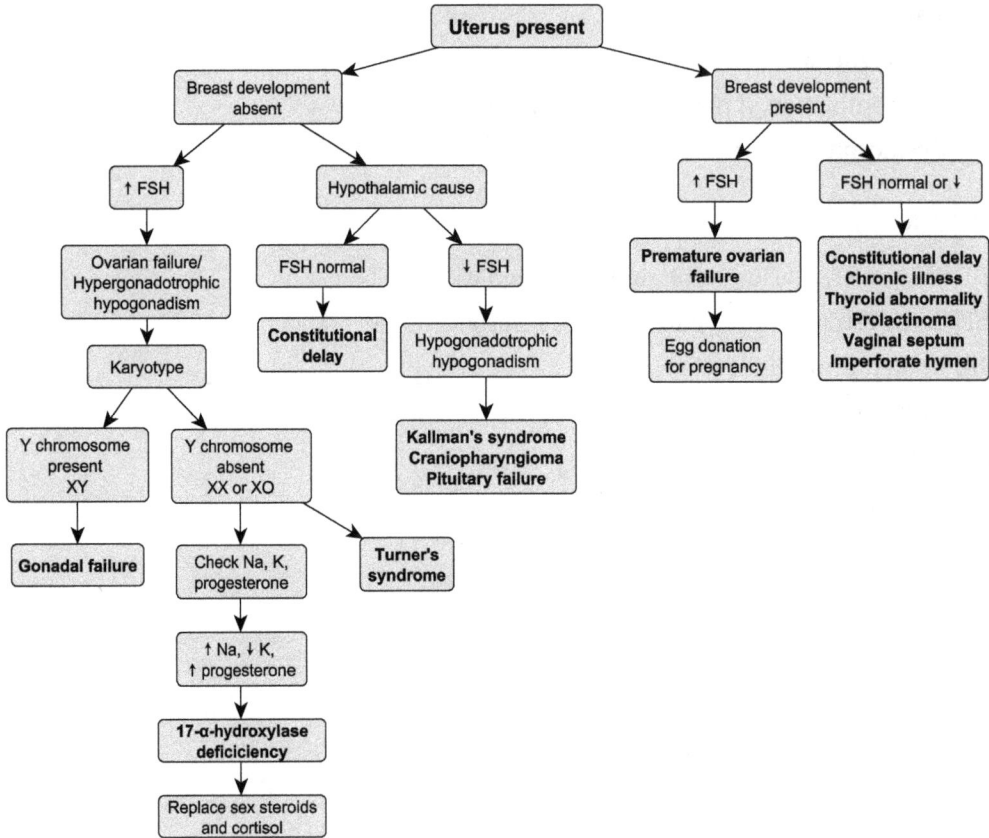

Figure 2.2. Algorithm for the diagnosis of primary amenorrhoea when the uterus is present

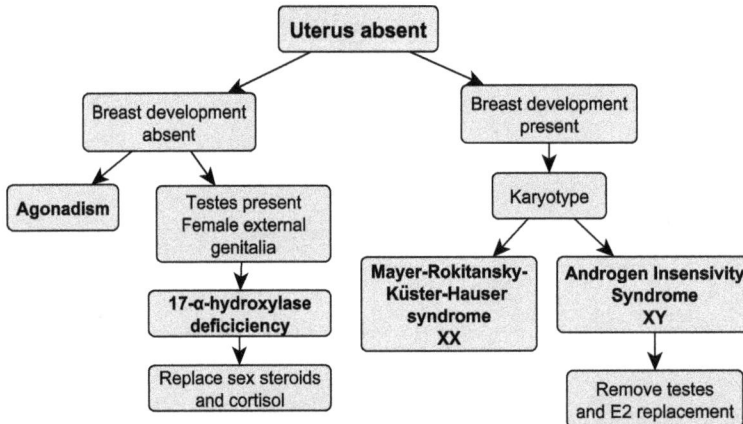

Figure 2.3. Algorithm for the diagnosis of primary amenorrhoea when the uterus is absent

Short-Answer Questions

Question 1

A 17-year-old girl complains of never having a period. She has absence of secondary sexual development. She never had sexual intercourse.

Part a

List your differential diagnoses.

Answer:

The differential diagnoses in the absence of secondary sexual development are as follows:

- Uterus present:
    - Ovarian failure
        - Gonadal dysgenesis
        - Mosaicism
        - Turner's syndrome
        - 17-α-hydroxylase deficiency
    - Hypothalamic failure secondary to inadequate GnRH release—constitutional delay
    - Pituitary failure
- Uterus absent:
    - 17-α-hydroxylase deficiency
    - 17,20-desmolase deficiency
    - Agonadism

Part b

What investigations will you order?

Answer:

As written in the text above.

Question 2

Point out the differences between androgen insensitivity syndrome (AIS) and Mayer-Rokitansky-Küster-Hauser syndrome.

Answer:

	AIS	MRKH syndrome
Development	Genetically inherited	Developmental accident
Karyotype	XY	XX
Testosterone level	Within normal male range	Within normal female range
Estrogen level	Low	Within normal female range
Pubic hair	Absent	Present
Breasts	Present	Present
Uterus	Absent	Absent
Vagina	Absent/rudimentary	Present
Gonads	Testes	Ovaries

Table 2.3. Difference between AIS and MRKH syndrome

Question 3

A 16-year-old presents with primary amenorrhoea.

Part a

What will you ask in the history?

Answer:

Although there is no legal requirement, if the girl is too shy to speak, it may be easier and better to speak with her mother. Questions relating to sexual habits, pregnancy, and the use of recreational drugs should not be asked when the mother is present. The following areas will be covered in the history:

- The age when secondary sexual characteristics started to develop
- Recent changes in weight
- Life stressors, exercise regimes, eating habits
- Smoking, alcohol intake, and the use of recreational drugs
- Any possibility of pregnancy
- Chronic illnesses: thyroid, kidney, prolactinoma, cystic fibrosis
- Medications
- Surgical history

- Ambiguous genitalia, hirsutism, virilism (for congenital adrenal hyperplasia and PCOS)
- Cyclical pelvic pain (may indicate imperforate hymen, vaginal septum, or absent vagina)
- History of head injury, blurring of vision, galactorrhoea (may indicate hypothalamic-pituitary axis disorder)
- Family history of late menarche

Part b

What areas will you focus on in the examination?

Answer:

Examine the girl in the presence of her mother or a chaperone.

- General examination: height, weight, arm span
- Features of Turner's syndrome: short stature, webbed neck, wide carrying angle
- Development of secondary sexual characteristics: breast development, pubic and axillary hair
- Hirsutism and acne, indicating PCOS
- External genitalia: male/female, presence of a normal vagina or rudimentary vagina
- Vaginal examination if the girl is willing: imperforate hymen, haematocolpos

Part c

What investigations will you do and why?

Answer:

- Serum β-hCG to exclude pregnancy
- FBE to check for anaemia and assess her general state of health
- UEC, especially Na and K to exclude 17-α-hydroxylase deficiency
- Autoimmune antibodies to exclude autoimmune causes of ovarian failure (galactosaemia, Addison's disease)
- TSH to exclude hypothyroidism
- Prolactin to exclude prolactinoma (not immediately after an examination as it may be unduly raised)
- FSH and LH to indicate hypothalamic-pituitary axis and ovarian function
- Oestradiol to assess ovarian function
- Testosterone: if in the male range, it will indicate XY karyotype or androgenisation on the gonadal streak
- Pelvic ultrasound scan: to find out the presence of uterus, ovaries, abdominal or inguinal testes, cervix, vagina, haematometra, haematocolpos
- Renal ultrasound and X-ray of spine for MRKH syndrome
- MRI brain if the prolactin is very high or absent breast development to exclude pituitary or hypothalamic neoplasia
- Karyotypes for XX, XO, XXX, XY, mosaicisms, or deletions
- X-ray left wrist to establish bone age

Part d

You diagnose Turner's syndrome in the girl. Briefly describe your principles of management.

Answer:

In Turner's syndrome, the levels of oestradiol and progesterone are very low due to the maldevelopment of the ovaries. A very small proportion will have some oocytes in their ovaries, and hence may ovulate and become pregnant. In the absence of any oocytes, she will need to receive an oocyte donation to become pregnant.

These women also need incremental dosages of oestradiol with progesterone to promote the development of secondary sexual characteristics and to prevent osteoporosis and endometrial hyperplasia.

Multiple-Choice Questions

Q1. In a case of primary amenorrhoea, which one of the following investigations should be done to exclude AIS?

    A. Pelvic ultrasound

    B. Diagnostic laparoscopy

    C. Serum thyroxine level

    D. Karyotype

Answer: D

Q2. Which one of the following is most consistent with 46XY gonadal dysgenesis (Swyer syndrome)?

    A. Ambiguous external genitalia

    B. Normal female infantile phenotype

    C. Small testes in the inguinal canal

    D. Circulating testosterone in the male range

Answer: B

Q3. A 19-year-old woman presents, never having had a spontaneous period. She has had vaginal bleeding following the administration of a combined contraceptive pill. She has Tanner stage 1 breast development. Which of the following would be least useful?

    A. Karyotyping

    B. Estrogen assay

    C. Prolactin assay

    D. FSH and LH assay

Answer: B

Q4. A 16-year-old tall, athletic girl presents with primary amenorrhoea. She has been diagnosed with AIS. Which of the following statements is correct in this context?

   A. Thelarche occurs normally due to peripheral conversion of testosterone to oestrogen.
   B. Axillary and pubic hair develops normally due to peripheral conversion of testosterone to oestrogen.
   C. Menstruation is irregular, 1–2 times in a year.
   D. Vulva, vagina, and ovaries are normally present.

Answer: A

Q5. A 15-year-old girl presents with primary amenorrhoea and features of masculinisation. She was taller than her peers in childhood. Pubic hair began to grow at 6 years of age. Excessive facial hair was noticed at 8 years, and she now shaves her facial hair twice a week. Her height is 160 cm, blood pressure is 120/80, and she has prominent muscle mass. Breast development is at Tanner stage 2. Her clitoris is enlarged, and labia are partially fused. On ultrasound scan, a uterus is seen, and no abnormal mass is seen in the pelvis. Her karyotype is most likely:

   A. 47, XXY
   B. 47, XYY
   C. 46, XY
   D. 46, XX

Answer: A

Q6. A 17-year-old presents with short stature and severe oligomenorrhoea. What is the most likely diagnosis, based on the following lab results?

Test	Value		Reference range
LH	8		4–25
FSH	9		3–25
17-hydroxyprogesterone	11.5	H	< 5.5
Testosterone	2.9	H	0.5–2.5
DHEAS	13.8	H	0.9–11.7

   A. Sertoli-Leydig cell tumour
   B. Late-onset congenital adrenal hyperplasia
   C. Cushing's syndrome
   D. Adrenal cortical adenoma

Answer: B

Q7. A 15-year-old with primary amenorrhoea weighs 50 kg and measures 170 cm in height. She is phenotypically female with no somatic abnormalities. Breasts are Tanner stage 2, and pubic hair is Tanner stage 3. Her external genitalia are infantile. Ultrasound shows a vagina and a small uterus. Her karyotype has been reported as 46XY. Her FSH is raised but LH, TSH, and prolactin are normal. She should undergo:

A. Bilateral gonadectomy

B. Hysterectomy

C. Hysterectomy with bilateral salpingo-oophorectomy

D. Diagnostic laparoscopy and gonadal biopsy

Answer: A (This patient has AIS, but it is possible for Müllerian structures such as the uterus to develop despite the XY karyotype.)

Q8. Daily application of oestriol cream to the vulva of a young girl is the treatment of which of the following conditions?

A. Lichen sclerosus

B. Labial adhesions

C. Atopic dermatitis

D. Acrodermatitis enteropathica

Answer: B

Q9. Which of the following is least common in Klinefelter's syndrome?

A. Low FSH

B. Azoospermia

C. Tall stature

D. Eunuchoidism

Answer: A

Q10. Which of the following conditions does **not** have the correct karyotype next to it?

A. Androgen insensitivity   46XY

B. True gonadal dysgenesis   46XY

C. Turner's syndrome   46XO

D. Female adrenogenital syndrome   46XX

Answer: C

Q11. Which of the following is the most important physical finding in establishing a diagnosis in a 14-year-old girl with primary amenorrhoea?

A. Acanthosis nigricans

B. Arm span exceeding height

C. Normal visual fields

D. Tanner stage 3 thelarche

Answer: D

Q12. Which of the following is **not** a part of Klinefelter's syndrome?

    A. Testicular hypoplasia

    B. Azoospermia

    C. Impotence

    D. High FSH

Answer: C

Q13. An 18-year-old with primary amenorrhoea and Müllerian agenesis will have which of the following features?

    A. Uterus present, breasts undeveloped

    B. Uterus present, breasts developed

    C. Uterus and breasts both undeveloped

    D. Uterus absent, breasts developed

Answer: D

Q14. A 16-year-old presents with primary amenorrhoea. Her breasts are developing. She does not have a uterus, but ovaries are present. Which of the following investigations will you **not** do in this clinical context?

    A. Renal ultrasound

    B. X-ray spine

    C. Progesterone challenge test

    D. Hearing test

Answer: C

Q15. Müllerian and Wolffian ducts are present in all of the following, except:

    A. AMH deficiency

    B. FSH receptor mutation

    C. Ovotestis

    D. Mixed gonadal dysgenesis

Answer: A

Q16. A 20-year-old with primary amenorrhoea has normal breasts and pubic hair, but the uterus and vagina are not present. Which of the following is **not** a likely diagnosis?

    A. Klinefelter's syndrome

    B. Testicular feminisation syndrome

    C. Gonadal dysgenesis

    D. Müllerian agenesis

Answer: D

Q17. Which of the following is **not** oestrogen-dependent?

A. Thelarche

B. Menarche

C. Adrenarche

D. Precocious puberty

Answer: C

Q18. How will you induce ovulation in an 18-year-old girl who had pituitary ablation for the treatment of craniopharyngioma?

A. Clomiphene

B. Pulses of GnRH

C. Cyclical oestrogen and progesterone

D. HMG followed by hCG

Answer: D

Q19. Which of the following is correct regarding androgen insensitivity syndrome?

A. The testosterone is lower than a normal male.

B. The risk of malignant transformation is high until 20 years of age.

C. Onset of puberty is delayed because of the absence of endogenous hormones.

D. The syndrome is X-linked recessive.

Answer: D

Q20. The absence of breast development indicates a lack of:

A. Progesterone

B. Testosterone

C. Prolactin

D. Estrogen

Answer: D

Q21. Which of the following is most important in the onset of menstruation?

A. Total body weight

B. Body composition

C. Ratio of body weight to lean body weight

D. Ratio of fat to total body weight and lean body weight

Answer: D

Q22. Which of the following statements is incorrect about menarche?

A. Moderately obese women have earlier onset of menarche.

B. Malnourished women have delayed menarche.

C. International athletes have delayed menarche because of stress.

D. Leptin affects GnRH and LH pulsatility.

Answer: C

Q23. Stress causes amenorrhoea because:

    A. It directly increases FSH secretion.

    B. It promotes increased secretion of corticotropin-releasing hormone, which inhibits GnRH.

    C. It directly decreases insulin-like growth factor binding protein 1.

    D. It increases insulin-like growth factor.

Answer: B

Options for Q24 and Q25.

    A. Start of episodic pulsatility of LH during sleep

    B. Episodic pulsatility of LH is absent before puberty

    C. Episodic pulsatility of LH occurs day and night after menarche

    D. Activation of the positive gonadotropin response to increase oestrogen

Q24. Which of the above is the initial hormonal change at the onset of puberty?

Answer: A

Q25. Which of the above is the last hormonal change of puberty?

Answer: D

Q26. Which of the following groups of conditions are most prevalent in women with primary amenorrhoea?

    A. Breasts absent but female internal reproductive organs present

    B. Breasts present and female internal reproductive organs present.

    C. Breasts present but female internal reproductive organs absent.

    D. Breasts absent and female internal reproductive organs absent

Answer: A

Q27. What is the most common association of primary amenorrhoea?

    A. Absent breasts

    B. Absent uterus

    C. Gonadal dysgenesis

    D. Pituitary failure

Answer: D

Q28. Primary amenorrhoea is a common feature in which of the following?

    A. Pregnancy

    B. Anorexia nervosa

    C. PCOS

    D. Premature menopause

Answer: B

Q29. A 15-year-old girl presents with severe lower abdominal pain. The pain is intermittent and commenced 12 months ago. Her periods have not started yet. She has normal secondary sexual characteristics. Her BMI is also normal. Her twin sister has regular periods. What is the most likely diagnosis?

    A. Polycystic ovarian syndrome

    B. Androgen insensitivity

    C. Hyperthyroidism

    D. Imperforate hymen

Answer: D

Q30. An 18-year-old never had a spontaneous period. She has had vaginal bleeding following administration of the oral contraceptive pill. She has little breast development. Which of the following will be least useful in making a diagnosis?

    A. Chromosomal analysis

    B. Estrogen assay

    C. Prolactin assay

    D. FSH and LH assay

Answer: B

Chapter 2.7.   Secondary Amenorrhoea

Definition

Secondary amenorrhoea is the absence of menses for at least six consecutive months, on a background of normal, regular menses.

Causes

The description below does not include the contributions from physiological causes and excessive prolactin, androgen, and cortisol production to secondary amenorrhoea.

Anatomical sites	Features	Diseases	Endocrine changes
Hypothalamus (62%)	Negative Progesterone Challenge Test (PCT)	Stress Sudden change in weight Neoplasm	Low FSH, LH, and oestradiol levels
Pituitary (16%) – hypogonadotropic amenorrhoea	Negative PCT	Chromophobic, basophilic, and acidophilic adenomas Necrosis	Low FSH, LH, and oestradiol levels
Ovary (12%) – hypergonadotropic hypogonadism	Negative PCT	Premature ovarian failure	Elevated FSH and LH
Uterus (7%)	Uterus cannot be sounded Negative PCT	Asherman syndrome Tuberculosis of the endometrium	No endocrine abnormality
Endocrinopathies		Hypothyroidism	High TSH and prolactin
		Cushing's disease	Low FSH, LH, elevated cortisol
		Late Onset Congenital Adrenal Hyperplasia (LOCAH)	Elevated 17-hydroxyprogesterone and DHEAS

Table 2.4. Causes of secondary amenorrhoea

Hypothalamic Causes

An estimated 62% of the secondary amenorrhoea causes fall into this group:

- Neoplastic
  - Craniopharyngiomas.
  - Granulomatous diseases from tuberculosis, sarcoidosis.

- Drugs
  - Phenothiazines.
  - Combined oral contraceptives.
  - Some antihypertensives.

- Stress and exercise
  - Stressful life situations—such as death of a close family member, divorce, sudden change of place, or stress from competitive exercise—can cause amenorrhoea.
    - This effect is thought to be mediated by GnRH suppression by the elevated levels of catecholamines, oestrogen, and β-endorphins.

- Weight loss
  - A sudden loss of 15–20% of weight below the ideal body weight can cause amenorrhoea due to inhibition of GnRH release from the hypothalamus due to a reduced frequency of GnRH pulses.
  - Pituitary and end-organ function remains unaffected until very sudden weight loss occurs.
  - Anorexia nervosa, a psychiatric disorder with significant weight loss (common in adolescent girls), also causes secondary amenorrhoea due to the inhibition of GnRH release. The following hormonal changes occur in anorexia nervosa:
    - Decreased levels of T3 (characteristic), ACTH, DHEAS
    - Increased levels of T4, GH, cortisol
  - A normal menstrual cycle is restored when the ideal body weight is reached.

- Functional hypothalamic amenorrhoea
  - This group of disorders includes all those women with secondary amenorrhoea who do not have any abnormality listed in the categories above.
  - This group of women have an abnormality of the cyclic variations of GnRH pulsatility, possibly due to a defect of the CNS neurotransmitter secondary to elevated opioid activity.
  - A positive PCT in this group of women will mean normal levels of endogenous oestrogen.

Pituitary Gland Causes

The pituitary disorder may affect multiple systems, such as thyroid, adrenal, growth hormone, in addition to FSH and LH, whereas primary disorders of the hypothalamus only affect one hormone. The pituitary gland disorders are broadly neoplastic or hypotensive in origin.

- Neoplastic
  - Chromophobe adenoma—most common, nonprolactin-secreting tumour
  - Basophilic adenoma—secretes excessive ACTH
  - Acidophilic adenoma—secretes excessive GH
- Hypotensive
  - Sheehan's syndrome—pituitary necrosis due to hypotension at childbirth
  - Simmonds disease—pituitary necrosis due to hypotension without pregnancy

Ovarian Causes

It primarily results from premature ovarian failure (premature menopause), which is usually transient or intermittent in the beginning and then becomes permanent. It usually results from chemotherapy or radiotherapy, or it is secondary to autoimmune diseases (e.g., hypoparathyroidism, Hashimoto's disease, Addison's disease). It can also result from the surgical depletion of ovarian follicles, such as ovarian cystectomies, tubo-ovarian abscess, or benign ovarian neoplasm. A high serum FSH will indicate an ovarian aetiology for amenorrhoea. Further tests, such as karyotyping, antinuclear antibodies, TSH, antithyroid antibodies, and DHEAS, will indicate the reason for premature ovarian failure. (This is also discussed in the Menopause chapter.)

Uterine Causes

Complete endometrial destruction from any cause will result in amenorrhoea. The two common causes of endometrial destruction are Asherman's syndrome and tuberculosis of the endometrium.

- Asherman's syndrome (intrauterine synechiae) if amenorrhoea starts after curettage.
  - Asherman's syndrome (Fritsch syndrome) is a rare condition involving intrauterine adhesions or fibrosis obliterating the endometrial cavity. It can also affect the myometrium and invariably results after a surgical curettage or multiple curettages.
  - There is a high incidence (30%) of Asherman's syndrome after curettage for:
    - Missed abortion
    - Pregnancy failure
    - Retained placenta
    - D&C
    - Myomectomy
    - Metroplasty
    - Caesarean
  - The diagnosis is established by a suggestive history, inability to sound the uterus, and an unsuccessful hysteroscopy.
- Tuberculosis of the endometrium.
- Schistosomiasis of the endometrium.

History

A detailed history covering the following areas must be taken:

- Age, parity, menstrual history
- Current drug use, chemotherapy, or radiotherapy
- Recent surgery, especially involving the uterus
- Weight loss, stress, strenuous exercise
- Menopausal symptoms
- Decreasing breast size
- Dryness of the vagina
- Symptoms of other systems, such as androgenisation, hypothyroidism, Cushing's syndrome, hypoparathyroidism

Examination

- Systemic examination including the following:
  - General appearance
  - BMI
  - CNS
  - Thyroid
  - Breasts
  - Excessive hair, acne, virilisation
- Abdominal examination, looking particularly for masses
- Uterine size, to check for pregnancy
- Vaginal and cervical examination for atrophic changes

Investigations

- β-hCG to rule out pregnancy
- FBE, UEC and urinalysis to rule out systemic disease
- Serum prolactin to rule out hyperprolactinaemia
- TSH, T4, T3 to rule out hypothyroidism and anorexia nervosa if suggestive history
- DHEAS to rule out any adrenal causes
- FSH, LH, and oestradiol to rule out hypothalamic causes or primary ovarian failure (POF)
- MRI of the CNS to rule out hypothalamic/pituitary neoplasms
- Pelvic ultrasound to rule out any uterine or adnexal pathology
- Karyotype and antinuclear antibodies to further investigate POF

A woman with secondary amenorrhoea who requests investigation should always be investigated, even when the duration is less than 6 months.

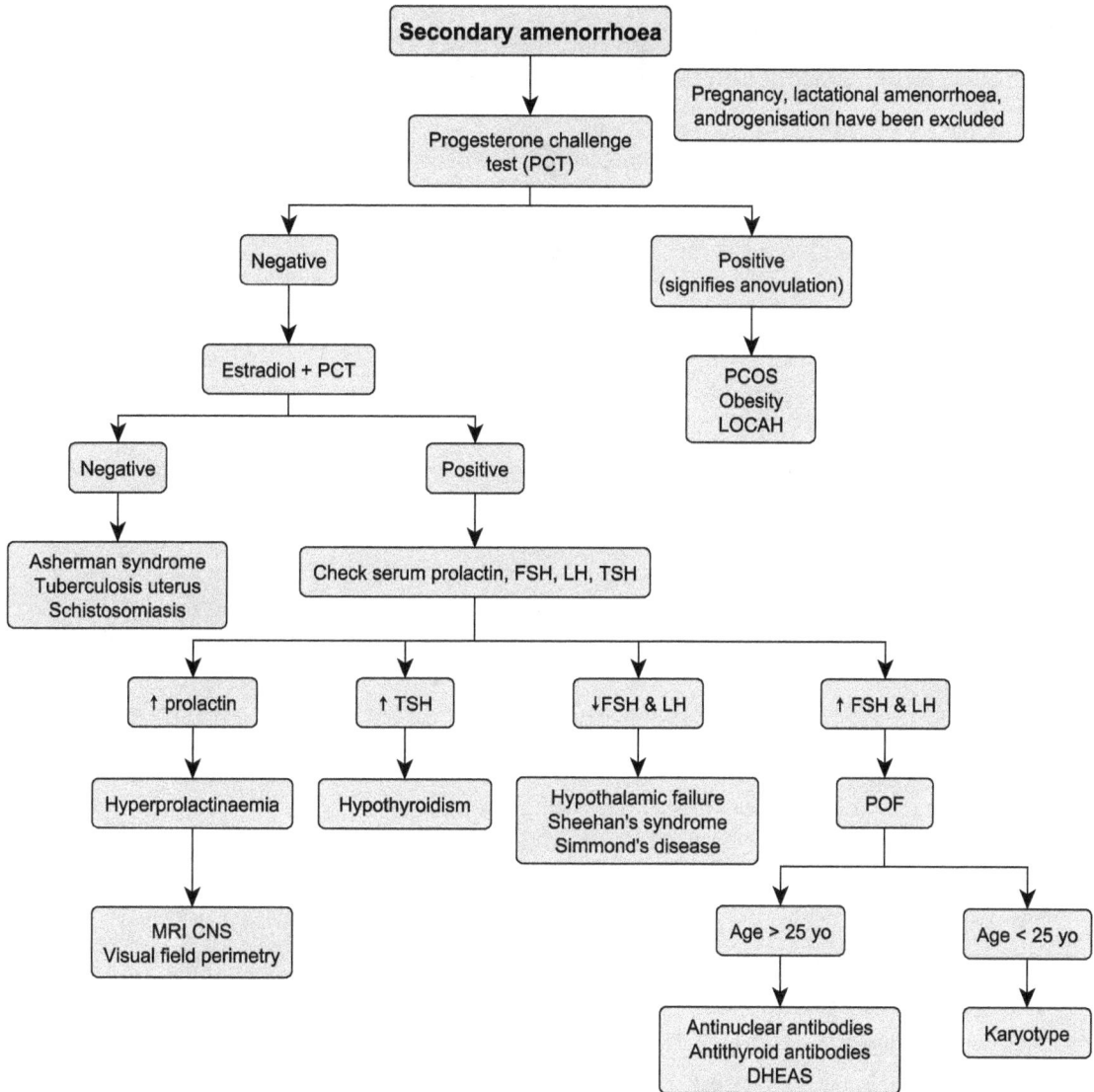

Figure 2.4. Algorithm for the diagnosis of secondary amenorrhoea

The treatment of secondary amenorrhoea should be instituted. Weight loss and stress should be managed by appropriate behavioural modifications. Drug use should be reviewed. Hypothalamic and pituitary gland disorders are usually self-limiting. Oestrogen and progesterone replacement should be given when the oestradiol level is low or the prolactin level is high, to prevent the development of osteoporosis. Non-prolactin-secreting pituitary neoplasms or prolactin macroadenomas require surgery.

In women with hypothalamic-pituitary dysfunction who are not desirous of pregnancy, cyclical progesterone will prevent endometrial hyperplasia. If this group of women desire pregnancy, ovulation should be induced by clomiphene. When the oestradiol level is low, clomiphene is not successful in inducing ovulation; hence, human menopausal gonadotropin (HMG) should be used. Women with POF wishing to achieve a pregnancy can use donor eggs.

Multiple-Choice Questions

Q1. Which is the most frequent cause of Asherman's syndrome?

    A. Curettage for miscarriage

    B. Metroplasty

    C. Prolonged use of hormonal IUCD

    D. Retained placenta following a ventouse delivery

Answer: A

Q2. Secondary amenorrhoea from strenuous exercise is due to:

    A. Weight loss

    B. Dietary reduction

    C. Stress

    D. A decrease in the level of β-endorphin

Answer: C

Q3. In anorexia nervosa, which of the following endocrine changes is consistently seen?

    A. Decreased T4

    B. Decreased T3

    C. Decreased GH

    D. Decreased cortisol

Answer: B

Q4. With respect to the oestradiol level in a failed (negative) progesterone challenge test, which of the following is correct?

    A. The E_2 level is < 40 pg/mL.

    B. The E_2 level is > 80 pg/mL.

    C. Progesterone level is < 40 pg/mL.

    D. Progesterone level is > 80 pg/mL.

Answer: A

Q5. The most frequent cause of secondary amenorrhoea is:

    A. POF

    B. Hypothalamic neoplasms

    C. Pituitary neoplasms

    D. Functional hypothalamic amenorrhoea

Answer: D

Q6. What is the most common histological finding in the ovaries of women with POF?

A. Fibrosis

B. Thecosis

C. Sclerosis

D. Stromal hyperplasia

Answer: C

Q7. In a woman with prolonged amenorrhoea, which of the following investigations is necessary?

A. Serum hCG

B. Serum prolactin

C. Skull X-ray

D. Pelvic ultrasound scan

Answer: A

Chapter **3**
Disorders of Puberty

Definitions

Puberty is defined as a cascade of synchronised morphological and endocrinological developments leading to reproductive and sexual maturity.

Adrenarche	Increase in adrenal androgen production, which occurs at the age of 6 years old in both boys and girls
Menarche	Time of the first menstrual bleed, which is often not associated with ovulation
Pubarche	Appearance of pubic hair, due to the effects of adrenal androgens
Spermarche	Time of first sperm production in boys, often heralded by nocturnal sperm production and appearance of sperm in the urine
Thelarche	Appearance of breast tissue in girls

Table 3.1. Chapter 3, Definitions

Chapter 3.1. Delayed Puberty

Clinical Physiology

Before puberty, the CNS-hypothalamic axis is inhibited by even a low level of circulating oestrogen. With weight gain and increased fat in the body, the CNS-hypothalamic axis becomes less inhibited by oestrogen. GnRH pulsatility of FSH and LH increases at night, initially, and then in the day as well at a later stage. Adipocytes secrete leptin, which correlates well with body weight, exerts a positive feedback on GnRH and LH pulsatility, and binds to the ovaries and endometrium. Increased secretion of GnRH and gonadotropins (FSH and LH) leads to increased synthesis of oestrogen from the ovaries. This step is the endocrinological milestone of puberty physiology. Oestrogen is essential for breast development. However, it is not essential for Müllerian duct development and regression of Wolffian ducts. Hence, even with low or absent oestrogen, the external and internal genitalia are phenotypically female.

Development of pubic and axillary hairs requires a small amount of androgens. The first clinically visible change that precedes this cascade of morphological and hormonal progression (puberty) is the development of breast buds. The mean interval between breast budding and the onset of menses is 2–3 years. It is very important to find out whether the absence of menses is due to a constitutional delayed puberty (CDP, or delayed menarche) or is pathological.

Characteristics

- There is wide variation in age of onset and progression of pubertal development.
- Genetics is the major determinant of the timing of puberty.
- But other factors influence the time of onset and the rate of progression of puberty:

  - Geographic location
  - Exposure to light
  - General health and nutrition
  - Psychological factors
  - Family history

- Normally, girls in the United States attain puberty by 13 years of age.

Diagnosis

- Investigation should be done when patients or parents are concerned.
- If puberty has not developed, a pathological cause should be considered, rather than simply attributing it to physiological delay.
- Physiologically delayed puberty tends to be familial.

Classification

- Hypergonadotropic hypogonadism—43%

  - Ovarian failure, with or without normal karyotype

- Hypogonadotropic hypogonadism—31%

  - Reversible causes: physiological delay, hypothyroidism, Cushing's syndrome, prolactinoma
  - Irreversible causes: GnRH deficiency, hypopituitarism, craniopharyngioma, malignant pituitary tumour

- Eugonadism—26%

History

- Helps determine if pubertal development is absent or stalled. An idea of the girl's growth pattern up to the time of evaluation is critical.
- Patients with constitutional delay have delayed growth, adrenarche, and sexual development.
- Nutritional habits, such as extreme dieting.
- Exercise intensity.
- Prior medical illness:

  - Inflammatory bowel disease (IBD)
  - Hypothyroidism

- Psychosocial deprivation.
- Medication usages.

- Neurologic symptoms suggestive of a CNS disorder:
  - Headache
  - Visual disturbances
  - Anosmia
  - Dyskinesia
  - Seizures
  - Mental retardation
- A positive family history of either constitutional delay or congenital GnRH deficiency can be a useful clue. However, it is nonspecific and is common in both constitutional delay and idiopathic hypogonadotropic hypogonadism due to mutations in FGFR1, which is an autosomal-dominant condition.

Examination

- Body measurements of height, weight, and arm span. Arm span exceeding height by more than 5 cm suggests delayed epiphyseal closure, secondary to hypogonadism. Serial standing height should be plotted on a growth chart.
- Tanner staging of secondary sexual characteristics. The breast bud is the earliest sign of pubertal development.
- Search for signs of hypothyroidism, gonadal dysgenesis, hypopituitarism, and chronic illnesses.
- Perform a neurological examination, including visual field, anosmia, and intracranial disease.
- Persistent deciduous teeth indicate hypothyroidism.
- Absence of pubic hair indicates hypopituitarism.
- Absence of pubic hair with vaginal pouch indicates androgen insensitivity.
- Associated congenital abnormalities, such as midline facial defects, cryptorchidism, and cleft palate, indicate congenital GnRH deficiency with or without other hypothalamic defects.

Investigations

Blood Tests

- FBE: 20% of women with sickle cell disease will have delayed puberty.
- ESR and LFT.
- Random FSH, LH, oestradiol
  - Distinguishes between hyper/hypogonadotropic states.
  - These measurements should not be corrected or scaled for age.
  - FSH level provides the greatest discriminative value at this time.
  - Low gonadotropins indicate constitutional delay and/or congenital GnRH deficiency.
- GnRH stimulation tests:
  - Not helpful in differentiating between constitutional delay and GnRH deficiency because of significant overlap of LH and FSH responses.
  - Can be resolved only with time and serial observation.

- Further tests for nutritional disorders and chronic illnesses:
    - Occult chronic illnesses may affect hypothalamic GnRH pulse generator.
    - Random serum prolactin:
        - May present as stalled puberty.
    - Can arise from prolactinomas or any hypothalamic or pituitary disorder that interrupts hypothalamic inhibition of prolactin secretion.
- TSH for hypothyroidism:
    - Delays puberty by unknown mechanism.
    - Growth velocity suddenly slows down.
    - Bone age is markedly delayed.
- DHEAS:
    - May help to distinguish between congenital GnRH deficiency and delayed puberty.
    - Normal in GnRH deficiency because of normal adrenal maturation and low in constitutional delayed puberty.
    - Values may overlap.
- Karyotype:
    - Turner syndrome.

Imaging

- Left hand and wrist X-ray to evaluate bone age:
    - Should be repeated serially.
    - Provides valuable information about the relationship between chronological age and skeletal maturation.
- Pelvic ultrasound scan—to confirm the presence of a uterus.
- MRI brain, if neurological symptoms, to look for hypothalamic/pituitary disease.
- Most of these disorders have in common a functional defect in GnRH secretion. Hence, no single test reliably distinguishes constitutional delay from other causes of delayed puberty. Constitutional delay forms only 10% of all cases of delayed puberty. Hence, all cases of delayed puberty must be investigated.

Management

- Treat the underlying disorders, such as hypothyroidism or IBD.
- Distinction between congenital GnRH deficiency and CDP remains uncertain and can only be resolved with longitudinal observation.
    - In constitutional delay, provide watchful observation with reassurance and psychological support.
    - Early hormonal treatment reduces anxiety and stress.
    - Girls with CDP will continue to develop pubertal changes when the bone age has reached 13 years.

- Estrogen:
  - Dose—0.5 mg oestradiol orally daily or 0.3 mg conjugated oestrogen orally daily.
  - Estrogen will not induce menstruation but will help attain full height potential and secondary sexual characteristics.
  - Cyclical progestin should not be added until there is substantial breast development, which usually takes 6–12 months.
  - Discontinue progestin for 1–3 months if breast growth has plateaued and menstruation has established to determine if spontaneous menstruation occurs, which should happen in CDP.
  - Gonadectomy in XY individuals around 20 years of age because of the increased risk of malignancy.
- Growth hormone:
  - Of controversial value without documented growth hormone deficiency.
  - Patients with congenital GnRH deficiency are not growth-hormone deficient and do not benefit from growth hormone therapy.

Multiple-Choice Questions

Q1. What is the earliest sign of puberty development?

    A. Appearance of pubic hair

    B. Appearance of breast bud

    C. Appearance of axillary hair

    D. Enlargement of the clitoris

Answer: B

Q2. What is the last sign of puberty development?

    A. Breast development Tanner stage 5

    B. Pubic hair development Tanner stage 5

    C. Menarche

    D. Enlargement of the vagina

Answer: C

Q3. Which of the following changes precede menarche?

    A. Peak height velocity

    B. Enlargement of the clitoris

    C. Enlargement of the vagina

    D. Enlargement of the labia majora

Answer: A

Q4. Approximately how many ovarian follicles does a girl have when she attains puberty?

    A. 30,000

    B. 60,000

    C. 100,000

    D. 400,000

Answer: D

Q5. In an adolescent, which of the following is a manifestation of a defect in the migration of primary germ cells?

    A. Pubertal delay

    B. Pubertal failure

    C. Congenital absence of vagina

    D. Precocious puberty

Answer: B

Q6. What is the approximate incidence of delayed puberty in girls?

    A. 0.1%

    B. 0.25%

    C. 1.0%

    D. 2.5%

Answer: D

Chapter 3.2.   Precocious Puberty

Definition

Precocious puberty (PP) is either the onset of secondary sexual characteristics before a girl reaches 8 years of age, or menarche before reaching 10 years of age. The incidence is 1 in 500 girls.

The steps of puberty development follow a normal sequence. There are two major concerns with PP:

- Social stigma of looking taller and heavier than her peers
- Short stature due to premature closure of the epiphyses

Causes

- GnRH-dependent (true PP)—most common type of PP (70%)
  - The exact cause is unknown.
  - The hypothalamic-pituitary-ovarian axis (HPOA) matures prematurely and results in normal menses, ovulation, and even pregnancy.
  - 30% of GnRH-dependent PP is due to the following CNS disorders:
    - Inflammatory: tuberculosis, encephalitis
    - Degenerative: secondary hydrocephalus, irradiation
    - Neoplastic: granulomas, hamartomas, teratomas
    - Congenital: hydrocephalus, cysts
  - Most CNS lesions are located in the region of the 3rd ventricle or mammillary bodies.
  - The mechanism by which these lesions produce PP is poorly understood. Hamartomas are known to secrete GnRH.
  - Most of these girls are under a lot of social pressure due to their "matured look" and hence become shy and withdrawn. However, their intellectual and behavioural development follows their chronological age.

- GnRH-independent (pseudo-PP)
  - o The most common cause of this type of PP is a granuloma cell tumour. Most of these are big enough to be palpated abdominally.
  - o Other oestrogen-secreting neoplasms: thecomas, luteoma, teratoma, choriocarcinoma.
  - o McCune-Albright syndrome: café-au-lait spots, fibrous dysplasia, cysts of the skull and long bones.
    - ▪ 40% of girls with this condition have PP.
  - o Congenital adrenal hyperplasia (CAH)
    - ▪ If diagnosed and treated in the neonatal period, normal puberty will develop.
    - ▪ However, if left untreated, the girl develops heterosexual PP due to excessive adrenal androgens.
    - ▪ If diagnosed late in childhood, isosexual PP develops.
  - o Hypothyroidism
    - ▪ Very rarely, PP develops due to a primary thyroxine deficiency. It is the only cause of PP in which bone age is retarded.
  - o Exogenous oestrogen
    - ▪ PP can develop when a girl uses someone else's (usually a family member's) oestrogen tablets, creams, or patches.
    - ▪ PP regresses after discontinuation of oestrogen.

History

A thorough history of PP should include the following:

- Onset and progression of pubertal changes and growth pattern in comparison to her siblings
- Headache, visual disturbances, abdominal pain, seizures with inappropriate laughter (gelastic seizures)
- Drug use, especially use of androgens and oestrogens
- Family history of PP

Examination

- Measurement of height, weight, and growth velocity
- Neurological examination: visual field, intracranial diseases, and neoplasms
- Café-au-lait spots
- Tanner staging of secondary sexual characteristics, virilisation
- Abdomen: any palpable mass

Investigations

- Endocrinological studies
    - FSH, LH, and oestradiol to distinguish central from peripheral causes
    - DHEAS, 17-hydroxyprogeterone, and testosterone to distinguish isosexual from heterosexual PP
    - TSH, T4, and T3 for hypothyroidism
    - Prolactin
    - Tumour markers: hCG and α-fetoprotein for ovarian neoplasm
    - GnRH stimulation test: distinguishes true from pseudo PP
- Imaging studies:
    - Left hand and wrist X-ray to estimate bone age
        - Should be repeated every 6 months
    - Pelvic ultrasound scan for uterus and ovarian enlargement
    - CT scan abdomen for adrenal neoplasm
    - MRI brain if suggestive history or clinical findings

Management

The aims of management are the following:

- To reduce gonadotropin secretion
- To reduce the peripheral effect of oestrogen and androgens
- To decrease the growth rate to normal
- To reduce skeletal maturation

Treatment depends upon the cause and the stage of disease at diagnosis.

Psychological support and education to the girl and her family should always be a part of the treatment plan.

Options for medical treatment include:

- GnRH agonist for both types of PP.
    - Monthly or 3-monthly injections or intranasal doses until the median age of puberty.
    - This should be started as soon as the diagnosis is made to reverse the changes and maximise adult height.
    - Its impact on adult height depends on the chronological age when treatment began.
    - Side effects: reaction at the injection site, vaginal bleeding
- For McCune-Albright syndrome: aromatase inhibitors, which prevent the conversion of androgens to active oestrogens.
- For hypothyroidism: thyroxine.
- For CAH: oestrogen to counteract adrenal androgens.

Surgery is required for CNS, ovarian, or adrenal neoplasms.

Short-Answer Questions

Question 1

A 6-year-old is brought to you by her mother with the complaint of vaginal bleeding for 10 days.

Part a

How will you take a history? What special considerations must you make in a history like this?

Answer:

I will conduct the conversation in a sensitive and non-judgmental fashion, ensuring complete privacy. If possible, I will have a female nurse present as a chaperone. The history will focus on possible causes of vaginal bleeding in this age group, and relevant information will be obtained from both the mother and the child, if possible. I will inquire about the following:

- Genital trauma
- Foreign body in the vagina
- Vaginal discharge: if present, duration, colour, odour
- Pain or burning during micturition
- Vaginal/cervical sarcoma botryoides
- Abdominal pain may indicate an ovarian tumour
- Sexual abuse: information about sexual abuse is very difficult to obtain
- History of bleeding disorders, precocious puberty in the family or in the child
- Drug use, either prescribed or accidental

Part b

What will you be looking for in your clinical examination?

Answer:

I will explain to the child and her mother regarding the need for the clinical examination and obtain their verbal consent. I will be sensitive and gentle, and I will ensure privacy at all times. If needed, I will also have a female nurse for chaperoning.

- General examination:
  - Vital signs
  - Pallor
  - Any marks, bruises, or scars suggesting abuse
  - Café-au-lait spots
- Tanner staging of secondary sexual characteristics.
- Abdominal examination for tenderness or masses.
- Perineal examination: Trauma to hymen or fourchette with or without a haematoma may indicate sexual abuse.
- A vaginal and rectal examination should only be done under anaesthesia.

Part c

How will you investigate this patient?

Answer:

- FBE.
- Vulvar bacterial swabs for microscopy and culture.
- Ultrasound scan of abdomen and pelvis for pelvic or vaginal tumours or vaginal foreign bodies.
- Examination under anaesthesia for:
  - Extent of vaginal injury, if suspected
  - Foreign body removal, if present
  - Atrophy
- If signs of precocious puberty are seen, I will perform the investigations listed in this chapter to make a diagnosis.

Part d

How will you treat her?

Answer:

I will treat the girl in consultation with a paediatrician. I will treat the cause:

- Remove foreign body, if found.
- Repair any vaginal or perineal lacerations.
- If vaginal atrophy is present, I will prescribe topical oestrogen cream.
- Bacterial or parasitic infections will be appropriately treated with an antibiotic or antihelminthic agent.
- If a vaginal or ovarian neoplasm is present, I will refer to a paediatric gynaecological oncologist.
- If precocious puberty is present, it will be treated with a GnRH agonist, and if there is a GnRH-independent cause, the primary disorder may also need to be treated.

Question 2

An 8-year-old girl is brought to you by her mother with the complaint of regular vaginal bleeding for the last 6 months.

Part a

How will you take a focused history?

Answer:

I will take a focused history in a sensitive and nonjudgmental fashion, ensuring complete privacy. I will obtain information around the possible causes of regular vaginal bleeding in this age group. I will seek information as follows:

- Duration, frequency, heaviness of bleeding and any associated pain
- History of easy bruising in the girl or her parents/siblings
- A detailed idea of the pattern of pubertal changes and growth velocity, as well as duration and development of thelarche and adrenarche
- Rule out CNS causes of pseudoprecocious puberty:
  - Any headache, visual disturbances, or seizures
  - Past history of brain disease, infection, or trauma
- Ingestion of any drug, especially oestrogen tablets

The most common cause of regular vaginal bleeding in a prepubertal girl is GnRH-dependent precocious puberty. In 30% of cases, puberty is GnRH-independent.

Part b

What will you look for in the examination?

Answer:

- Café-au-lait spots—McCune-Albright syndrome.
- Generalised tubercles—neurofibromatosis.
- Tanner staging of secondary sexual characteristics:
  - Presence of thelarche and adrenarche will indicate precocious puberty.
- Height, weight, and serial plotting of growth velocity.
- Abdominal examination to exclude hydrocephalus, cerebral tumours, hamartomas, infection.
- Visual field perimetry.
- Absence of pubertal changes indicates accidental use of oestrogen or regular vaginal trauma.

Part c

List the causes of precocious puberty.

Answer:

- GnRH-dependent PP
  - Cause mostly unknown
  - CNS disorders
    - Inflammatory: tuberculosis, encephalitis
    - Degenerative: irradiation, secondary hydrocephalus
    - Neoplastic: hamartomas, teratomas
    - Congenital: hydrocephalus, arachnoid, and suprasellar cysts
- GnRH-independent PP
  - McCune-Albright syndrome
  - Congenital adrenal hyperplasia
  - Hypothyroidism
  - Exogenous oestrogen
  - Granulosa cell tumour of the ovary
  - Other ovarian neoplasms: thecoma, luteoma

Multiple-Choice Questions

Q1. What is the best treatment for precocious puberty in a 7-year-old?

    A. Medroxyprogesterone acetate

    B. GnRH agonists

    C. Combined oral contraceptive pill

    D. Clomiphene citrate

Answer: B

Q2. Which of the following is **not** a feature of McCune-Albright syndrome?

    A. Bony dysplasia

    B. Café-au-lait spots

    C. Cysts of the skull bone

    D. Primary amenorrhoea

Answer: D

Q3. Normal height with minimal pubertal development may be seen in:

    A. Turner syndrome

    B. Pure gonadal dysgenesis

    C. Testicular feminisation

    D. Kallmann syndrome

Answer: D

Q4. Which of the following is used to treat idiopathic central precocious puberty?

    A. Exogenous gonadotropins

    B. GnRH antagonists

    C. GnRH agonists

    D. Ethinyl oestradiol

Answer: C

Q5. A 9-year-old consults you with regular vaginal bleeding. She had adrenarche at 8 years and thelarche at 7 years. What is the most likely diagnosis?

    A. Gonadal tumour

    B. McCune-Albright syndrome

    C. Idiopathic (GnRH dependent) precocious puberty

    D. Hypothyroidism

Answer: C

Q6. Which of the following is the least probable to be the cause of precocious puberty?

A. Hydrocephaly

B. McCune-Albright syndrome

C. Fröhlich's syndrome

D. von Recklinghausen's disease

Answer: C

Q7. A 6-year-old girl has persistent blood-stained vaginal discharge. What would you do as her treating gynaecologist?

A. Consider child abuse

B. Conduct a thorough vaginal and rectal examination

C. Arrange an examination under anaesthesia

D. Arrange an ultrasound scan to exclude foreign body and vaginal cancer

Answer: C

Q8. A young boy presents with delayed puberty. Investigations show low FSH, LH, and testosterone. Which of the following conditions is **not** a part of the differential diagnosis?

A. Kallmann syndrome

B. Constitutional delay

C. Klinefelter syndrome

D. Dax–1 gene mutation

Answer: C

Q9. A 3-day-old male baby has a swollen left breast with a discharge. The initial management should be:

A. Urgent surgical referral.

B. Urgent neonatal referral.

C. Get an ultrasound scan of the left breast.

D. Explain that it is physiological and reassure.

Answer: D

Q10. A 14-year-old girl with menarche 6 months ago complains of unpredictable vaginal bleeding with menses despite using tampons. The most likely explanation is:

A. Vesicovaginal fistula

B. Vaginal agenesis

C. Rectovaginal fistula

D. Duplication of vagina, cervix, and uterus

Answer: D

Chapter 4
Early Pregnancy Complications

Definitions

Abortion	Synonymous with miscarriage
Anembryonic pregnancy (blighted ovum)	When the mean gestational sac diameter is 25 mm or more, and the sac does not contain a fetal pole (embryo)
Blastocyst	Early embryonic stage of development, with cells having differentiated into an outer cell mass and inner cell mass, with a central fluid-filled cavity
Clinical miscarriage	When there is sonological or histological evidence of miscarriage
Decidua	The modified endometrium that exists during pregnancy; it forms the maternal part of the placenta under the influence of oestrogen.
Embryo	Conceptus up to 9 weeks of pregnancy
Gestational sac	Fluid-filled elliptical or oval sac with an echogenic rim at least 2 mm thick, eccentrically placed within the decidua
Mean sac diameter	The sum of the internal sac diameter in three planes, divided by three
Miscarriage	Either the failure of an intrauterine pregnancy before 20 completed weeks of pregnancy (or age of viability as determined by the country's law), or the loss of pregnancy with a fetal weight of 400 g when the gestational age is not known
Preclinical miscarriage	Pregnancy where implantation started but failed
Pregnancy of unknown location	When the pregnancy test is positive, but there is no sonological evidence of an intra- or extrauterine pregnancy
Pseudosac	A collection of fluid, centrally placed in the endometrial cavity and surrounded by the endometrium with a positive pregnancy test, without the features of a true gestational sac
Recurrent miscarriage	Three or more consecutive miscarriages
Subchorionic haematoma	Sonographically visible haematoma separating the gestational sac from the decidua

Table 4.1. Chapter 4, Definitions

Chapter 4.1.　　Miscarriage

Clinical Physiology of Miscarriage

Assessing Gestational Age

The duration of a normal pregnancy is 240 days or 40 weeks from the first day of the last menstrual period (LMP) of a 28-day menstrual cycle. The gestational age is always calculated from the first day of the LMP and not from the date of conception. The expected date of delivery is calculated by adding 9 months and 7 days to the LMP, or by subtracting 3 months and adding 7 days to the LMP (Naegele's rule).

The determination of gestational age by LMP is inaccurate in 11–42% of cases (Evidence Level II). An ultrasound scan dating has a margin of error of 4 days in first-trimester scans.

Human Chorionic Gonadotropin

Human chorionic gonadotropin (hCG) is a glycoprotein consisting of a smaller alpha subunit and a larger beta subunit, bound together by a disulphide bond with a half-life of 24 hours. Structurally, it is similar to LH, FSH, and TSH. It is secreted by syncytiotrophoblasts, which are the placental functioning units, consisting of a continuous, multinuclear layer on the surface of the villi. The secretion of hCG starts just after implantation occurs. It is detectable in blood or urine a week after conception. The level keeps rising by at least 66% every 48 hours (85% confidence interval) until 11 weeks of gestation. The level starts decreasing after 11 weeks and plateaus at 20 weeks of gestation at 10,000–20,000 IU/L for the rest of the pregnancy. The levels vary so widely that the estimation of gestational age on the basis of hCG is inaccurate.

To detect hCG, most laboratories employ a monoclonal antibody that is specific to the beta subunit of hCG. This is to ensure that tests do not make false positives by confusing with LH, FSH, and TSH. hCG is also detected in the blood in gestational trophoblastic disease, germ cell ovarian tumours, and testicular cancers.

Mechanism of Miscarriage

In a normal pregnancy, after the blastocyst has implanted, the extravillous cytotrophoblast erodes the vascular walls and enters the lumen of the spiral arteries. The muscle layer of these arteries is slowly replaced by fibrous tissue. These become the uteroplacental arteries, which eventually supply oxygen and nutrition to the developing embryo. At the same time, the cytotrophoblastic cells also partially plug the lumen of the spiral arteries, reducing the blood flow to the intervillous space (IVS). The IVS disappears by the end of the first trimester.

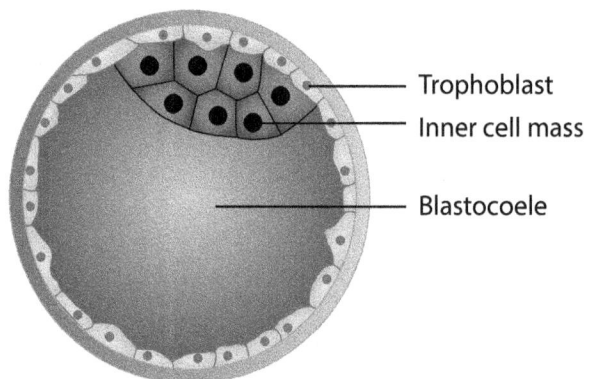

Figure 4.1. Large, well-expanded blastocyst. The outer cell mass and inner cell mass can be easily seen.

Altered trophoblastic invasion of the spiral arterioles could damage uteroplacental arteries and the IVS and cause pregnancy failure. Premature and diffuse onset of intervillous blood flow is abnormal and may increase the oxidative stress on the early placental tissue. This may lead to impaired placental development and pregnancy failure (Jauniaux E et al., 2003).

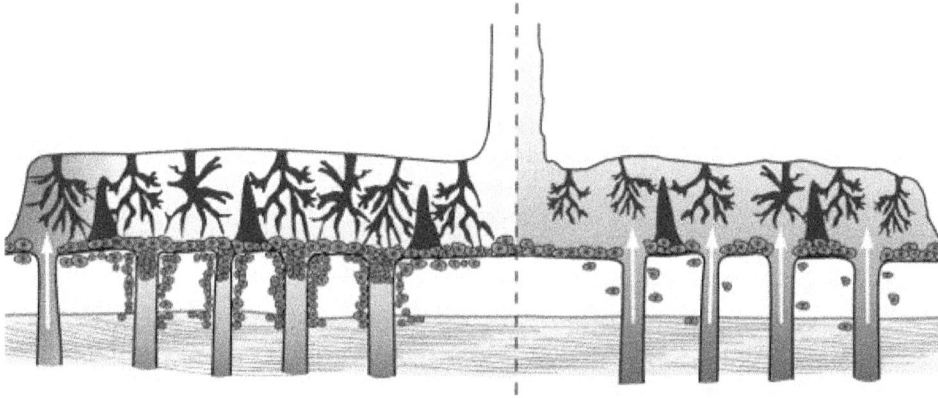

Figure 4.2. Comparison between placental vessels in normal pregnancy (left) and abnormal vessel development that may lead to miscarriage (right) (Jauniaux E et al., 2003)

A resistive index (difference in the blood velocity in an artery between systole and diastole, divided by systolic velocity) of > 0.55 in the uteroplacental circulation in very early pregnancy (gestational sac diameter < 12 mm) or very active intervillous blood flow predicted pregnancy failure, with a sensitivity of 88% and specificity of 90% (Merce et al., 1997).

Risk Factors

- Chromosomal abnormalities:
  - Aneuploidy of the conceptus is a major factor leading to miscarriage. The prevalence of chromosomal abnormalities in miscarriage varies from 50–60%. Its incidence is higher in chorionic villi (70–85%) compared with the embryo. These abnormalities largely result due to errors of gametogenesis (meiotic nondysjunction) in males and females, fertilisation, or cleavage of the zygote. The incidence of these errors increases after 36 years of age in the female. The following is a list of common chromosomal abnormalities in the conceptus of miscarriage (in the order of decreasing frequency):
    - Autosomal aneuploidy (50–65%).
    - Monosomy 45X (7–15%).
    - Triploidy (15%).
    - Tetraploidy (10%).
- Maternal age:
  - Increasing maternal age leads to an increased incidence of aneuploidy.

- Uterine and cervical abnormalities:
  - Up to 25% of females with the congenital abnormalities of the uterus and cervix miscarry. The congenital abnormalities are listed below in the order of decreasing frequency:
    - Unicornuate uterus (50%).
    - Bicornuate and septate uterus (25%).
    - Cervical incompetence.
  - The acquired abnormalities, such as submucous myoma or an endometrial polyp, are uncommon factors.

- Endocrine factors:
  - Progesterone deficiency due to decreased synthesis in the corpus luteum in the first 7 weeks of pregnancy.
  - Thyroid abnormalities:
    - Presence of antithyroid antibodies (odds ratio triples).
    - Hypothyroidism, although the evidence is conflicting.
  - Uncontrolled diabetes mellitus increases fetal anomalies.
  - Insulin resistance:
    - It causes a preinflammatory state in the uterus. The level of plasminogen activator inhibitor I is increased, which acts as a procoagulant and thrombophilic agent.
  - It has also been shown that the incidence of miscarriage is higher in women with PCOS, hypersecreting LH on day 8.

- Immunological factors:
  - Sharing of major histocompatibility locus antigens (HLA) between males and females.
  - Coeliac disease—antibodies are toxic to the trophoblast.

- Thrombophilias, both acquired and inherited cause placental vascular thrombosis.

- Infection:
  - *Staphylococcus.*
  - *Streptococcus.*
  - *Neisseria.*
  - *Ureaplasma urealyticum.*
  - *Mycoplasma hominis.*
  - *Toxoplasma gondii.*

- Behavioural:
  - Smoking—smoking more than 14 cigarettes a day increases the miscarriage risk 1.7 times.
    - It only affects euploid fetuses.
  - Alcohol—consuming alcohol 2 days a week doubles the risk of miscarriage.
  - Caffeine—more than 2 cups of coffee a day increases the risk of miscarriage.
  - Exposure to anaesthetic gases.
  - Stress.

Epidemiology

The incidence of miscarriage is about 15% in the normal population. Miscarriages before 10 weeks are mostly due to chromosomal problems, and late miscarriages are due to anatomical problems of the uterus and cervix.

Human reproduction is a very inefficient process. 30% of pregnancies are lost in between fertilisation and implantation, and another 30% between implantation and the first missed period. The rate of miscarriage decreases as the pregnancy advances.

Types

1. Threatened miscarriage:
   - Uterine bleeding with or without mild pain with a closed cervix and live fetus(es). About 50% of these pregnancies will be lost. There is an increased incidence of preterm labour, fetal growth restriction, and increased perinatal death if the pregnancy continues.
2. Missed miscarriage:
   - Fetal death with a closed cervix and often no uterine bleeding, pain, or passage of any pregnancy tissue through the cervical os.
3. Incomplete miscarriage:
   - Uterine bleeding with some pain, passage of pregnancy tissue through the cervical os, and the fetus is not identifiable or not alive.
4. Complete miscarriage:
   - Spontaneous passage of all fetal and placental tissue, with cessation of pain and bleeding, and an empty uterus.
5. Septic miscarriage:
   - Any miscarriage resulting from uterine infection.
6. Inevitable miscarriage:
   - Heavy vaginal bleeding and pain due to uterine contraction, with an open cervix.

History

A focused history should be obtained about the severity and duration of uterine bleeding and lower abdominal cramps or pain, the first day of the LMP, any positive pregnancy test, and the quantitative level of serum β-hCG, if available. Information about previous miscarriage(s) and risk factors as mentioned above should also be obtained. A good history can lead to the presumptive diagnosis, such as:

- History of pain and bleeding in early pregnancy, followed by the passage of products of conception through the open cervix = incomplete miscarriage.
- History of strong lower abdominal cramps or pain, and heavy uterine bleeding, with an open cervix = inevitable miscarriage.
- History of lower abdominal pain and uterine bleeding, with the passage of grapelike vesicles through the cervix = molar pregnancy.

Examination

- Haemodynamic compromise, depending upon the severity of symptoms.
- Lower abdominal tenderness may or may not be present.
- Speculum examination:
  - Normal in missed miscarriage.
  - Internal os may be open.
  - Products of conception/blood may be seen at the os or in the vagina.
- Bimanual examination:
  - Cervical dilation could be confirmed if it admits a finger.
  - Uterine size should be assessed.
  - Palpate for any adnexal mass.

Differential Diagnosis

- Very early normal pregnancy when the yolk sac or fetal pole are not visible sonographically
- Anembryonic pregnancy
- Ectopic pregnancy
- Gestational trophoblastic disease (molar pregnancy)

Investigations

- FBE.
- Blood group and antibodies.
- Serum quantitative β-hCG may need to be repeated after 48 hours.
  - Less than a 66% rise, or a decline in serum β-hCG levels on two samples at least 48 hours apart confirms a diagnosis of miscarriage before 11 weeks of pregnancy.
- Transvaginal/translabial ultrasound scan.
  - Absence of fetal heartbeat when crown-rump length (CRL) > 7 mm = missed miscarriage. No other investigation is required.
  - Absence of fetal pole when mean sac diameter > 25 mm = anembryonic pregnancy. No other investigation is required.
  - Empty uterus with normal endometrium and cessation of uterine bleeding and pain = complete miscarriage.
  - Uterus with tissues of mixed echogenicity in the endometrial cavity, with uterine bleeding and some lower abdominal cramps = incomplete miscarriage.
  - A normal intrauterine gestational sac with a live fetus and mild pain/bleeding = threatened miscarriage.

Role of Ultrasound in Miscarriage

The pelvic ultrasound scan is the mainstay of the investigation of miscarriage. It detects the size and number of gestational sac(s), viability of pregnancy, presence of a live fetus, gestational age, chorionicity and amnionicity, and it also shows predictors or definite signs of a miscarriage, including its type. In early pregnancy, a transvaginal scan, on account of a better resolution, has higher sensitivity than a transabdominal scan and bimanual examination.

Failure to visualise an intrauterine gestational sac by a transvaginal ultrasound scan, when the serum β-hCG is > 1500 IU/L, suggests an extrauterine pregnancy.

Gestational (Chorionic) Sac

A true gestational sac is ovoid or elliptical and is surrounded by an echogenic rim (double decidual reaction). It is seen in the upper half of the endometrium and is eccentrically situated. It is first seen at 4 weeks and 3 days from the LMP. The mean sac diameter grows at a rate of 1 mm/day between the 5th and 6th weeks of gestation. Once a normal uterine gestational sac is seen, the chance of a subsequent miscarriage is around 11% (Goldstein, 1994).

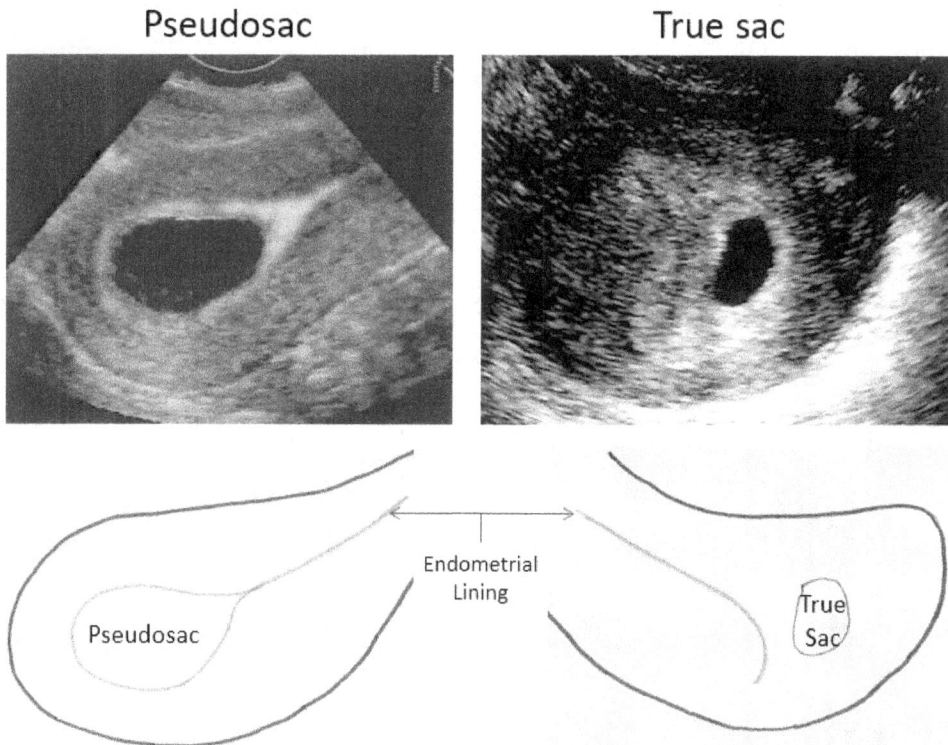

Figure 4.3. Sonological and diagrammatic illustrations of a pseudosac and a true sac

Crown-Rump Length

The fetal pole is first seen at 5 weeks and 2 days from the LMP. CRL is the distance between the top of the fetal head and the rump, and is measured in the midsagittal plane when the fetus is in a neutral position. CRL is used to date the early pregnancy. Dating of the pregnancy is most accurate when the CRL is measured between 6 and 10 weeks of gestation, since the growth of CRL is linear in this period and there is less biological variation.

In early pregnancy, CRL of twins and triplets is the same as in a singleton pregnancy. However, the fetuses in a multiple gestation often have different CRLs. When this happens, the smaller CRL should be used to date the pregnancy.

Yolk Sac

It is the ringlike, spherical structure seen inside the gestational sac in early pregnancy. The embryological primary yolk sac is not visible sonologically. The sonologically visible yolk sac is a secondary yolk sac. It becomes visible at 5½ weeks of pregnancy (mean gestational sac diameter = 8 mm) and is eccentrically located inside the gestational sac. In a normal pregnancy, it is the precursor of the embryo, which becomes visible on its margin. The diameter of the yolk sac increases steadily from 3 to 6 mm between 5½ and 10 weeks of pregnancy. It supplies nutrition to the embryo and also participates in erythropoiesis of the embryo. On 3-D ultrasound with surface rendering, its surface appears like a honeycomb. It disappears around 12 weeks of pregnancy, either by self-decay or after being compressed by the growing amniotic membrane. It serves the following very important diagnostic functions:

- Landmark for detecting the embryo within the gestational sac.
- A normal yolk sac within a normal gestational sac is a predictor of a normal pregnancy, when the fetal pole has not appeared.
- Marker of amnionicity.

Amniotic Cavity

The amniotic cavity is the ringlike structure containing the developing embryo. It starts to develop at the margin of the yolk sac. It is visible at 7 weeks of gestation, and is larger than the yolk sac. Around 8 weeks, its diameter is equal to the CRL. It keeps expanding in all directions, obliterating the extraembryonic coelom and ultimately fuses with the gestational (chorionic) sac by about 12 weeks of pregnancy.

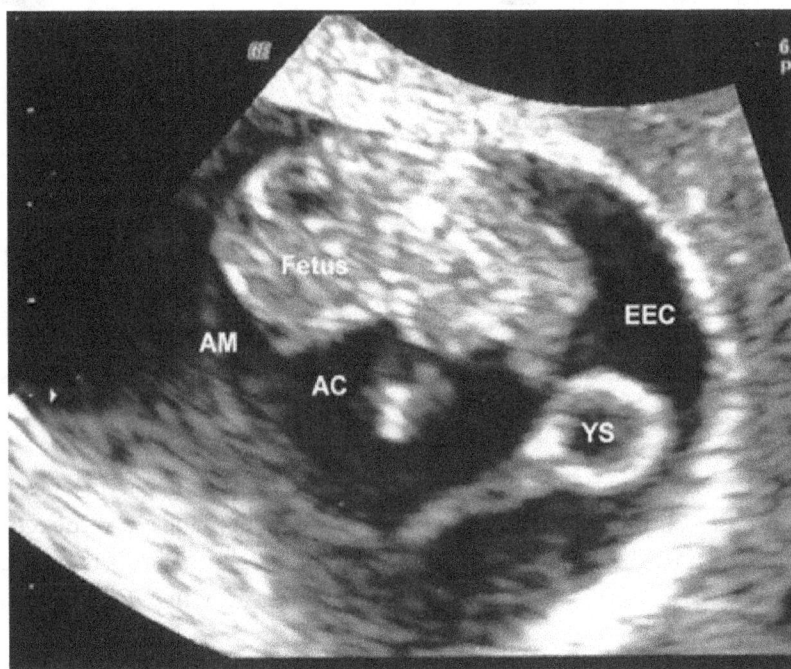

Figure 4.4. Sonogram of 7-week pregnancy, demonstrating fetus, amniotic membrane (AM), amniotic cavity (AC), yolk sac (YS), and extraembryonic coelom (EEC). The amniotic cavity obliterates the extraembryonic coelom as it expands.

Subchorionic Haematoma

Otherwise known as an intrauterine haemorrhage, a subchorionic haematoma is a haematoma between the gestational sac and decidua. It may be the first sign of a defective placentation and associated oxidative stress to the fetus (Jauniaux, 2005). Its volume and site are predictors of pregnancy failure.

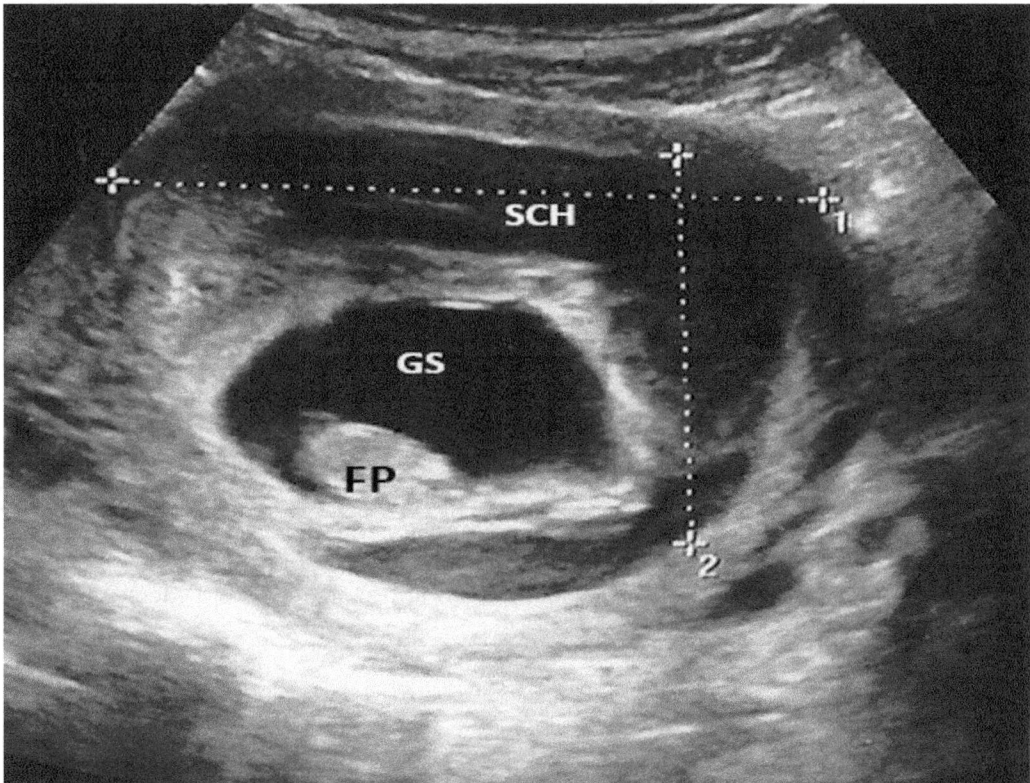

Figure 4.5. Sonogram showing subchorionic haematoma (SCH) detaching the gestational sac (GS) with a live fetus (FP) from the uterine wall on three sides

Sonological Predictors of Miscarriage

Feature	Predictors of miscarriage
Gestational sac	Irregular, small, or empty.
Yolk sac	Abnormal shape, size, calcified, hyperechoic, or double.
CRL	Miscarriage rate decreases with increasing CRL: | CRL	Miscarriage rate | |---|---| | Empty sac | 12% | | 5 mm | 7.2% | | 6–10 mm | 3.3% | | > 10 mm | 0.5% | A CRL deficit exceeding 2 standard deviations increases the risk of miscarriage (Mukri, 2008).
Fetal heart rate	A fetal heartbeat must be seen when the CRL > 7 mm, but in most normal cases, the embryonic heartbeat is first seen by a transvaginal ultrasound scan at a CRL of 2 mm. A consistently low fetal heart rate of 85 bpm, at a gestation of greater than 7 weeks, indicates a poor prognosis. A heart rate less than 1.2 standard deviations from the mean indicates a poorer outcome (Falco, 1995).
Subchorionic haematoma (SCH)	An SCH near the umbilical cord insertion into the placenta or a volume of 50% of the gestational sac volume indicates a poor prognosis. Spontaneous loss rate in the presence of an SCH is approximately 9% (Pedersen JF et al., 1990).

Table 4.2. Predictors of miscarriage

Diagnosis

Key:
POC - Products of conception
CRL - Crown-rump length
MSD - Mean sac diameter
Y - Yes
N - No

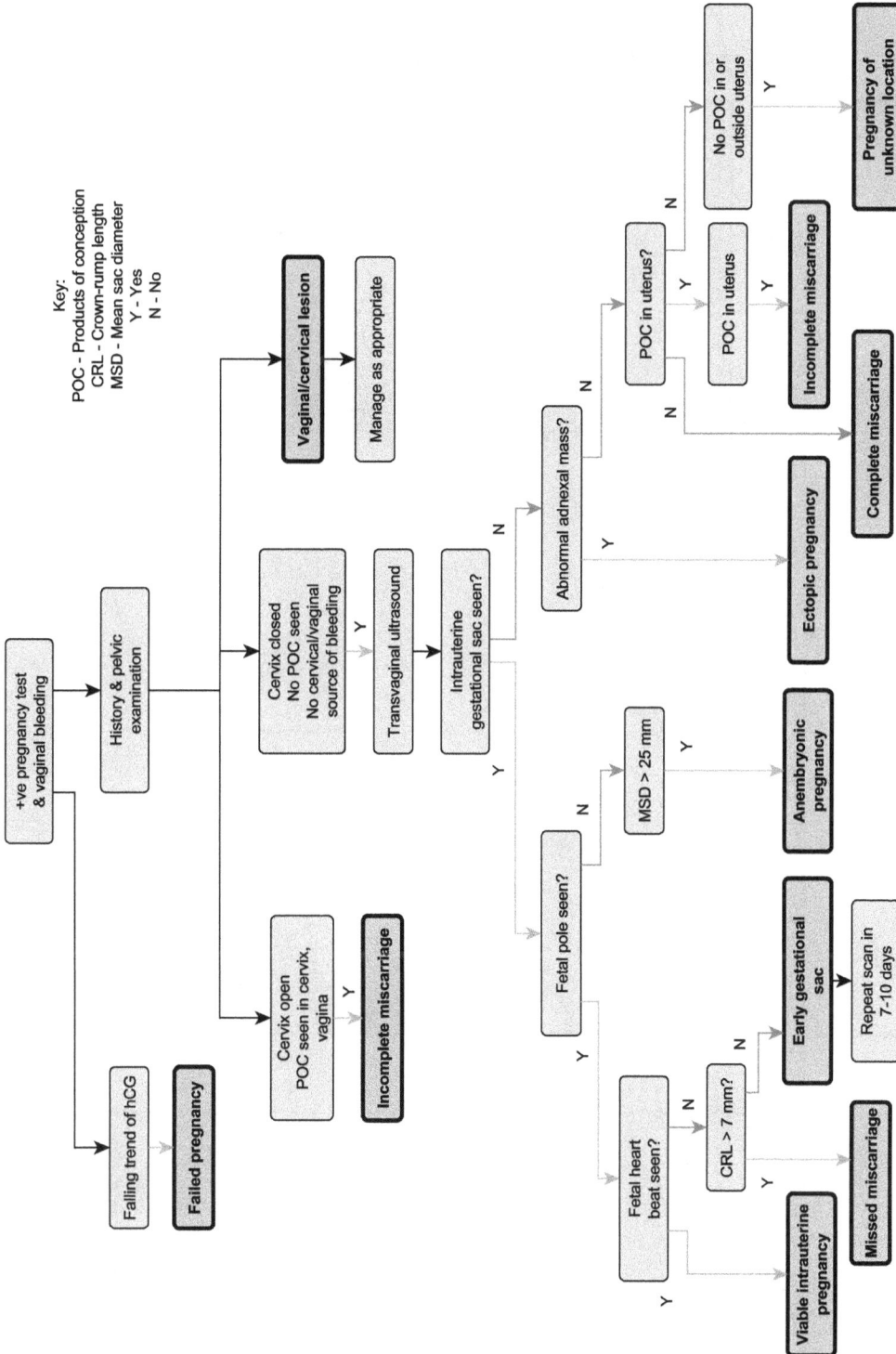

+ve pregnancy test & vaginal bleeding

History & pelvic examination

Falling trend of hCG

Failed pregnancy

Cervix open POC seen in cervix, vagina

Incomplete miscarriage

Vaginal/cervical lesion

Manage as appropriate

Cervix closed No POC seen No cervical/vaginal source of bleeding

Transvaginal ultrasound

Intrauterine gestational sac seen?

Abnormal adnexal mass?

POC in uterus?

No POC in or outside uterus

Pregnancy of unknown location

POC in uterus

Incomplete miscarriage

Ectopic pregnancy

Complete miscarriage

Fetal pole seen?

MSD > 25 mm

Anembryonic pregnancy

Early gestational sac

Repeat scan in 7-10 days

Fetal heart beat seen?

CRL > 7 mm?

Missed miscarriage

Viable intrauterine pregnancy

Figure 4.6. Diagnostic algorithm of miscarriage

Management

Type	History	Examination	Transvaginal Sonography	Management	Anti-D administration if female is Rh-negative and has no antibodies	Anti-D after 12 weeks
Threatened	Mild bleeding (spotting) and minimal pain	Cervical os closed No POC seen	Normal intrauterine pregnancy, with a live fetus (FHR present)	Exclude other causes of early pregnancy bleeding Reassure parents and advise rest Repeat scan in 2 weeks if still symptomatic		Anti-D after 12 weeks
Missed	Asymptomatic, or spotting ± mild pain	Cervical os closed No POC seen	Normal intrauterine pregnancy with a dead fetus	Expectant, medical, or surgical management, depending on size of gestational sac		
Inevitable	Heavy vaginal bleeding and severe pain	Cervical os open Ballooning of lower uterus No POC seen	Intrauterine gestational sac present but may be displaced inferiorly Fetus may be alive or dead	Emergency evacuation of the retained POC		
Incomplete	Bleeding and pain	Cervical os open Some POC seen in cervix or vagina	Intrauterine retained POC	Expectant, medical, or surgical management, depending on amount of retained POC		
Complete	Bleeding and pain improving or resolved	Cervical os closed (It may be open if expulsion of POC was recent.)	No intrauterine gestational sac Endometrial thickness <15 mm	Reassurance		
Septic	Fever, bleeding, and significant pain in the lower abdomen and pelvis	Cervical os open or closed Malodourous, pink, vaginal discharge Pyrexia and tachycardia Tender lower abdomen and boggy, tender uterus	Variable	High vaginal or cervical swab Blood culture if temperature >38.4°C Antibiotics – ampicillin + metronidazole + gentamicin Curettage 12 hours after antibiotics if haemorrhage is severe and uterus not empty		
Pregnancy of unknown location	Asymptomatic, or spotting ± mild pain	Cervical os closed	No sign of intrauterine or extrauterine pregnancy	Serial serum β-HCG and scan Methotrexate		

Table 4.3. Summary of types of miscarriage

A developing miscarriage cannot be stopped. The aim of the treatment is to reduce pain, suffering, bleeding, and infection, and to expedite the evacuation of the uterus. The treatment of miscarriage should be individualised, and the patient's preference must be taken into account.

Anti-D immunoglobulin should be administered intramuscularly within 72 hours to all Rh-negative women who have no antibodies, except women with a threatened miscarriage before 12 weeks of pregnancy.

There are three methods of treatment, which are equally effective: expectant, medical, and surgical.

Expectant

- Prerequisites
  - Patient's consent
  - No sign of infection
  - Haemodynamically stable

- Duration
  - Review in 10–14 days
  - 37% expel POC in 1 week and 50% in 1 month
  - Could be prolonged if the patient is well and happy to continue
- Advantages
  - High patient satisfaction
  - No need for medical or surgical treatment, if successful
  - Infection rate similar in all forms of treatment
  - More successful in incomplete miscarriage

- Disadvantages
  - More blood loss
  - Less successful in missed miscarriage
  - No guarantee that it will be successful

Medical

Medical treatment is by the prostaglandin E_1 analogue misoprostol, which increases uterine contraction, promotes cervical ripening, and hence reduces the expulsion time. According to NICE, mifepristone should not be routinely used because there is no proportional increase in the success rate.

- Prerequisites
  - As in expectant.

- Dose
  - 400–800 µg administered vaginally or orally.
  - Vaginal administration causes a sustained higher serum level than the oral route, and gastrointestinal side effects are fewer.

- Advantages
  - Avoids expectant or surgical treatment and need for hospitalisation.
  - Shorter duration of treatment compared with expectant.
  - Success rate is 80%.
  - Cost-effective strategy.
- Disadvantages
  - No guarantee that it will work.
  - Side effects of misoprostol, such as fever, nausea, and diarrhoea.
- Predictors of success
  - Incomplete miscarriage with AP diameter of POC < 30 mm.
  - Gestational sac size < 35 mm.
  - CRL < 23 mm.

Surgical

Surgery is the treatment for women who are haemodynamically unstable, when there are signs of infection, or at the patient's request. It is done by surgically evacuating the POC under anaesthesia by suction curettage, which is safer and easier to do (Evidence Level I). Haemodynamically unstable women should first be resuscitated. A blood transfusion may be required if the haemoglobin count is low. Tissue removed from curettage should be histologically examined to exclude an ectopic or molar pregnancy (Evidence Level IV). All women should receive a full explanation of the operative findings, follow-up of histological examination, and contraceptive and cervical cytological advice. In the absence of a recurring cause for miscarriage, if the woman wants to conceive in the near future, she should be advised to have at least one normal period before she tries to conceive. She should also start folic acid supplementation at least one month prior to conception and continue until 10 weeks after conception. The folic acid supplementation reduces the incidence of spina bifida by about 70%.

- Prerequisites
  - Patient's consent.
  - Not suitable for expectant or medical management.
- Advantages
  - No waiting, shorter duration of procedure.
  - Patient can get back to her activities the very next day.
  - POC are histologically examined to confirm the presence of chorionic villi and to exclude gestational trophoblastic disease and placental thrombosis (Evidence Level IV).
- Disadvantages
  - Inherent risks of surgery, including those from anaesthesia.
    - Oxytocin reduces blood loss by a statistically significant amount.
  - Risk of cervical trauma.
  - Uterine perforation 1: 250 cases.
  - Failure rate is 1–5%.
  - Intrauterine adhesions in 40% of cases.
  - Pelvic infection rate is 3%, similar to other methods.
    - Routine antibiotic prophylaxis is not beneficial (Evidence Level IB).

Long-term follow-up of all women undergoing these different treatment modalities have shown a similar live-born pregnancy rate of 80% after 5 years.

Short-Answer Questions

Question 1

How will you manage a woman with pregnancy of unknown location?

Answer:

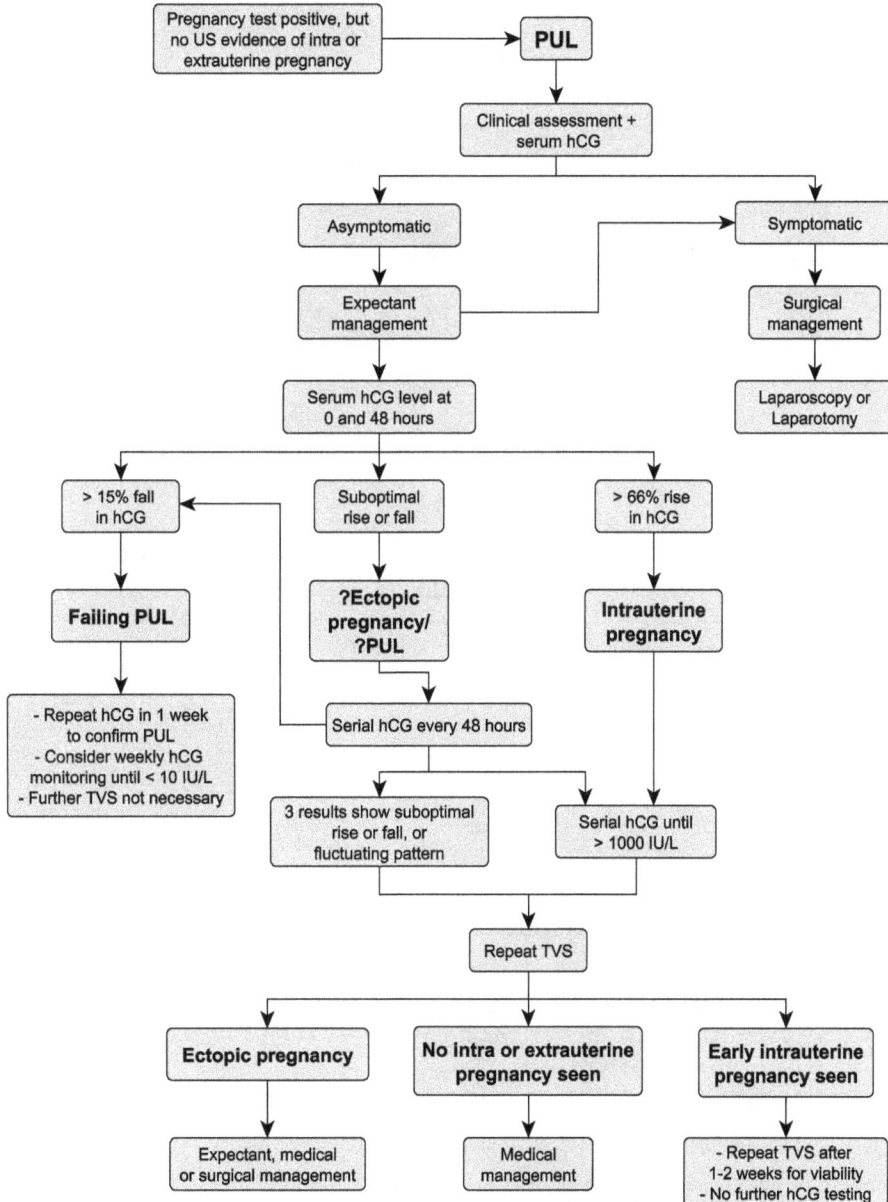

Figure 4.7. Management algorithm for PUL

Question 2

A 21-year-old presents to you with light vaginal bleeding. She is otherwise well, without any pain. Her LMP was 6 weeks ago, and the pregnancy test is positive. On examination, she has a bulky uterus, closed cervix, and no tenderness.

Part a

List your differential diagnoses.

Answer:

- Threatened miscarriage
- Missed miscarriage
- Ectopic pregnancy
- Gestational trophoblastic disease
- Physiological bleeding of pregnancy
- Infection (cervicitis, vaginitis)
- Cervical ectropion
- Polyps
- Fibroids – unlikely

Part b

Discuss the investigations you would order for this patient, to narrow down the diagnosis and assist with your treatment.

Answer:

I would order a transvaginal ultrasound scan. I would also want serial β-hCG levels at 0 and 48 hours.

Part c

A transvaginal ultrasound scan confirms a live intrauterine pregnancy. However, the patient presents 3 days later with heavy vaginal bleeding. What is your initial management?

Answer:

1. Ensure the patient is haemodynamically stable.
   - Monitor vital signs (hypotensive, tachycardic), patient appearance (pallor, cool peripheries), fluid balance.
2. Establish venous access.
   - Take bloods for blood group and cross-match, and also check if patient is Rh-negative.
   - If the patient is febrile, do blood cultures.
3. Give IV fluids if needed, correct anaemia if present, oxygen.
4. Put in a urinary catheter to monitor output if needed.
5. Prescribe analgesia for any pelvic pain.
   - Not NSAIDs.

Part d

On speculum examination, you see many large clots around the cervix, with an open external os. You see products of conception coming out of the cervix. What is your diagnosis, and how would you manage this woman?

Answer:

Incomplete miscarriage.

If products are present in the os, they must be removed promptly; otherwise, the patient may have a vasovagal response, more bleeding, or pelvic pain.

- Remove digitally.

Or

- Remove with sterile ovum/sponge-holding forceps.
    - If bleeding continues, give patient misoprostol to aid complete uterine evacuation.
    - Monitor the bleeding and prevent complications.
    - Perform a follow-up scan to ensure the uterus is empty.

If products are not present in the os, management is different:

- Conservative
    - As long as the patient is happy and there is no vaginal discharge, excess bleeding, pyrexia, or abdominal pain, follow-up scan twice weekly until complete (but make sure it does complete).
- Medical
    - If vaginal bleeding is relatively mild. If heavy, the patient needs surgical management.
    - Misoprostol (prostaglandin analogue).
    - May use OxyContin/PG analogues with either surgical procedure to facilitate uterine evacuation and prevent postprocedure bleeding.
    - In the case of bleeding, can use bimanual uterine compression to reduce and manage it.
- Surgical
    - Suction evacuation (preferred).
    - Dilatation and curettage:
        - Complications—GA cx, uterine perforation, infection, bleeding, etc.

Multiple-Choice Questions

Q1. Of the following, which is the smallest gestational-sac diameter at which a confident diagnosis of an anembryonic pregnancy can be made by a transvaginal ultrasound scan?

A. 15 mm

B. 20 mm

C. 25 mm

D. 30 mm

Answer: C

Q2. A 20-year-old lady presents with vaginal bleeding and lower abdominal pain with 7 weeks of amenorrhoea. What would you expect your junior doctor to do first?

    A. Check abdomen for signs of peritonism.

    B. Do a urine pregnancy test.

    C. Check haemoglobin.

    D. Check pulse, blood pressure, temperature, and respiratory rate.

Answer: D

Q3. Which of the following statements regarding spontaneous miscarriage is correct?

    A. Bacterial vaginosis is associated with increased incidence of first-trimester miscarriage.

    B. Among chromosomally abnormal spontaneous conceptuses, the most common abnormality is triploidy.

    C. DES exposure increases risk of spontaneous miscarriage.

    D. The karyotypic abnormalities in spontaneous conceptuses are similar to those in live-born neonates.

Answer: C

Q4. The photobiologic basis for action of the CO_2 laser on tissue is absorption of CO_2 laser energy by:

    A. Mitochondria

    B. Cell membrane

    C. Intracellular water

    D. Intracellular proteins

Answer: C

Q5. Which of the following statements is incorrect about the value of the yolk sac in the clinical practice?

    A. A normal yolk sac is a precursor of the embryo.

    B. With the help of the yolk sac, the embryo could be located inside the gestational sac.

    C. It is a marker of chorionicity in a multiple pregnancy.

    D. In 3-D surface rendering mode, it has a honeycomb appearance.

Answer: C

Q6. You are seeing a female miscarrying at 19 weeks of gestation. On vaginal examination, you feel the fetal legs in the vagina. The rest of the fetal body is inside the cervix and uterus. How will you manage this female?

    A. Gently pull out the rest of the fetus from the cervix

    B. Provide analgesia and support with expectant management in the hospital

    C. Perform a dilatation and evacuation under GA

    D. Try to gently push the fetus back into the uterus, if still alive, and perform an emergency cervical cerclage

Answer: B

Q7. You are seeing a 20-year-old lady with an intrauterine gestational sac with a CRL of 6 mm with no fetal cardiac activity. What will you do?

A. Treat her for missed miscarriage

B. Treat her for threatened miscarriage

C. Do serial quantitative β-hCG 48 hours apart and then review

D. Perform a transvaginal ultrasound scan in 2 weeks and then review

Answer: C

Q8. You are seeing a 23-year-old lady with an intrauterine gestational sac with a CRL of 8 mm with no fetal cardiac activity and no vaginal bleeding. When will you administer anti-D immunoglobulin to her?

A. Immediately, if her blood group is Rh-negative

B. Immediately, if she is Rh-negative and has not had anti-D immunoglobulin within last 3 weeks

C. As in B above, with no preformed antibodies

D. As in C above, as soon as possible but definitely within 72 hours, intramuscularly

Answer: D

Chapter 4.2. Recurrent Miscarriage

Definition

Recurrent miscarriage, also known as habitual miscarriage, is defined as 3 spontaneous and consecutive miscarriages.

Epidemiology

The incidence is 2–5%. The risk of a further miscarriage after 2 consecutive miscarriages is 25%, and after 3 consecutive miscarriages, it is 45%.

Risk Factors

The risk factors are the same as those described in the Miscarriage chapter. Most recurrent miscarriages happen later in gestation, indicating that maternal or environmental factors are more commonly at play.

History

One should adopt a sympathetic and caring attitude, as such women are extremely traumatised. Care should be provided in a dedicated unit, as this improves outcomes (Evidence Level IV).

History should explore the following:

- Details and gestational age of each miscarriage
- Medical problems, e.g., diabetes, hypertension
- History of pelvic infection

- Cervical or uterine surgery
- Family history of recurrent miscarriages

Investigations

These could be started after any number of miscarriages, at the woman's request. In 60% of cases, a cause can be found.

- Screening for antiphospholipid antibodies
- Karyotyping of the conceptus and both partners (Evidence Level III)
- 3-D pelvic ultrasound, or hysteroscopy and laparoscopy, for uterine and cervical abnormalities (Evidence Level III)
- Screening for thrombophilias, especially Factor V Leiden, prothrombin gene mutation, and protein S deficiency
- HbA1C
- Thyroid autoantibodies
- Varicella and rubella antibodies

Management

Nonpharmacological

- Optimise BMI
- Avoid smoking, caffeine, and alcohol
- Reduce stress, e.g. relaxation techniques, meditation
- Start folic acid supplementation at least one month before the next conception

Medical and Surgical Treatment

If a cause has been found, that should be treated.

Antiphospholipid syndrome (APS) is present in 15% of women with recurrent miscarriages and in less than 2% of the general population. It affects trophoblastic function and differentiation in early miscarriages and uteroplacental thrombosis in late miscarriages. Its effective treatment reduces the risk of miscarriage and increases the live pregnancy rate. It should be treated with low-dose aspirin and fractionated heparin (Evidence Level I) after a pregnancy is confirmed, and it should be continued for the rest of the pregnancy and even for 6 weeks postpartum. Randomly starting aspirin and fractionated heparin has no benefit.

The finding of an abnormal karyotype in the parents or conceptus should lead to a referral for genetic counselling. There is a 3–5% incidence of balanced structural chromosomal abnormalities in couples with recurrent miscarriages. Miscarriage can result from an unbalanced chromosomal abnormality. An unbalanced chromosomal abnormality in a fetus is usually inherited from a parental balanced structural abnormality, usually either reciprocal or Robertsonian translocation. There is a 50–70% chance of a healthy live birth in the future. Preimplantation genetic diagnosis is an option for translocation carriers (Evidence Level IV), but it does not improve the rate of live births. Other options include gamete donation or adoption.

Uterine abnormalities usually result in late miscarriages. The evidence is not strong in favour of uterine septum resection to improve pregnancy rates; however, transfundal metroplasty (surgery to resect septum and restore endometrial contour) is worth considering.

Women with a history suggestive of cervical incompetence should have serial cervical length surveillance from 16–24 weeks of subsequent pregnancies. A cervical cerclage should be offered, if a cervical length of 25 mm or less on transvaginal sonography is found before 24 weeks of pregnancy (Evidence Level I).

The evidence to support the use of progesterone as a treatment for recurrent miscarriage is not strong (Evidence Level I). However, it is still being widely used in clinical practice.

With unexplained recurrent miscarriage, the prognosis is excellent for the future if supportive care is offered in a dedicated unit (Evidence Level I). The prognosis worsens with the number of miscarriages and increasing maternal age.

Short-Answer Questions

Question 1

Discuss the role of inherited thrombophilias in recurrent miscarriage.

Answer:

- Factor V Leiden (the most common inherited thrombophilia) mutation is associated with recurrent first-trimester miscarriage, nonrecurrent miscarriage after 19 weeks, and recurrent fetal loss after 22 weeks' gestation. Factor V Leiden mutation involves substitution of glutamine for arginine at position 506 on the factor V gene. This results in partial inhibition of factor V. Women who are homozygous for the Factor V Leiden mutation have a much higher chance of adverse pregnancy outcomes and recurrent miscarriages compared with heterozygous women.

- Protein S and antithrombin III deficiencies are associated with recurrent and nonrecurrent fetal demise after 22 weeks of gestation and also early and recurrent miscarriages.
  - Protein S is an acute-phase reactant, and its level decreases by higher concentration of oestrogen, pregnancy, surgery, and trauma. Hence, it should only be assayed nearly 2 months after pregnancy has ended.

- Activated protein C resistance is associated with recurrent first-trimester miscarriages.

- Prothrombin gene mutation, which is seen in 5% of the Caucasian population, results in a higher serum concentration of prothrombin. It is associated with recurrent first-trimester miscarriages (relative risk 2.56) and late fetal demise. It is diagnosed by gene analysis.

- Homocysteinemia causes pregnancy loss in two ways:
  - Homocysteine, an essential amino acid, damages the vascular endothelium when in higher concentrations, promoting clot aggregation in the placental vasculature.
  - It also causes pregnancy loss by its direct teratogenic effect.
  - Methylenetetrahydrofolate reductase (MTHFR) enzyme reduces the level of homocysteine. With the mutation of this enzyme, it is not able to reduce the level of homocysteine, which in turn causes placental thrombosis. Maternal MTHFR homozygosity is weakly associated with fetal neural-tube defects.

- o Surprisingly, studies have shown an association between miscarriages and MTHFR mutations and not with homocysteine levels.
- o The level of homocysteine also fluctuates with diet and menstrual cycle. Oestrogen reduces the level of homocysteine.
- o MTHFR is diagnosed by gene-mutation testing.
- o MTHFR activity is increased by folic acid 4 mg and vitamin B12 500 μg daily periconceptually, which is continued until well after puerperium.
- o It reduces miscarriage rate, pregnancy complications, and fetal malformation.

Question 2

A 36-year-old woman comes to you at 8 weeks of pregnancy with mild crampy pain and uterine bleeding. She had a vaginal delivery at 29 weeks of pregnancy 3 years ago, after painless dilatation of the cervix. Since then, she had 2 miscarriages at 8 and 12 weeks of pregnancy. A transvaginal ultrasound scan shows an intrauterine gestational sac with a CRL of 10 mm with no fetal heartbeat.

Part a

What will you be asking for in the history?

Answer:

- For the current pregnancy
    - o LMP, cycle regularity, and duration
    - o Severity and duration of pain and bleeding
    - o Smoking, alcohol, recreational drugs, allergies
    - o Patient's recent mood
    - o Social support, including that of immediate family
    - o Dental hygiene
    - o Nutritional status

- For previous miscarriages
    - o Details of each pregnancy
    - o Any pain or bleeding preceding the miscarriage
    - o Results of ultrasound scans and histology reports following the miscarriage
    - o Any karyotype of the prior conceptuses or patient or partner

- For delivery at 29 weeks
    - o Vaginal discharge, bleeding, fever, uterine contractions preceding the delivery
    - o History of spontaneous rupture of membranes
    - o Use of cocaine
    - o Was fetal fibronectin test performed?
    - o Details of antenatal screen, ultrasound scan results, and any vaginal swab microscopy
    - o Birth weight of the baby and subsequent health of the child
        - ▪ Breastfeeding
- Medical and surgical history
    - o Diabetes, thyroid problems, autoimmune diseases, thrombophilias
    - o Uterine and cervical surgery

- Family history
  - o Especially of DVT or recurrent miscarriages

Part b

Which investigations will you order for the future?

Answer:

- FBE, blood group, and antibody screen
- Histology and karyotype of the product of conception
- Karyotype of both partners, if not previously done
- HbA1C, TSH, and thyroid autoantibodies
- APS screen
- Thrombophilia screen
- FSH, LH, SHBG, and free androgen index when not pregnant
- Transvaginal ultrasound scan to exclude any Müllerian abnormality, submucous myoma(s), endometrial polyps, or polycystic ovaries

Part c

Discuss the treatment and evidence behind it that could improve the prognosis for future pregnancies.

Answer:

- Behavioural changes:
  - o Weight optimisation.
  - o Avoidance of smoking, alcohol, and recreational drugs.
  - o Dental hygiene: strong association with disease and adverse outcome; no evidence of benefit from treatment.
- Medical optimisation:
  - o Stabilise diabetes and thyroid function.
  - o Start metformin if PCOS (insufficient evidence to evaluate its benefits).
  - o Aspirin and heparin if APS; reduces miscarriage rate by 54% (Evidence Level I).
- Uterine abnormalities:
  - o Surgery if abnormalities present:
    - Transfundal metroplasty
    - Resection of uterine septum (insufficient evidence that it improves pregnancy rate) or recurrent myoma
    - Endometrial polypectomy
- Cervical abnormality (incompetence or short cervix < 25 mm):
  - o Fortnightly transvaginal ultrasound scan for cervical length surveillance in between 16 and 24 weeks of gestation.
  - o Cervical cerclage if cervical shortening is progressive (Evidence Level I).
- Progesterone treatment does not improve pregnancy rate in recurrent miscarriage (Evidence Level I).

- Psychological support and :
  - There is strong evidence that in case of unexplained recurrent miscarriage, outcomes for future pregnancies are improved and a live birth rate of 86% is achieved without pharmacological treatment with proper psychological support and counselling (Evidence Level II).
- Abnormal karyotype of the POC:
  - Genetic counselling: 50–70% chance of a normal birth in the future.
- Parents are carriers of translocations:
  - Preimplantation genetic diagnosis, but it does not improve pregnancy rates (Evidence Level IV).
  - May need gamete donation or adoption.
- hCG supplementation:
  - Evidence is insufficient to evaluate its value in the treatment of recurrent miscarriage.
- Unexplained recurrent miscarriage:
  - Excellent prognosis if supportive care is offered in a specialised unit (Evidence Level I). The prognosis worsens with the number of miscarriages and increasing maternal age.

Question 3

A 35-year-old patient consults you at 6 weeks of pregnancy with light vaginal bleeding. A transvaginal ultrasound scan shows an intrauterine gestational sac with a fetal pole of 4 mm with no heartbeat.

Part a

What is the earliest CRL at which an embryonic heartbeat could be seen?

Answer:

By a transvaginal scan, the embryonic heartbeat is the first embryonic structure seen adjacent to the yolk sac. The CRL at this stage is 2 mm.

Part b

At what CRL can a diagnosis of missed miscarriage be confidently made?

Answer:

CRL = 7 mm.

Since the CRL is 4 mm, a diagnosis of missed miscarriage cannot be made only on the basis of just one ultrasound scan. Unless there is a suboptimal rise in serum quantitative β-hCG over a 48-hour period, no growth of CRL, or the appearance of the fetal heartbeat a week later on transvaginal ultrasound scan, a diagnosis of missed miscarriage cannot be made. Hence, the diagnosis at this stage is either very early intrauterine pregnancy of uncertain viability.

Part c

Will you prescribe anti-D, if this patient is Rh-negative?

Answer:

Evidence shows that there is no advantage in anti-D administration at this gestation in a case of threatened miscarriage. Despite this, I would still prescribe 250 IU of anti-D immunoglobulin intramuscularly to this patient if there are no serum anti-D antibodies, so as to avoid isoimmunisation.

Part d

Briefly discuss your management of the patient.

Answer:

My management will include the following:

- Supportive care and reassurance.
- Detailed history of pain, bleeding, LMP, regularity of the menstrual cycle, any associated medical problems, and previous history of any miscarriage or pregnancy.
- Any chromosomal abnormality that runs in the family.
- Blood tests: FBE, blood group, antibody screen, quantitative β-hCG.
- Review in 48 hours with another serum quantitative β-hCG.
- Get hold of any prior ultrasound scans or serum quantitative β-hCG in this pregnancy.

The further management will be on an outpatient basis.

- Advise patient to report to the nearest emergency department if the vaginal bleeding becomes heavy or the pain worsens.
- Review in 48 hours with another serum quantitative β-hCG.
  Please see Figure 4.8. for the management algorithm at the time of this review.

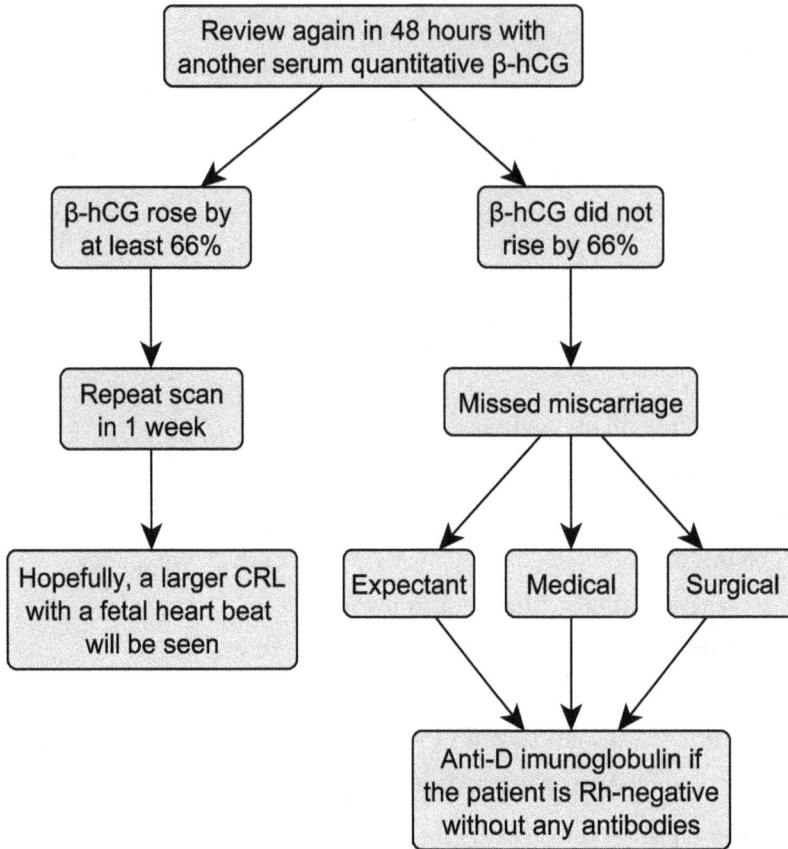

Figure 4.8. Management of miscarriage based on serum β-hCG

Question 4

Discuss the clinical features and management of a suspected septic miscarriage at 9 weeks in a 24-year-old who is not in a stable relationship.

Answer:

Symptoms:

- Lower abdominal pain
- Malodorous vaginal discharge
- Fever
- Sweaty (may also be cold and clammy)

Signs:

- Febrile (hypothermia if in Gram-negative septicaemia)
- Tachycardia, hypotension, tachypnoea; may be delirious
- Tender lower abdomen; may also show signs of peritonitis, such as guarding, rigidity, and rebound tenderness

- Vaginal examination:
  - o Bloody, malodorous discharge
  - o POC may be seen in the external os or vagina
  - o Cervix may be open (admits a finger)
  - o Bulky and tender uterus
  - o Tender adnexa

Investigations:

- FBE, CRP, and blood culture
- Blood group, antibody screen
- UEC, LFT, group and hold, coagulation screen
- Transvaginal ultrasound scan
- High vaginal swab

Treatment:

- If a miscarriage is seen on the transvaginal ultrasound scan, and/or POC is seen in the vagina or cervix, and the clinical features and investigations show evidence of infection, then a diagnosis of septic miscarriage is established.
- Resuscitate if in septic shock.
- Commence broad-spectrum antibiotics (combination of cephazolin, metronidazole and gentamicin) and continue for one week.
- Arrange an evacuation of the retained products of conception as soon as possible under general anaesthesia. Have a low threshold to use ergometrine to control bleeding.
- Transfuse blood if low haemoglobin preoperatively or excessive intraoperative bleeding.
- ICU admission may be needed if in shock.
- Potential complications of surgery, immediate and late, should be explained to the patient at the time of obtaining consent.
  - o Immediate complications: haemorrhage, uterine perforation, incomplete emptying of the uterus, septicaemia, hysterectomy
  - o Delayed complications: Asherman's syndrome, subfertility
- Administer anti-D immunoglobulin if Rh-negative.

Posttreatment counselling:

- Explain the surgery and surgical findings.
- Follow-up on histology of products of conception.
- Emphasise safe sex and the use of contraception, and encourage regular cervical cytology screening.

Question 5

What are the chances of a further miscarriage in a 38-year-old woman with three consecutive early miscarriages with no prior live birth?

Answer:

The incidence of miscarriage increases with increasing age. At 38 years of age, the risk of miscarriage is 20–25%. The risk of a fourth miscarriage after 3 consecutive miscarriages is about 45%. The combinations of increasing age and recurrent miscarriages increases the risk of a fourth miscarriage. Not having a live birth also affects her miscarriage rate adversely.

Question 6

Discuss the evidence and role of progestogens in the prevention of miscarriage.

Answer:

Progesterone secreted by the corpus luteum decidualises the endometrium for the blastocyst to implant. It is postulated that in some women, the cause of miscarriage is the lack of progesterone from the corpus luteum. Hence, it is inferred that progestogen supplementation in the early stages of pregnancy could help continue the pregnancy.

There is no evidence from randomised controlled trials that routine progestogen therapy to healthy women can prevent a miscarriage in the first trimester of pregnancy. However, there is evidence of some benefit from progestogen therapy in recurrent miscarriages. A meta-analysis (Haas and Ramsey, 2013) showed that with progestogen therapy, the rate of miscarriage was lower in the treatment group. It also showed that there was no increased incidence of adverse effects in either the mother or the baby due to progestogen therapy.

There is some evidence that progestogen therapy reduces the incidence of miscarriage in a case of threatened miscarriage. Exogenous synthetic progestogens significantly increased the pregnancy rates in IVF.

Ongoing research to seek stronger evidence is continuing.

Question 7

Justify the investigations for antiphospholipid syndrome (APS) in a woman who consults you for recurrent miscarriages (RM).

Answer:

The justifications of investigations for APS are as follows:

- The prevalence of APS in women with recurrent miscarriages is nearly 15%, whereas the prevalence in the general population is only 2%.
- There are definite indicators of APS in the history of RM, such as three consecutive early miscarriages.
- There are evidence-based tests for the clear diagnosis of APS, such as antiphospholipid antibodies and anti-β_2-glycoprotein I. These tests are easily available, reproducible, and not expensive.

- Once diagnosed, there is definite evidence of better outcome in women with RM. For example, starting aspirin before conception or just after conception reduces the risk of miscarriage, and starting enoxaparin following establishing fetal viability decreases pregnancy complications and thrombosis. These treatments also reduce the risks of other pregnancy complications such as, IUGR, PET, DVT, and stillbirth.

Multiple-Choice Questions

Q1. Which of the following is the most common aetiological factor for recurrent miscarriage?

A. Immunologic

B. Anatomic

C. Genetic

C. Endocrine

Answer: A

Q2. What is the most common explanation of recurrent miscarriage in the presence of antiphospholipid antibodies?

A. Placental infarction

B. Defective trophoblast invasion

C. Placental vasculopathy

D. Decreased apoptosis of trophoblasts

Answer: B

Q3. Which of the following is **not** correct for recurrent miscarriage due to coeliac disease?

A. Coeliac disease antibodies have direct antitrophoblast properties.

B. Coeliac disease antibodies have anticoagulant properties.

C. Coexistent nutritional deficiencies play a role.

D. Improvement in pregnancy rates occur with treatment.

Answer: B

Q4. Which is the most prevalent genetic abnormality in a woman with recurrent miscarriage?

A. Balanced reciprocal translocation

B. Robertsonian translocation

C. Sex chromosome mosaicism

D. Inversions

Answer: A

Q5. In which of the following is embryonic cardiac activity still visible by a transvaginal ultrasound scan?

A. Pregnancy of unknown location

B. Incomplete miscarriage

C. Threatened miscarriage

D. Missed miscarriage

Answer: C

Q6. A 25-year-old woman with 3 consecutive miscarriages under 12 weeks and no prior children consults you for further management. All routine investigations for recurrent miscarriage are normal. Which of the following would you recommend at 7 weeks of her next pregnancy?

A. Heparin and aspirin

B. Serial progestogen level or empirical progestogen therapy

C. Pelvic ultrasound scan

D. Serial quantitative hCG levels

Answer: C

Chapter 4.3. Ectopic Pregnancy

Definitions

An ectopic pregnancy is one occurring outside the endometrial cavity.

A chronic ectopic pregnancy is nonviable pregnancy tissue secondary to either tubal rupture or abortion. It may cause chronic abdominal pain due to adhesions, and there may be a reduced/normal hCG level.

Cornual pregnancy	Pregnancy in the cornual area of a uterus, usually bicornuate
Culdocentesis	Aspiration of fluid from the pouch of Douglas through the posterior fornix of the vagina
Fimbrioplasty	Opening the blocked fimbrial end of the fallopian tube and restoring fimbrial anatomy and function
Heterotopic pregnancy	Simultaneous pregnancy in the endometrial cavity as well as outside the endometrial cavity
Interstitial pregnancy	Pregnancy in the interstitial part of the fallopian tube; this term is often used synonymously with cornual pregnancy
Salpingectomy	Removal of a fallopian tube surgically, either fully or partially
Salpingitis isthmica nodosa	Diverticulum of the inner layer of the fallopian tube passing through the muscularis layer
Salpingolysis	Dividing the peritubal adhesions
Salpingostomy	Making an artificial opening in the fallopian tube along its length, but not closing the opening with a suture
Salpingotomy	Making an artificial opening in the fallopian tube along its length, and closing the opening with a suture
Tubal abortion	Expulsion of products of conception into the peritoneal cavity, through the fimbrial end

Table 4.4. Chapter 4.3. Definitions

The description below is of acute ectopic pregnancy. It has been modified from Luciano and Jain (2004).

Epidemiology

Incidence

2%—The incidence is rising due to increased incidence of assisted reproductive technique (ART) and PID.

Mortality

3.4 per 10,000 ectopic pregnancies. Ectopic pregnancy is the leading cause of first-trimester pregnancy-related deaths.

Location

- Tubal—97–98% of cases. Of these:
  - Ampullary: 55–75%
  - Isthmic: 20–25%
  - Fimbrial: 17%
- Cornual/interstitial: 2–4%
- Ovarian: 0.15–0.5% (increasing, 1: 7,000 pregnancies—a random event, no risk factors)
- Cervical: 0.1%
- Abdominal: 0.3–1.4%
- Hysterotomy scar: 1 in 2,000 pregnancies, 6% of ectopics in women with previous lower uterine segment caesarean section
- Heterotropic pregnancy: 1 in 4,000 to 1 in 15,000 ectopic pregnancies, incidence increasing due to ART

Clinical Physiology

A tubal, cornual, or interstitial pregnancy develops because of one or the other of the following two pathologies:

1. Problems with the propulsive mechanism of the fallopian tube ("tube")
   - This may result due to damage to the tubal architecture and endosalpinx by salpingitis. The incidence of tubal pregnancy increases with the number of episodes of salpingitis and increasing age of the woman.
   - High levels of serum progesterone from minipills, levonorgestrel-containing IUCD, clomiphene, or HMG-induced ovulation reduce tubal motility.
   - Salpingitis isthmica nodosa (SIN) causes dysfunction of the tubule transport mechanism without anatomic obstruction.
   - Adhesions between the tube, peritoneum, or bowel may cause tubal dysfunction and anatomic obstruction.
   - Tubal surgery, such as salpingectomy and anastomosis, can traumatise the endosalpinx and muscular layer of the tube, and hence can lead to a tubal pregnancy.

2. Problems with the zygote/morula

- o It is hypothesised that either structural or genetic (aneuploidy) problems in the fertilised egg adversely affect propulsion into the endometrial cavity.
- o According to another hypothesis, the relatively poor blood supply to the tube results in inappropriate signalling to the corpus luteum, causing low progesterone synthesis. This leads to slow or absent growth of the conceptus, which fails to be propelled into the endometrial cavity.
- o Transmigration of the ovum from the contralateral ovary has also been blamed for tubal pregnancy.
- o Unfortunately, evidence is not strong for any of the above hypotheses.

Chapter 4.3.1. Tubal Pregnancy

Risk Factors

Degree of risk	Risk factors	Odds ratio
High	Previous ectopic pregnancy	9.3–47
	Previous tubal surgery	6.0–11.5
	Tubal ligation	3.0–139
	Tubal pathology	3.5–25
	In utero DES exposure	2.4–13
	Current IUCD use	1.1–45
Moderate	Infertility	1.1–28
	Previous cervicitis (gonorrhoea, chlamydia)	2.8–3.7
	History of pelvic inflammatory disease	2.1–3.0
	Multiple sexual partners	1.4–4.8
	Smoking	2.3–3.9
Low	Previous pelvic/abdominal surgery	0.93–3.8
	Vaginal douching	1.1–3.1
	Early age of intercourse (< 18 years)	1.1–2.5

Table 4.5. Risk factors and odds ratio for ectopic pregnancy

Effect of Contraception on Tubal Pregnancy

Users of intrauterine or oral hormonal contraception are at low risk of conceiving. However, if they do conceive, there is an increased risk of an ectopic gestation when compared with women not using contraception:

Contraceptive method	Ectopic pregnancy/All pregnancies
Levonorgestrel intrauterine device	1:2
Tubal sterilisation	1:3
Progesterone intrauterine device	1:4
Copper intrauterine device	1:16
Norethindrone-only pill	1:20
Norgestrel-only pill	1:21
Combination pills	0
All women	1:50

Table 4.6. Ratio of incidence of ectopic pregnancy compared with all pregnancies with use of different contraceptive methods

Natural History

- Tubal abortion
  - Migration of the gestational sac from the tube into the peritoneal cavity through the fimbrial end. Sometimes this becomes an abdominal pregnancy. Otherwise, the pregnancy is gradually resorbed.
- Tubal rupture usually around 8 weeks of gestation
  - Pain and haemoperitoneum.
- Pregnancy failure and resorption
  - The pregnancy remains in the tube and is gradually resorbed.
  - It may lead to a chronic ectopic pregnancy at that site.

History

The classic triad of pain, amenorrhoea (with a positive pregnancy test), and vaginal bleeding is present in only 50% of patients—most commonly in patients with a ruptured ectopic. There is no pathognomonic pain of ectopic pregnancy. Shoulder-tip pain signifies a haemoperitoneum secondary to tubal rupture. In the author's experience, a haemoperitoneum can also result from bleeding through the affected fimbrial end with an intact tube. The blood irritates the diaphragm and hence the sensation of pain is referred to the shoulder tip. Both the diaphragm and the shoulder tip have the same innervation by the phrenic nerve (C3, C4 and C5).

Examination

Physical examination findings prior to rupture are generally nonspecific, and vital signs are normal. Postrupture, the patient may be haemodynamically unstable, with a postural drop in blood pressure, and signs of peritonism and cervical excitation (a nonspecific finding and only indicates mild peritoneal irritation). Pain may improve initially after rupture as distension of the tube resolves, but pain will recur due to haemoperitoneum. An adnexal mass may be palpated in up to 50% of cases (may be the corpus luteum). Sensitivity of the bimanual pelvic examination is very low.

Differential Diagnosis

- Threatened/incomplete miscarriage
- Ruptured corpus luteum
- Endometriosis
- Torted adnexal mass
- PID
- Degeneration of fibroid
- Septic miscarriage

Investigations

Blood Tests

- Full blood examination
- Blood group and antibody screen
- Group and hold
- Serum quantitative β-hCG
    - Levels increase exponentially over first 6 weeks of amenorrhoea.
    - A 66% rise in β-hCG over 48 hours represents the lower limit of normal values for viable intrauterine pregnancies.
    - The β-hCG pattern most predictive of an ectopic pregnancy is when the rise in the level is very slow (doubling time of > 7 days).
    - For falling levels, a half-life of less than 1.4 days is rarely associated with an ectopic pregnancy.
    - Serial levels are required when the results of initial ultrasound scan are indeterminate.
    - Single measurement of β-hCG has limited utility; it is only useful in excluding a pregnancy.
- Serum progesterone
    - Less than 5 ng/mL is highly suggestive of an abnormal pregnancy (risk of normal pregnancy 1:1,500).
    - 70% of patients with viable intrauterine pregnancies have serum progesterone of greater than 25 ng/mL, but only 1.5% of patients with ectopic pregnancies.
    - This test is rarely used because of the difficulty in interpreting results between 5 and 25 ng/mL, higher costs, and length of time needed to get the result from the laboratory.

Ultrasound

- Intrauterine pregnancy can be diagnosed one week earlier with transvaginal (TV) scanning compared with transabdominal (TA) scanning.
- All viable intrauterine pregnancies can be seen on transabdominal scanning when the β-hCG is greater than 2000 IU/L.
- All viable intrauterine pregnancies can be seen on transvaginal scanning when the β-hCG is greater than 1500 IU/L.
- If there is no sign of an intrauterine gestation, and the β-hCG is less than 1500 IU/L, the differential diagnoses include the following:
  - Normal intrauterine pregnancy, too early for visualisation
  - Abnormal intrauterine gestation
  - Recent miscarriage
  - Ectopic pregnancy
  - Nonpregnant patient—β-hCG originating from elsewhere (e.g. tumour)
- A pseudogestational sac (collection of fluid in the endometrial cavity, see Figure 4.3.) may be confused with a true sac, which occurs in 8–29% of patients with ectopic pregnancy.
  - The eccentrically placed double-decidual reaction (hyperechoic double-decidual ring) is the characteristic feature of a true gestational sac and can help to distinguish between a true and a pseudogestational sac.
  - The appearance of a normal yolk sac within the gestational sac is another reassuring feature of an early normal intrauterine pregnancy.
- The presence of cardiac activity within the uterine cavity is definitive evidence of an intrauterine pregnancy, but fetal cardiac activity is also seen in some ectopic gestational sacs (10%).
- A transvaginal ultrasound scan has a sensitivity of 95% and specificity of 100% for the diagnosis of an ectopic pregnancy. A transvaginal ultrasound scan with serum quantitative hCG measurement allows a confident diagnosis of ectopic pregnancy in many women without a laparoscopy (Evidence Level IIA).

Operative

- Dilatation and curettage (rare)
  - Only performed when the pregnancy has been confirmed to be nonviable, and the location of the pregnancy cannot be determined by ultrasonography.
  - Absence of chorionic villi in the uterine curettings excludes an intrauterine pregnancy.
  - On the other hand, presence of Arias-Stella reaction on histological examination of the uterine curettings indicates an ectopic pregnancy.
- Culdocentesis—rarely done
- Laparoscopy—both diagnostic and therapeutic
  - False negative rate is 3–4%, and the false positive rate is 5%.
  - False positivity is due to tubal dilation or discolouration that is misinterpreted as an ectopic pregnancy, resulting in unnecessary damage or removal of the tube.

Management

The principles of treatment are:

- Anti-D immunoglobulins, 250 IU, if the woman is of Rh-negative blood group without any antibodies (Evidence Level IV).
- Haemodynamically unstable patients need a laparotomy (evidence level IV) or a laparoscopy in skilled hands.
- Medical therapy with methotrexate is safe, cost-effective, and preferred in certain situations.
- Laparoscopy for salpingostomy or salpingectomy is the main alternative.
- Expectant management is rarely appropriate (asymptomatic, no haemoperitoneum, and serum hCG falling normally).

Medical

Methotrexate is as effective in selected cases (up to 94% success) as laparoscopic treatment (Evidence Level IIA). At least 15% of women treated by methotrexate will require more than one dose, and 7% will have tubal rupture during follow-up (Evidence Level IIA).

Success is predicted by low initial β-hCG and by at least a 15% fall in β-hCG between day 4 and day 7. The exact threshold varies between individual institutions, and is based on the comfort level with risk of failure or rupture.

Mechanism of Action

Methotrexate is a folic acid antagonist and inhibits DNA synthesis and cell reproduction, primarily in actively proliferating cells, such as malignant cells, trophoblasts, and fetal cells. Methotrexate is a structural analogue of folic acid that competitively inhibits the binding of dihydrofolic acid (FH2) to the enzyme dihydrofolate reductase (DHFR). DHFR is responsible for reducing FH2 to folinic acid (FH4), the active intracellular metabolite. Thus, methotrexate decreases the amount of intracellular FH4 available and affects the metabolic pathways within the cell that are FH4-dependent. These pathways include purine and pyrimidine metabolism and amino acid and polyamine synthesis.

Criteria

- Haemodynamically stable (Evidence Level IV)
- No pelvic pain
- β-hCG < 5000 IU/L (varies between institutions)
- No fetal cardiac activity (Evidence Level IIA; presence of fetal cardiac activity should be a contraindication), an unruptured ectopic mass size < 3.5cm, and no fluid in the peritoneal cavity or pouch of Douglas on transvaginal ultrasound
- Compliant with regular follow-up
- Agrees to use reliable contraceptive for 3–4 months posttreatment
- Desires future fertility
- No preexisting severe medical condition or disorder
- No known contraindications to methotrexate
- No coexisting intrauterine pregnancy
- Not breastfeeding

Dose

The methotrexate dose is 50 mg/m² body surface area, given intramuscularly in a single injection. Multidose protocol for women with cornual or cervical ectopics is used where the dose is 1 mg/kg on alternate days, giving 4 doses with folinic acid rescue. Single and multidose regimens are equally effective for tubal pregnancies.

<u>Follow-up</u>

- Day 4: β-hCG.
- Day 7: β-hCG, FBE, UEC, and LFT.
- Day 14: FBE, β-hCG.
- Weekly follow-up, ideally in a dedicated clinic, until β-hCG is <5 IU/L. β-hCG can take several weeks to fall.
- An increase in β-hCG levels in the first three days following therapy (i.e., up to day 4) is not unusual. This is due to continued β-hCG production by syncytiotrophoblasts.
- If β-hCG does not fall by more than 15% between days 4–7:
- o Administer second dose of methotrexate (required in 15% of cases).
- If a second dose is administered:
  - o Day 7: confirm normal LFT. The second injection should be given in opposite gluteal muscle.
  - o Day 11: β-hCG.
  - o Day 14: FBE, β-hCG, LFTs, UEC.
- Women with evidence of rupture or significant pelvic/abdominal tenderness need surgery.
- The ectopic pregnancy is often noted to increase in size and may persist for weeks on serial ultrasound examinations. This probably represents haematoma, rather than persistent trophoblastic tissue, and is not predictive of treatment failure.
- Methotrexate can also be injected directly into ectopic.

<u>Side Effects and Precautions</u>

- The most common are stomatitis and conjunctivitis.
- Rare side effects include gastritis, enteritis, dermatitis, pneumonitis, alopecia, elevated liver enzymes, and bone marrow suppression.
- Approximately 30% of patients in the single-dose and 40% in multi-dose regimens will have side effects.
- Abdominal pain may occur as the pregnancy resolves, which responds mostly to simple analgesia.
- Avoid vaginal intercourse until follow-up is complete (to avoid rupture). Contraception should be recommended for 3 months.
- Avoid alcohol for 7 days.
- Avoid herbal remedies and vitamin preparations containing folate.
- Seek urgent medical help if severe abdominal pain and vaginal bleeding.

Surgical

<u>Indications</u>

- Ruptured ectopic pregnancy
- Contraindications to use of methotrexate (see criteria)
- Inability or unwillingness to comply with monitoring after medical therapy
- Lack of timely access to a hospital for management of tubal rupture, which can occur during medical therapy
- Failed medical therapy
- Previous tubal sterilisation
- Known tubal disease with planned in vitro fertilisation for future pregnancy
- Coexisting intrauterine pregnancy

The treatment of choice is salpingectomy if the contralateral tube is normal, as evidence suggests that there is no advantage for salpingostomy over salpingectomy in this situation (Evidence Level IIA). Laparoscopic salpingostomy should be the treatment of choice when the contralateral tube is abnormal and future fertility is desired (Evidence Level IIA), the patient is haemodynamically stable, and there is a reasonable chance of adequate tubal function in the future. The subsequent rate of live intrauterine pregnancies is similar in both salpingostomy and salpingectomy, but there is a higher risk of persistent or recurrent ectopic pregnancy in salpingostomy (Evidence Level IIA).

Both of these operations can be done by laparoscopy or laparotomy. Laparoscopy has significant advantages compared with laparotomy in terms of a shorter operative time, less intraoperative blood loss, shorter hospitalisation, less analgesic requirement, and shorter recovery time (Evidence Level IA)—but at the cost of higher rates of persistent trophoblastic tissue. There was no difference in overall tubal patency rates (RR 0.89, 95% CI 0.74–1.1) between a laparoscopy and laparotomy (Evidence Level IA). There is no difference in terms of future pregnancy outcomes or rates of ectopic recurrence between the two approaches.

Persistent disease occurs in 4–15% of cases. β-hCG levels should be monitored postsalpingostomy, given the higher risk. These patients should be treated with single-dose methotrexate (if not contraindicated) and then be monitored with β-hCG and ultrasound. Repeat surgery may be indicated.

Chapter 4.3.2.   Cornual Pregnancy

A true cornual pregnancy is in the cornu of a unicornuate or bicornuate uterus. It presents later compared with a tubal pregnancy and often results in massive intraperitoneal bleeding, causing increased morbidity and mortality.

On transvaginal ultrasound scan, a gestational sac is seen high and into the cornual area of the uterine fundus.

Difference between Interstitial and Cornual Pregnancy

An interstitial pregnancy is in the interstitial part of the tube and is surrounded by at least 5 mm of thick myometrium on all sides. It is separated from the endometrial cavity by a hyperechoic line. Because of the myometrial covering, an interstitial pregnancy can distend to a far greater size than a tubal pregnancy.

A myometrial envelope of less than 5 mm all around is suspicious of a cornual pregnancy.

Treatment

- Methotrexate if unruptured and asymptomatic.
- Surgery if ruptured (90% rupture).
  - The type of surgery, such as laparotomy, laparoscopy (Trivedi & Roman, 1998), cornual resection, or hysterectomy, depends upon the gynaecologist's expertise and the facilities available.

Chapter 4.3.3.   Ovarian Pregnancy

Most ovarian pregnancies cause massive intraperitoneal bleeding. Occasionally, the diagnosis is made only at surgery. An ovarian pregnancy is diagnosed if the following criteria are met:

- The tube, including the fimbria, is separate from the ovary and normal.
- The ectopic sac is densely attached to the ovary.
- Ovarian tissue is present in the wall of the ectopic gestational sac.

Treatment

Ovarian resection either by a laparotomy or laparoscopy. The affected ovary can be saved in almost all cases.

Chapter 4.3.4.   Abdominal Pregnancy

Abdominal pregnancies mostly result from tubal abortion or sometimes from tubal rupture. Abdominal pregnancies have also been reported after a hysterectomy due to the presence of a abdomino-vaginal fistula. The prognosis for the fetus is poor, and fetal survival rate is nearly 11%. Diagnosis is often late and difficult. An ultrasound scan will show an empty uterus and normal adnexa. A fetus is seen separate from the uterus, often with a heartbeat.

Treatment

Once the diagnosis is suspected or made, the fetus is removed by a laparotomy. A delay in the treatment may result in serious intraperitoneal bleeding. The placenta should also be removed as much as possible. Partial removal of the placenta can sometimes cause serious bleeding. Methotrexate will help in the dissolution of any placental tissue that remains in the abdominal cavity.

Chapter 4.3.5. Cervical Pregnancy

This presents with vaginal bleeding without cramping pain. Risk factors include multiparity, miscarriage, and cervical instrumentation. A cervical pregnancy is diagnosed if the following criteria are met:

- Soft, extremely vascular, and dilated cervix.
- Gestational sac with increased surrounding vascularity and containing either a yolk sac or an embryo, which may show a heartbeat. The sac could be round or hourglass-shaped.
- Closed internal os and empty endometrial cavity.

This presentation can be easily confused with a failing intrauterine pregnancy, when the gestational sac is in the process of being expelled through the cervix. A comparison with a previous ultrasonogram, if available, will allow differentiation between these two diagnoses.

Differential Diagnosis

- Incomplete miscarriage
- Degenerating cervical myoma
- Carcinoma of the cervix

Treatment

- Methotrexate, either systemically or through local injection.
- Surgery: evacuation of the gestational sac following bilateral uterine artery embolisation. A hysterectomy is needed in nearly 50% of cases, especially if the gestation is advanced.

Outcome

After an ectopic pregnancy, 38–89% of women will achieve a subsequent intrauterine pregnancy. Recurrent ectopic pregnancy occurs in 15% (range 4–28%); the recurrence risk rises to 30% following two ectopic pregnancies. If the woman does not conceive in the first 12 to 18 months after surgical therapy of ectopic pregnancy, or her contralateral tube is damaged or absent, referral for in vitro fertilisation is appropriate.

Short-Answer Questions

Question 1

You are seeing a 25-year-old nulliparous woman with a β-hCG of 1500 IU/L, following a period of amenorrhoea of 7 weeks. She is asymptomatic and haemodynamically stable. A transvaginal ultrasound scan shows an empty uterus, normal ovaries, no abnormal adnexal mass, and very little fluid in the pouch of Douglas. How will you manage this woman?

Answer:

History:

- Pain history: location, radiation, onset, duration, nature, course, worsening pain, any shoulder-tip pain
- Gestational age: LMP, regularity of menstrual cycle, serum quantitative β-hCG if available; conception spontaneous or assisted
- Bleeding history: frequency, volume, duration, passing any tissue or grapelike vesicle
  - Triggers to bleeding: postcoital, trauma, spontaneous; blood group if known
- Associated symptoms: symptoms of early pregnancy (nausea, vomiting, breast tenderness), dysuria, constipation
- Last meal, just in case surgery is required
- Past medical history: history of STI, PID, tubal or pelvic surgery, appendicitis, endometriosis, dysmenorrhoea, DVT, any other medical problems
- Last cervical smear
- Other: medications, allergies, smoking, alcohol

Examination:

- General appearance: consciousness, colour, pallor, breathing, sweating, cold and clammy
- Vital signs: pulse, BP, temperature, respiratory rate
- BMI
- General: thyroid, chest, CVS exam
- Abdominal exam: softness, tenderness, guarding and rigidity, any palpable mass, abdominal distension
- Vaginal bivalve speculum exam: quantity and colour of blood in the vagina, source of blood, cervical external os open or closed, any POC/grapelike vesicle in the vagina or cervix; Vaginal or cervical trauma or disease
- Bimanual exam: uterine size = dates, cervical os open, adnexal tenderness or mass, cervical excitation

Investigations

- FBE, UEC, LFT
- Serum quantitative β-hCG (already done in this patient)
- Pelvic ultrasound scan (already done in this patient)

Based on the given findings, the diagnosis is pregnancy of unknown location (PUL).

Management

- Expectant treatment
  - Since the woman is asymptomatic and hemodynamically stable
  - Prerequisites
    - β-hCG level shows a decreasing trend; keep monitoring serum quantitative β-HCG levels until they normalise.
    - Emphasise the need for compliance.
- Methotrexate
  - Indications
    - The woman does not want expectant management.
    - Serum β-hCG level static or slowly rising.
  - Discuss the benefits and risks of methotrexate treatment, as in the text.
- Future conception
  - At least one year after finishing methotrexate treatment, because of the risks of fetal malformation, miscarriage, and stillbirth (Evidence Level III).

Question 2

A 25-year-old G1P0 woman presents with vaginal bleeding and some mild lower abdominal pain after 8 weeks of amenorrhoea. Her pregnancy test is strongly positive.

Part a

What are the differential diagnoses?

Answer:

- Miscarriage—threatened
- Miscarriage—incomplete, complete, inevitable, missed
- Ectopic pregnancy
- Molar pregnancy
- Incidental bleeding
  - Postcoital
  - Cervical or vaginal origin—malignancy (cervical cancer), vaginal lesion, ectropion, polyps, trauma

Part b

Outline your initial plan of management.

Answer:

History:

- Gestational age: LMP, regularity of menstrual cycle, serum quantitative β-hCG if available. Conception spontaneous or assisted.
- Bleeding history: volume, duration, frequency, passing any tissue or grapelike vesicle.
  - Triggers: postcoital, trauma, spontaneous, blood group if known.
- Pain history: location, radiation, onset, duration, nature, course, worsening pain, any shoulder-tip pain.
- Associated symptoms: symptoms of early pregnancy (nausea, vomiting, breast tenderness), dysuria, constipation.
- Last meal, in case surgery required.
- Past medical history: history of STI, PID, tubal or pelvic surgery, appendicitis, endometriosis, dysmenorrhoea, DVT, any other medical problems.
- Last cervical smear.
- Other: medications, allergies, smoking, alcohol.

Examination:

- General appearance: consciousness, colour, pallor, breathing, sweating, cold and clammy.
- Vital signs: pulse, BP, temperature, respiratory rate.
- BMI.
- General: thyroid, chest, CVS exam.
- Abdominal exam: softness, tenderness, guarding and rigidity, any palpable mass, abdominal distension.
- Vaginal bivalve speculum exam: quantity and colour of blood in the vagina, source of blood, cervical external os open or closed, any POC/grapelike vesicle in the vagina or cervix. Vaginal or cervical trauma or disease.
- Bimanual exam: uterine size = dates, cervical os open, adnexal tenderness or mass, cervical excitation.

Investigations:

- FBE
- Blood group and antibodies
- Group and hold
- Serum quantitative β-hCG
- Transvaginal ultrasound scan
- Histology on any tissue expelled from vagina: POC/molar pregnancy, decidua.

Diagnosis:

Follow the algorithm Figure 4.6. from the "Miscarriage" chapter to make a diagnosis. If a diagnosis of a tubal pregnancy is reached, then the treatment is:

- Counselling: Discuss both medical and surgical treatments, their indications and contraindications, advantages and disadvantages, and the required follow-up. Emphasise that intrauterine pregnancy rates and tubal patency rates for both modes of treatment are similar.
- Blood group and anti-D: If mother is Rh-negative and not sensitised, then administer 250 IU of anti-D immunoglobulin IM to prevent isoimmunisation.
- Medical treatment with systemic methotrexate: only if the vital signs are normal, the patient is comfortable and not in distress, serum quantitative β-hCG < 5000 IU/L, ultrasound scan showing an adnexal mass with < 3.5 cm in diameter with no fetal cardiac activity and minimal fluid in the POD. Organise follow-up as per text.
- Surgical treatment: If the criteria for medical treatment are not met or the patient does not want medical treatment, in an uncomplicated woman with normal contralateral tube, the surgical treatment of choice is a laparoscopic complete salpingectomy.

If a diagnosis of miscarriage or molar pregnancy is made, treat them as described in the respective chapters.

Question 3

A 22-year-old sees you for a follow-up of a left laparoscopic salpingectomy for a tubal pregnancy of 3 cm in diameter with a live embryo. She wants to know why she did not receive methotrexate. She also wants to discuss her contraceptive options.

Answer:

This lady's situation satisfies one of the many contraindications for methotrexate treatment. A live embryo is a contraindication because it reduces the chance of success of methotrexate therapy (Evidence Level IIA). She might have had other contraindications as well, such as:

- Haemodynamic unstable
- In severe pain and vaginal bleeding
- Allergic to methotrexate
- Unwilling to submit to regular follow-up
- Breastfeeding
- Serum β-hCG > 5000 IU/L

15% of patients require a second course of methotrexate, and 7% have a tubal rupture.

Future contraception

- She should avoid IUCD, because of the increased risk of an ectopic pregnancy if a pregnancy were to occur.
- Apart from abstinence and barrier methods, the combined oral contraceptive pill is the most appropriate option.

- A depot medroxyprogesterone acetate injection or etonogestrel subdermal implant will also be suitable if she is happy about the side effects—most commonly irregular vaginal bleeding (20%).

- She should also be advised that if she were to miss her next period, she should have a pregnancy test. If this is positive, she should have an early transvaginal ultrasound.

- The risk of recurrence of ectopic pregnancy is 15%.

Question 4

You are seeing a 25-year-old haemodynamically stable and asymptomatic woman with a β-hCG of 2500 IU/L, a 3-cm complex right adnexal mass, and an empty uterus. She had a left partial salpingectomy 6 months earlier, for a tubal pregnancy. She is nulliparous. How will you counsel her for treatment?

Answer:

My counselling would cover the management of her current presentation and future fertility issues.

Management of her current problem:

Based on the above scenario, the diagnosis is an ectopic pregnancy.

- Inform the woman about ectopic pregnancy and its recurrence rate (15%).
- Give written information and answer her questions.
- Discuss the pros and cons of medical and surgical management as described above.
    - If she chooses to have surgery, laparoscopy is the best approach because she is haemodynamically stable.
    - Both surgical treatments (salpingectomy and salpingostomy) and methotrexate have comparable results.
    - With salpingostomy and methotrexate, she will require β-hCG follow-up until the level normalises.
    - An ectopic pregnancy can undergo molar transformation, the risk of which is increased with salpingostomy compared with salpingectomy. This then leads to requirement for further follow-up and the potential of increased morbidity from the subsequent methotrexate therapy.
- Since the woman is asymptomatic and haemodynamically stable, I will seek her informed and written consent for whatever treatment she chooses.

Future fertility issues:

- Recurrence of a tubal pregnancy increases the risk of infertility.
- There is a 54% chance that with conservation of the right tube with a salpingostomy, she may have a future successful pregnancy.
- If a salpingectomy is done, she will require IVF.
- Fertility rates are similar for salpingostomy and methotrexate.
- Recurrence of ectopic pregnancy rates are similar for both salpingostomy and methotrexate.
- Referral to a fertility centre for further counselling.

Question 5

Compare and contrast with evidence the treatments of a tubal pregnancy with methotrexate and laparoscopy.

Answer:

	Methotrexate	Laparoscopy
Mode of action	Decreasing intracellular folinic acid level, causing failure of trophoblasts	Removes gestational sac with or without the fallopian tube.
Indications	• Sac diameter < 3.5 cm, with no fetal heartbeat (Evidence Level IIA) and no excessive fluid in the pouch of Douglas • β-hCG < 5000 IU/L • Asymptomatic, haemodynamically stable (Evidence Level IV) • Willing to come for follow-up visits • Not breastfeeding	• Unsuitable for medical treatment • Haemodynamically unstable • Ruptured tube • In severe pelvic pain • Recurrent ectopic pregnancies • Woman's desire to have surgery
Advantages	• Safe, cost-effective, no hospitalisation required • No surgery, avoiding its complications and abdominal scars	• Provides definitive and immediate treatment • Histological confirmation is obtained • Woman can try to conceive again earlier • Shorter follow-up and recovery time (Evidence Level IA)
Disadvantages	• Prolonged follow-up • Side effects of methotrexate • 15% risk of subsequent dosing with methotrexate and 7% risk of tubal rupture (Evidence Level IIA) • Should not conceive for 1 year	• Risks from surgery and anaesthesia • False negative rate 3–4% • False positive rate 5% • Higher risk of persistent or recurrent ectopic pregnancy (Evidence Level IIA) and trophoblastic disease with salpingectomy (8%)
Success rate	94%	Equally comparable (Evidence Level IIA)
Tubal patency rate	Equal	Equal
Future pregnancy outcomes	Same	Same

Table 4.7. Comparison of methotrexate and laparoscopy as treatments for tubal pregnancy

Question 6

How will you counsel a woman who sees you for tubal reanastomosis surgery following prior sterilisation?

Answer:

I will counsel her as follows:

- A new relationship forms the basis of most such requests (Evidence Level III).
- Discuss comorbidities that could affect future fertility, such as obesity, diabetes, and hypertension.
- Assess ovulation status, male partner's semen quality, and his ability to perform successful intercourse.
- Previous ectopic pregnancy is a contraindication for this procedure.
- The best results are obtained if the sterilisation was done by a laparoscopy using clips, followed by Falope ring. If the length of residual fallopian tube is less than 4 cm, outcomes of reanastomosis are poorer.
- Success of tubal anastomosis varies according to the surgeon's skill, age of the woman, and time since sterilisation. Success rates are on the order of 31–92%.
- The rate of conception is highest within a year of tubal reanastomosis surgery.
- The incidence of tubal pregnancy following tubal reanastomosis surgery is 0–7%. She should have an ultrasound scan as early as possible in the next pregnancy.

Multiple-Choice Questions

Q1. Which of the following statements is **incorrect** regarding the development of persistent trophoblasts in a treated tubal pregnancy?

- A. Laparoscopic salpingostomy has a persistent trophoblast rate of 8%.
- B. Open salpingostomy has a persistent trophoblast rate of 4%.
- C. The incidence of persistent trophoblast increases when the starting hCG level is < 1500 IU/L.
- D. The incidence of persistent trophoblast is indicated by a rapid rise in preoperative hCG and the presence of active tubal bleeding.

Answer: C

Q2. A 25-year-old woman receiving methotrexate for a right tubal pregnancy has a serum hCG level of 1200 IU/L on day 7. Her starting serum hCG was 1000 IU/L. She had a caesarean section 1 year ago. How will you manage this woman?

- A. Review diagnosis
- B. Administer another dose of methotrexate
- C. Perform surgery
- D. Ignore because this rise is physiological

Answer: B

Q3. A woman, uncomplicated otherwise, has a diagnosis of a right tubal pregnancy with a complex adnexal mass of 4 cm. How will you treat her?

  A. By laparoscopic partial salpingectomy
  B. By laparoscopic salpingectomy
  C. By laparoscopic salpingostomy
  D. By laparoscopic salpingotomy

Answer: B

Q4. You are at home when you receive a call from the hospital about a woman with a bicornuate uterus who is nearly 10 weeks from her LMP and had a positive home urine pregnancy test 2 weeks ago. She is complaining of severe lower abdominal pain and some vaginal bleeding. Her BP is 90/60 and pulse rate is 110/minute. Abdominal ultrasound showed no intrauterine pregnancy and a 6-cm adnexal mass. What will you do?

  A. Arrange a laparoscopy and probable linear salpingostomy
  B. Arrange platelet count and LFT in preparation for methotrexate therapy
  C. Arrange a laparoscopy with a probable laparotomy
  D. Do nothing until I can see the patient myself in 40 minutes

Answer: C

Q5. How long does it take for the fertilised egg to implant?

  A. 5 days
  B. 6 days
  C. 7 days
  D. 8 days

Answer: C

Q6. What is the most common predisposing factor for a tubal pregnancy?

  A. DES exposure in utero
  B. Multiload copper intrauterine contraceptive device
  C. Levonorgestrel-containing intrauterine contraceptive device
  D. Salpingitis

Answer: D

Q7. You are consulting a G1P0 lady one week after termination of a pregnancy at 6 weeks gestation. She has no symptoms but has a positive pregnancy test and a uterine size equivalent to 6–7 weeks. The termination of pregnancy had yielded a small amount of tissue but was otherwise uneventful. The histology showed that the uterine curettings were decidual. The next step in the management of this patient is:

A. Transvaginal ultrasound scan

B. Progesterone challenge test

C. Repeat curettage

D. Exploratory laparotomy

Answer: A

(Absence of chorionic villi in the uterine curettings suggests either the patient had a complete miscarriage or the pregnancy is outside the uterus—that is, ectopic pregnancy. She needs an urgent scan to rule out an ectopic pregnancy.)

Q8. A 19-year-old, with an LMP 6 weeks ago, presents with sudden onset of pelvic pain and vaginal spotting. On examination, she has bilateral adnexal tenderness. The ultrasound scan shows no gestational sac in the uterus. Her serum β-hCG is 6000 IU/L. What will you do?

A. Laparotomy

B. Laparoscopy

C. Repeat β-hCG in 48 hours

D. Transvaginal ultrasound scan in 1 week

Answer: B

Q9. Which of the following is most suggestive of an ectopic pregnancy?

A. A transabdominal ultrasound scan shows no intrauterine gestational sac, and β-HCG is < 4000 mIU/mL.

B. A transvaginal ultrasound scan shows no intrauterine gestational sac, and β-HCG is < 600 mIU/mL.

C. β-hCG > 7000 mIU/ml, and serum progesterone is < 40 mg/mL.

D. Transabdominal ultrasound scan shows no intrauterine gestational sac, and β-HCG is > 7000 mIU/mL.

Answer: D

Q10. Which of the following has the highest risk of an ectopic pregnancy if the woman accidentally falls pregnant?

A. Condoms

B. Diaphragm

C. Combined oral contraceptive pills

D. Progestogen-only pills

Answer: D

Q11. A 17-year-old is having a laparotomy for a ruptured right tubal pregnancy. The right ovary is seen to have a 10-cm cyst. The left ovary is normal. The most appropriate management of this right ovarian cyst is:

A. Right ovarian cystectomy

B. Aspirate the cyst only

C. Cystectomy with wedge resection of the left ovary

D. Observe and rescan in 6 weeks

Answer: A

Chapter 4.4.   Gestational Trophoblastic Disease

Definitions

Choriocarcinoma	Aggressive and malignant proliferation of villous trophoblast with early and distant metastasis
Complete mole (CM)	Uncontrolled proliferation of diploid trophoblastic villi with hydropic transformation without a fetus, unless a multiple pregnancy
Epitheloid trophoblastic tumour	A variant of placental site trophoblastic tumour (PSTT)
Gestational trophoblastic disease (GTD) Also known as: • Hydatidiform mole • Molar pregnancy • Complete mole/partial mole • Choriocarcinoma	A spectrum of disorders of uncontrolled and abnormal proliferation of trophoblastic cells
Invasive mole (IM)	CM or PM that invades the myometrium
Partial mole (PM)	Uncontrolled proliferation of triploid/tetraploid trophoblastic villi with the presence of fetal tissue
Persistent trophoblastic disease Also known as: • Persistent trophoblastic neoplasia • Gestational trophoblastic neoplasia (GTN) Involving one of the following: • Invasive mole (IM) • Choriocarcinoma (CC) • Placental site trophoblastic tumour (PSTT) • Epitheloid trophoblastic tumour (ETT)	Uncontrolled and malignant proliferation of villous trophoblasts/intermediate trophoblasts with invasion of the myometrium and metastasis In the absence of histological confirmation, diagnosed by persistently high β-hCG after surgical evacuation of a molar pregnancy
Placental site trophoblastic tumour	Malignant proliferation of intermediate trophoblasts with slow and late metastasis through lymphatics
Theca lutein cyst	Multicystic, bilateral ovarian cysts with a soap-bubble or spike-wheel appearance due to high hCG level

Table 4.8. Chapter 4.4. Definitions

118

	CM	PM	IM	CC	PSTT	ETT
Definition	Derived from villous trophoblast No fetus, unless coexisting twin.	Derived from villous trophoblast Fetus present	CM or PM invading myometrium	Highly malignant trophoblastic tumour	Neoplasia from intermediate trophoblast	Neoplasia from intermediate trophoblast
Malignant	Premalignant	Premalignant	Malignant	Malignant	Malignant	Malignant
Incidence	0.5–1 in 1000 pregnancies Increased incidence in Asian women	3 in 1000 pregnancies	15–20% of CM and 1–5% of PM	1 in 50,000 pregnancies	Difficult to establish due to rarity, about 0.2% of all cases of GTD	Only a handful of cases described so far
Genetics	Androgenetic Monospermy 46XX (80%) Dispermy 46XX or 46XY (20%) Nuclear DNA paternal but mitochondrial DNA maternal Associated with mutations of NLRP7 and KHDC3L	Triploid 69XXY Dispermy Tetraploid	May originate from a CM or PM (less common), normal conception or tubal pregnancy PSTT more common after a normal pregnancy Incidence greatest in first year after pregnancy			
Risk factors	Maternal age <15 or >40 years Low intake of carotene and animal fat Prior molar pregnancy After 1st mole, the risk of 2nd mole = 1–2% After 2nd mole, the risk of a 3rd mole = 15–20% Risk does not increase by changing the partner				More common after a normal pregnancy	
Histology	Abnormal budding villous structure with hyperplasia, stromal karyorrhectic debris and collapsed blood vessels	Patchy villous hydrops, abnormal irregular villi, trophoblastic pseudo-inclusions and patchy trophoblast hyperplasia		hCG-producing malignant epithelial tumour with central necrosis and both cytotrophoblastic and syncytiotrophoblastic cells; mononuclear cells predominate; no formed chorionic villi; myometrial invasion	Invasive tumour consisting of mononucleate and multinucleate trophoblastic cells at the implantation site with inflammatory reaction	

	CM	PM	IM	CC	PSTT	ETT
hCG	Very high > 200,000 IU/L	Slightly high	hCG	Subtypes of β-hCG exist: free β-hCG, β-core, nicked free β, C-terminal peptide; false positives excluded by measuring urinary β-hCG	Low levels of β-hCG Positive for HPL	
Metastasis	4% incidence	0.5% incidence	Lungs	Early blood metastasis to lungs, brain, and pelvic organs	Metastasise later and slower, mainly through lymphatics to uterine wall, pelvic lymph nodes, lungs, and brain	
Presentation	Vaginal bleeding prior to 16 weeks					
	Excessive uterine size Anaemia Hyperemesis Pre-eclampsia Theca lutein cysts Hyperthyroidism Passing grapelike vesicles	Less common Oedematous villi May have fetal tissue	Heavy vaginal bleeding Lower abdominal pain Intraperitoneal haemorrhage	SOB Brain or intraperitoneal haemorrhage	Vaginal bleeding after any type of pregnancy Amenorrhoea	
Diagnosis	Presence of symptoms Very high β-hCG level Characteristic ultrasound findings Diploid karyotype, positive for p57 on immunostaining	Presence of symptoms Slightly high or normal β-hCG level Characteristic ultrasound findings Histological examination of POC Triploid/tetraploid karyotype	Presence of symptoms Persistent or rising β-hCG level after evacuation of a molar pregnancy and ultrasound findings	Presence of symptoms Rising β-hCG level after evacuation of a molar pregnancy Characteristic ultrasound features may not be visible	Presence of symptoms, mostly after a normal pregnancy β-hCG level not very high, but high levels of free β-hCG fragments Increased HP1 volume of radiological disease Characteristic ultrasound features may be seen	

Table 4.9. Summary of types of gestational trophoblastic disease

Clinical Physiology

Gestational trophoblastic disease (GTD) is a spectrum of abnormalities of trophoblastic proliferation and hydropic transformation. The human trophoblasts share some of the features of a malignant cell, such as rapid cell division, local invasion, and metastasis. The molar fluid is either derived from the diffusion of maternal plasma or from synthesis in the trophoblasts. The hydropic transformation of the villous mesenchyma results from an absence, maldevelopment, or regression of the villous vasculature, which makes drainage of fluid impossible.

The terms *partial mole* and *complete mole* describe the premalignant variations of a spectrum of disorders. Partial moles are biparental, mostly triploid, as a result of dispermic fertilisation of a normal ovum. In this condition, only some chorionic villi are swollen, and the fetal tissue, cord, and amniotic membrane are present in some form. The fetus is triploid with congenital abnormalities and is never viable.

Complete moles are androgenic and diploid, as a result of the fertilisation of an ovum with no chromosomes (empty ovum), followed by the duplication of the DNA (46XX) or, in 20% of cases, by dispermic fertilisation of an empty ovum (46XY). Although nuclear DNA is entirely paternal, mitochondrial DNA is maternal. Mutations in two genes, NLRP7 and rarely KHDC3L, are associated with this condition. With a complete mole, all placental villi are swollen, and the fetus, cord, and amniotic membrane are absent.

Choriocarcinomas are malignant, hCG-producing epithelial neoplasms with a central necrosis and compromising both syncytiotrophoblasts and cytotrophoblasts invading the myometrium. Invasive moles are those partial (less common) and complete moles (more common) which deeply invade the myometrium and very rarely metastasise into the lungs.

Placental site trophoblastic tumours develop from intermediate trophoblasts after any type of pregnancy and are less virulent in their malignant behaviour compared with the choriocarcinoma. They produce HPL, less hCG (more variants and fragments of β-hCG, such as hCG-H, free β subunit, β-core, nicked free-β, and C-terminal fragments), and metastasise slowly by the lymphatics.

An epithelioid trophoblastic tumour is a variant of the above, with similar behaviour pattern but distinctive hyalinisation.

Gestational trophoblastic disease is a unique spectrum of disorders that produce only one specific marker, hCG. This is easily and accurately measured in blood and urine. The level of hCG reflects the disease volume. Because of the early presentation, often classical clinical and histological features are not seen, and the treatment is aimed at the normalisation of the hCG level. In the absence of a clear histological diagnosis, differentiation between a complete or partial mole can be made through ploidy analysis by flow cytometry, in-situ hybridisation or molecular genotyping, and immunostaining of the p57 gene.

Management

The aim of treatment is complete hCG remission and not necessarily radiological remission.

- Suction curette with up to a 12 mm suction catheter:
  - No prolonged use of cervical ripening agent, i.e., misoprostol (Evidence Level IV).
  - No intraoperative oxytocic agent because of the risk of trophoblastic embolism (Evidence Level II).
  - Oxytocic, preferably ergometrine, should be used after the completion of curettage to prevent trophoblastic embolisation.
  - All cases must be registered with the molar registry.
  - Follow up with serum hCG levels fortnightly, until the level is normal. Thereafter, monthly urine hCG for 6 months.
  - Avoid getting pregnant during the period of surveillance. Oral contraceptive pills should only be commenced after the serum level has returned to normal, as oestrogen may act as a growth factor for trophoblastic tissue.
  - In future pregnancies, check hCG levels 6 and 10 weeks after delivery.
  - A second curettage due to the persistence of symptoms should be avoided because most patients will still need chemotherapy.
  - Anti-D to Rh-negative women with PM.
  - There is no evidence of benefit from mifepristone (Evidence Level III).

- Twin-molar pregnancy:
  - If the fetus is normal, a pregnancy is allowed to continue until term.
  - The woman should be counselled about increased perinatal morbidity.
  - There is a 25% chance of a live birth and a 36% chance of a premature delivery (Evidence Level III).
  - The incidence of preeclampsia is variable.

FIGO Scoring	0	1	2	3
Age (years)	< 40	> 40	—	—
Antecedent pregnancy	Mole	Abortion	Term	—
Interval months from end of index pregnancy to treatment	< 4	4 – > 7	7 – < 13	≥ 13
Pre-treatment serum hCG (IU/L)	< 103	103 – < 104	104 – < 105	≥ 105
Largest tumour size, including uterus (cm)	< 3	3 – < 5	≥ 5	—
Site of metastases	Lung	Spleen, kidney	Gastrointestinal	Liver, brain
Number of metastases	—	1 – 4	5 – 8	> 8
Previous failed chemotherapy	—	—	Single drug	2 or more drugs

Table 4.10. FIGO scoring system to establish risk in GTN

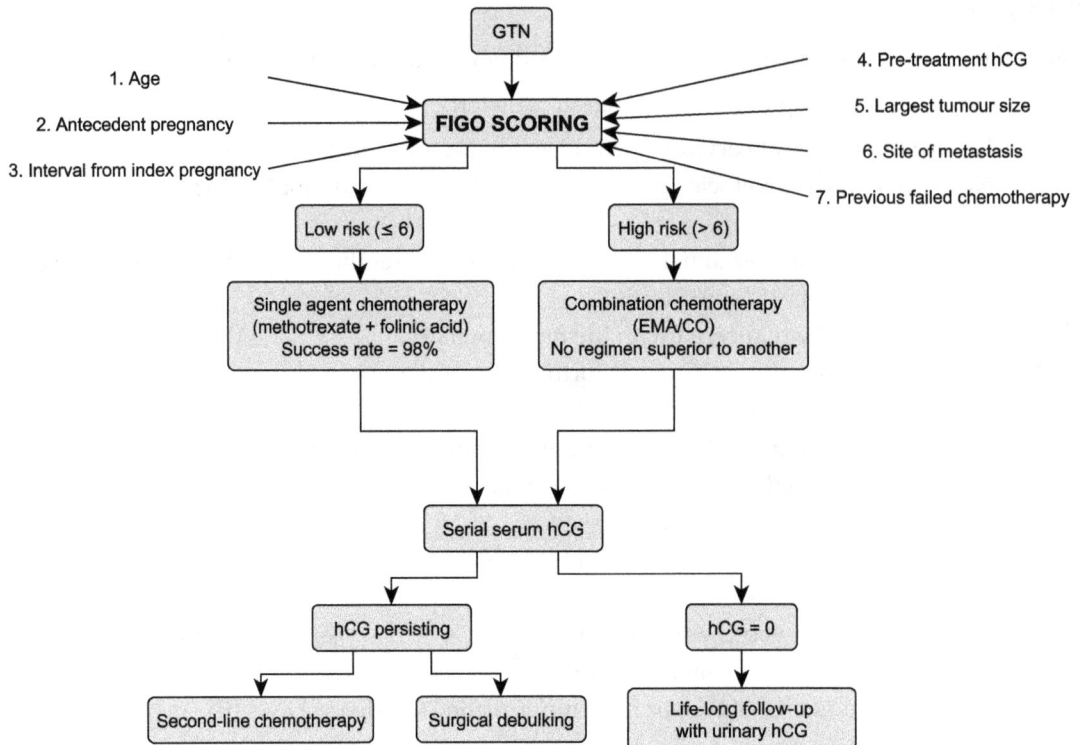

Figure 4.9. Algorithm for treatment of GTD, according to FIGO scoring

A complete hCG response is an essential component of successful treatment, but the complete disappearance of the ultrasound finding is not.

The prognosis for females with GTN after a nonmolar pregnancy may be worse, due to a delayed diagnosis or advanced disease with distant metastasis (Evidence Level II).

Risks of Chemotherapy

- Risk of relapse is 3%, greatest in the first year.
- Risk of a second malignancy, e.g., AML, colon cancer, breast cancer (Evidence Level III).
- Menopausal age is lowered by 3 years (Evidence Level III).
- Risk of teratogenicity and masking of signs of relapse if pregnancy occurs within a year.

Treatment of PSTT

This tumour is chemo-resistant, and hence, treatment is surgery, which involves a hysterectomy and pelvic lymphadenectomy with conservation of the ovaries. The best prognostic indicator is the interval from the index pregnancy. An interval of less than 4 years has 100% survival. The overall 5-year survival is 75%.

Short-Answer Questions

Question 1

What are the risks of complete mole and partial mole?

Answer:

	Complete mole	Partial mole
Ongoing bleeding	Present	Present
Fetal risks	No fetus	Fetal malformation, IUGR
Chemotherapy	15%	0.5%
Development of choriocarcinoma	15%	0.5%
Metastasis	4%	0.5%
Hyperthyroidism and pre-eclampsia	Rare	Even rarer

Table 4.11. Comparison of risks of complete mole and partial mole

Question 2

A histology report of a uterine curetting, performed for miscarriage, shows a partial mole. How will you manage this woman?

Answer:

- Counsel the woman about molar pregnancy.
- Provide any written information, if available.
- Refer to molar registry.
- Fortnightly serum quantitative hCG until the level becomes 0.
- Thereafter, monthly urinary hCG for 6 months.
- Administer anti-D immunoglobulin if the woman is Rh-negative, if not already administered.
- Advise against a pregnancy in the follow-up period. Can use COC once hCG is normalised.
- Plateauing or rise in hCG indicates GTN.

The management of GTN in this case will be as follows:

- Staging by CXR:
  - MRI brain and CT chest, abdomen, and pelvis if the CXR shows any lesions.
- Risk score according to FIGO risk scoring system (shown in the algorithm above).

- If low risk (≤ 6):
  - o 50 mg methotrexate IM on alternate days for 4 doses.
  - o Folinic acid rescue on intervening days for 4 days.
  - o The methotrexate/folinic acid regimen is continued every 2 weeks until 6 weeks after hCG has become 0.
  - o Explain the side effects of methotrexate: headache, rash, sun sensitivity, gum and GIT irritation.

- If high risk (> 6) or methotrexate resistance:
  - o EMA/CO (etoposide, methotrexate, actinomycin D, cyclophosphamide, vincristine/ oncovine)
  - o Follow up, up to 6 months, as above.
  - o Follow up after 6 months:
    - Urine hCG weekly for 1 year, then 6-monthly for the next 5 years, then yearly for the rest of her life.

- If a pregnancy ensues, check serum hCG at 6 and 10 weeks after delivery.

Question 3

What are the physiological and nonphysiological functions of hCG? What problems do you envisage in hCG surveillance of GTN?

Answer:

Functions of hCG:

1. Promote continued secretion of oestrogen and progesterone from the corpus luteum. This leads to the cessation of the first menses after conception.
2. Used to diagnose and monitor the treatment of GTD/GTN, ectopic pregnancy, and a failed pregnancy.
3. Used as a tumour marker for germ cell tumours.
4. Used as a marker of fetal aneuploidy.
5. Used in IVF for follicular maturation.

Problems in hCG surveillance of GTN:

Initiation or cessation of chemotherapy and the need for surgery depend upon the accurate measurement of β-hCG. An increase in the sensitivity of hCG assays and the discovery of β-hCG variants and fragments, such as hCG-H, free β-subunit, β-core, nicked free-β, and C-terminal fragments, pose the following problems:

1. False negative results: the assay should be able to detect all forms of β-hCG; otherwise false negative results will occur.
2. False positive results: this is due to the cross reactivity of the assay with circulating heterophile antibodies, making the molecules too large for glomerular filtration. This possibility is eliminated by measuring urinary hCG.

3. Persistent low-level elevation of β-hCG without evidence of disease: this is increasingly happening due to the increasing sensitivity of hCG assays without clinical or radiological evidence of the disease. Possible explanations of this phenomenon are quiescent GTN, nongestational neoplasia, and a physiological elevation in some women.

Question 4

How would you confirm a diagnosis of choriocarcinoma? Discuss the indications of chemotherapy in molar pregnancy.

Answer:

Confirmation of choriocarcinoma diagnosis:

Suggestive history:

- A history of normal, ectopic, or molar pregnancy. The risk of choriocarcinoma is highest when the antecedent pregnancy is a complete mole (15%).

Symptoms:

- Vaginal bleeding.
- Dyspnoea.
- Haemoptysis.
- Stroke.
- Intraperitoneal bleeding.
- Hyperemesis.
- Hyperthyroidism.

Signs:

- Enlarged uterus.

Investigations:

- Markedly increased serum quantitative β-hCG.
- CXR and MRI brain, abdomen, and pelvis may identify metastatic disease.
- A transvaginal ultrasound scan may show a complex, hyperechoic vascular mass in the uterine cavity, which is possible with theca lutein cysts.
- Histology of the POC will show choriocarcinoma, if present.

Indications for chemotherapy:

- Stationary/elevated serum β-hCG.
- Vaginal bleeding in the presence of abnormal β-hCG.
- Evidence of metastasis in lungs, brain, liver, or kidneys.
- Choriocarcinoma on the histology of uterine curettings.

Question 5

What would you advise a woman with GTD regarding when she can try to conceive again? Briefly discuss the outcome of such a pregnancy.

Answer:

The woman should be advised to try to conceive when the 6-month follow-up period has ended. If she had been on chemotherapy, she should wait at least one year after completion of treatment due to the increased risk of fetal malformation, miscarriage, and stillbirth (Evidence Level III). The risk of a second molar pregnancy is 1 in 80. If a second molar pregnancy did occur, it will be of the same histological type.

However, 98% of women will have a normal pregnancy without an increase in the rate of obstetric complications. An early ultrasound scan should be done to exclude recurrence. Serum hCG should be checked at 6 and 10 weeks after the birth of the baby, and the placenta should be sent for histological examination to exclude GTD.

Question 6

What will be your advice regarding contraception to a woman with the diagnosis of a molar pregnancy?

Answer:

- She should use barrier methods with a spermicidal agent until the hCG level has normalised.
- She may start using COC after this hCG level has normalised.
- Do not use an IUCD because of the risks of uterine perforation during insertion and vaginal bleeding after insertion.
- Do not use progesterone-only pills because of the risk of irregular vaginal bleeding, which may be confused as recurrence of GTN.
- Treatment of GTN does not affect fertility.
- Contraception should be continued for at least 6 months without chemotherapy and 12 months with chemotherapy.

Question 7

Will you administer anti-D immunoglobulin to a Rh-negative woman with a complete mole at 12 weeks of pregnancy?

Answer:

I will not administer anti-D immunoglobulin to this woman because chorionic villi are poorly vascularised and do not express D antigen in a complete molar pregnancy (Evidence Level IV).

Question 8

Tabulate the ultrasound features of different types of GTD.

Answer:

	CM	PM	IM/PSTT	CC
Appearance	Snowstorm	Swiss cheese	Focal, heterogenous, echogenic myometrial lesions with cystic spaces	Intrauterine blood lacunae surrounded by hyperechoic areas
Vascularity	Avascular	Avascular	Vascular	Vascular
Fetus	Absent, unless twins/triplets	Present, abnormal, IUGR	Absent	Absent
Uterine artery blood flow	Low resistance, high-peak systolic velocity	High resistance flow	Low resistance, high-peak systolic velocity	Low resistance, high-peak systolic velocity

Table 4.12. Ultrasound features of different types of GTD

The features of CM, as described in Table 4.12. are seen only after 9 weeks of pregnancy.

Theca lutein cysts are bilateral, multicystic ovaries with a soap-bubble or spoke-wheel appearance. They are seen in 50% of GTD cases, due to very high levels of hCG.

Multiple-Choice Questions

Q1. What is the most common feature of a molar pregnancy?

A. Regular vaginal bleeding

B. Irregular vaginal bleeding

C. Hyperemesis

D. Passing grapelike vesicles per vagina

Answer: B

Q2. A 23-year-old Asian woman had a suction curettage for a missed abortion in her first pregnancy. The histology of the products of conception showed a partial mole. Follow up β-hCG levels:

A. Should be continued for 6 months

B. Can be discontinued if hCG returns to normal at 8 weeks

C. Indicate persistent gestational trophoblastic disease if level plateaus over 3 weeks

D. Indicate persistent gestational trophoblastic disease if there is a 5% rise over 2 values

Answer: A

Q3. For which of the following conditions is pelvic lymphadenopathy required?

  A. Familial complete mole

  B. Invasive mole

  C. Choriocarcinoma

  D. Placental site trophoblastic tumour

Answer: D

Q4. While following up a woman with a complete mole, what will be your indication for chemotherapy?

  A. Constant quantitative hCG for 1 week

  B. hCG trending upward

  C. hCG normalising after 6 weeks

  D. Opaque shadows on CXR

Answer: B

Q5. You are following up a 30-year-old G1P0 woman after an evacuation of retained products for a miscarriage at 9 weeks. Histology of the curettings shows trophoblastic proliferation with hydropic changes and no fetal tissue. What will be your next action?

  A. Single-agent chemotherapy

  B. Hysterectomy

  C. Weekly hCG levels

  D. MRI of brain, chest, abdomen, and pelvis

Answer: C

Q6. The half-life of hCG is much longer compared with other glycoprotein hormones due to:

  A. a characteristic α-chain

  B. a characteristic β-chain

  C. increased content of fructose

  D. increased content of sialic acid

Answer: D

Q7. You are doing a repeat evacuation 3 weeks after the initial one for a miscarriage at 9 weeks. The histology of the POC was unremarkable. What will you do with the POC removed after the current evacuation?

  A. Send for karyotyping even if it was done last time

  B. Send for microbiological examination

  C. Send again for histological examination as GTN can develop at any time

  D. Not send for any examination

Answer: C

Q8. The need for chemotherapy following a complete mole is:

    A. 10%

    B. 15%

    C. 20%

    D. 30%

Answer: B (Evidence Level III)

Q9. The need for chemotherapy following a partial mole is:

    A. 0.5%

    B. 1%

    C. 2%

    D. 4%

Answer: A

Q10. A partial mole pregnancy will be:

    A. Completely maternal in origin

    B. Completely paternal in origin

    C. Biparental in origin

    D. Could be any of the above

Answer: C

Q11. Which of the following could be tetraploid?

    A. CM

    B. PM

    C. PSTT

    D. ETT

Answer: B

Q12. Which has a worse prognosis?

    A. Gonadal choriocarcinoma

    B. Gestational choriocarcinoma

    C. Epitheloid trophoblastic tumour

    D. Placental site trophoblastic tumour

Answer: A

Q13. How will you treat a theca lutein cyst?

    A. Laparoscopic cystectomy if ovarian diameter > 5 cm

    B. Aspiration of cyst fluid with ultrasound guidance

    C. Observe; will resolve once the molar tissue regresses

    D. Methotrexate

Answer: C

Q14. Which of the following is **not** correct regarding GTD?

    A. Complete hCG response and radiological response are needed for the successful treatment.

    B. Intervention is not needed for residual posttreatment masses outside the CNS.

    C. Women with relapsed disease still have a good chance of cure, despite multiple chemotherapy.

    D. Complete hCG response is needed for the successful treatment but not complete radiological response.

Answer: A

Q15. Which of the following is **not** used for ploidy analysis?

    A. Flow cytometry

    B. In-situ hybridisation

    C. Microarray

    D. Molecular genotyping

Answer: C

Q16. Which of the following is correct for p57 in the context of GTD?

    A. It is a paternally imprinted gene, expressed maternally.

    B. It is a maternally imprinted gene, expressed paternally.

    C. It is a paternally imprinted gene, expressed paternally.

    D. It helps to distinguish between GTD and GTN.

Answer: A

Q17. Which of the following genes are **not** associated with GTD?

    A. p54

    B. p57

    C. NALP7

    D. KHDC3L

Answer: A

Q18. Which of the following will be your treatment for a 26-year-old nulliparous lady with persistent nonmetastatic trophoblastic neoplasia?

    A. Multiagent chemotherapy

    B. Single-agent chemotherapy

    C. Pelvic irradiation

    D. Total abdominal hysterectomy

Answer: B

Q19. For constant levels of sensitivity and specificity, increasing the prevalence of the condition in the sample will:

A. Lower the positive predictive value

B. Increase the positive predictive value

C. Not alter the predictive value

D. Increase or decrease the positive predictive value, depending on other factors

Answer: B

Chapter 5
Gynaecological Infections

Chapter 5.1.   Sexually Transmitted Infections (STIs)

Definitions

Bacteria	Unicellular, prokaryotic organisms that have a cell wall but lack organelles and an organised nucleus
Fungus	Unicellular or multicellular, spore-forming, eukaryotic organisms that feed by decomposing and absorbing organic matter
Incubation	Period between time of infection and time when symptoms first appear
Obligate	Restricted to a particular function or mode of life, such as intracellular environment
Parasite	Organism that lives in or on another organism, deriving its food from the host, at the host's expense
Virus	Complex, nonliving infective agent that contains DNA or RNA strands within a protein coat; able to replicate within a host cell

Table 5.1. Chapter 5.1. Definitions

Common STIs and vaginal infections

	Causative organisms	Incubation	Incidence	Signs and symptoms
Chlamydia	*Chlamydia trachomatis*— obligate intracellular (columnar) bacterium Strains D–K cause genital infection	5 days	10% of women of childbearing age 25% in sub-fertile women	• Asymptomatic (80%) • Mucopurulent vaginal discharge • Vaginitis • Cervicitis • Urethritis • Laparoscopy: pelvic inflammation, violin string adhesions, Fitz Hugh Curtis syndrome
Lymphogranuloma venereum	*Chlamydia trachomatis* Strains L1-L3	3 days to 6 weeks	Seen in tropics More common in males	• Shallow, painless ulcer of the labia and vestibule • Painful lymphadenopathy in the inguinal and perianal area • Proctocolitis • Malaise, fever
Gonorrhoea	*Neisseria gonorrhoea* Gram negative intracellular diplococcus	3 weeks to 3 months	1% in reproductive age group	• Asymptomatic mucopurulent vaginal/urethral discharge • Can cause tonsillitis, conjunctivitis, proctitis
Syphilis	*Treponema pallidum* Spirochete, anaerobe	10 to 90 days		• Primary syphilis: painless ulcer (chancre) on the cervix, labia, site of inoculation, rubbery feel with inguinal lymphadenopathy • Secondary syphilis: maculopapular rash, symmetrical, involves palms and soles; condylomata lata and snail track ulcers on mucus membranes; alopecia, arthritis, meningitis • Tertiary syphilis: sensorineural deafness, stroke, insanity
Trichomoniasis	*Trichomonas vaginalis,* flagellate protozoa	4 to 28 days	5–13% in general population 9.4–29.5% in HIV positive women	• Asymptomatic • Itchy purulent foamy vaginal discharge • Vulvovaginitis • Inflamed cervix— 'strawberry cervix'

Investigations	Treatment without pregnancy	Implications for pregnancy	Treatment in pregnancy
PCR on columnar cervical cells, urine sample	Doxycycline 100 mg PO BD for 10 days Azithromycin 1 g IV/PO stat Treat sexual partners	May cause infertility by damaging tubes, neonatal conjunctivitis and pneumonia; preterm labour, chorioamnionitis, premature ROM, endometritis	Erythromycin 500 mg BD for 2 weeks Azithromycin 1 g stat
• Complement fixation test of the aspirate from a discharging lymph node • Antibody titre > 1:64 indicative of acute infection • "Groove sign"	Doxycycline 100 mg BD 3 weeks Azithromycin 1 g weekly for 3 weeks Ciprofloxacin 750 mg BD for 3 weeks	Painful perineum Fistula	As above
Examination of Gram-stained smear and culture of urethral, cervical or vaginal swab on Thayer Martin medium	Ceftriaxone 250 mg IM or Amoxycillin 2 g stat or Spectinomycin 2 g stat Treat sexual partners	Vertical transmission to the fetus at the time of vaginal birth	Same as nonpregnant
Screening tests: RPR, VDRL Diagnostic tests: TPHA, TPPA (particle agglutination) Demonstrating TP on dark field microscopy	Benzathine penicillin 2.4 MU IM, repeated after 1 week	Vertical transmission: abnormal teeth, skin scarring, Sabre Tibia, deafness, interstitial keratitis, fetal death	Same as nonpregnant
Vaginal pH > 5 Microscopy of vaginal secretion: 60% sensitivity, HVS culture	Metronidazole 400 mg BD for 5/7 or 2 g stat	Preterm birth	Same as nonpregnant

	Causative organisms	Incubation	Incidence	Signs and symptoms
Bacterial vaginosis	Anaerobic bacteria, e.g. *Gardnerella, Bacteroides Mobiluncus* species *Peptostreptococci* marked decrease in *Lactobacilli*	12 hours to 5 days	Most common cause of asymptomatic vaginitis	• Musty/fishy vaginal odour • Frothy grey-white vaginal discharge, sticking to the vaginal walls • No vaginal inflammation • May cause PID or endometritis
Vaginal candidiasis (not a STI) (Thrush)	*Candida albicans* in 80% of cases; *Candida glabrata* (fungus) Predisposing factors: • Immunosuppression • Tight undergarments • Vaginal douching • Antibiotic use • Hyperoestrogenic states	2–5 days	50–75%; most common in women of 20–30-year age group	• Asymptomatic • Curdlike white vaginal discharge which does not stick to the vaginal walls • Vulvovaginal itching and sometimes redness
Genital herpes	Herpes simplex usually type II but also Type I DNA virus	2–7 days	12%–twice as common in women of 35–44-year age group	• Vesicular lesions (dew drop appearance) surrounded by a zone of erythema on perineum, vagina, cervix, thigh • Very painful but recurrent infections less painful • Multiple vesicles join to form ulcers • Periurethral lesions may cause urinary retention and vulvar oedema
Genital warts (Condylomata acuminata)	Human papilloma virus (HPV) type 6, 11 May be infected simultaneously with more than one type	3 months	Peak incidence between 15 and 25 years; approximately 65% of individuals with an infected partner develop warts; 30% of infected women will have macroscopic recognisable lesions	• Warts could be present on vulva, vagina, cervix, perineal area; may be small or coalesce to form large balls Infection progresses by autoinoculation • Usually no pain or itching • Rarely verrucous squamous cell carcinoma

Investigations	Treatment without pregnancy	Implications for pregnancy	Treatment in pregnancy
• Presence of 'Clue cells' on wet smear microscopy • Vaginal secretion pH > 4.5 • Vaginal secretion when mixed with KOH, causes amine-like odour positive 'Whiff test' • High vaginal swab culture	• Single dose clindamycin • Metronidazole orally or vaginally • Introduction of oral or vaginal Lactobacillus • Concurrent treatment of male partner is not needed	Preterm ruptured membrane–fetal death	Metronidazole as in nonpregnant women
Normal pH of vaginal fluid, culture of vaginal fluid, check for diabetes and immunosuppression	Topical antifungals (clotrimazole, miconazole); oral and topical antifungals for recurrent disease or when predisposing cyclical factors	Can be isolated in 25% of women; can cause itchy discharge, tender and oedematous vulva; asymptomatic disease does not need treatment	Same as nonpregnant
• Serological tests for IgG and IgM • PCR from the vesicular fluid • Viral culture • Presence of IgG of the same type as the virus isolated from the affected area points to recurrent infection	• Aciclovir, famciclovir or valaciclovir • Analgesia • Lignocaine gel • Bathing in salt water	• Vertical transmission during vaginal birth • Incidence of neonatal infection in primary herpes = 41% (Evidence Level III); higher risk if primary infection occurs during last few weeks of pregnancy, as there is no time for development of protective maternal antibodies • Risk of neonatal transmission in recurrent infection = 3% (Evidence Level III)	Aciclovir for primary infection; it reduces viral shedding
• Diagnosis is by visual inspection • Histological confirmation may be obtained • Differential diagnoses: naevi, papillomatosis, seborrheic keratosis, condyloma lata, giant condyloma	• Podophyllin destroys wart cells • Imiquimod cream – acts by increasing host's production of interferon and TNF • Cryotherapy, Diathermy ablation/excision • Interferon α–2β injection into the base of the mucous membrane does not form scar	More common in pregnancy Very rarely, can be vertically transmitted to the baby at birth, causing vocal cord papilloma Presence of genital warts is not an indication for Caesarean section	Cryotherapy or diathermy in 3rd trimester

Table 5.2. Summary of sexually transmitted infections

Multiple-Choice Questions

Q1. Which of the following does not cause Fitz-Hugh-Curtis syndrome?

A. *Chlamydia trachomatis*

B. *N. gonorrhoea*

C. *T. pallidum*

D. Anaerobic *Streptococci*

Answer: C

Q2. Which of the following statements is **not** correct for syphilis?

A. It is caused by an anaerobic organism.

B. VDRL becomes negative after treatment after 2 years.

C. After treatment TPHA remains positive for years.

D. The serological tests are negative in secondary syphilis.

Answer: D

Q3. Which is the most sensitive and specific test for syphilis?

A. Fluorescent treponemal antibody test

B. TP haemagglutinin assay

C. TP particle agglutination test

D. Microscopy

Answer: A

Q4. Which of the following statements is true for a chancre?

A. It is usually painful.

B. It does not appear at the site of inoculation.

C. 5% of lesions occur in extragenital locations.

D. Chancres are usually multiple.

Answer: C

Q5. Which of the following is true for the RPR card test?

A. The test is used as an index of response to therapy.

B. Biological false positive results are quite common.

C. The test detects the antigen in a patient's blood.

D. The test is positive in the presence of an excess of anticardiolipin antibody.

Answer: A

Q6. Venereal Disease Research Laboratory slide test is not positive in which of the following conditions?

A. HIV

B. Acute Herpes simplex

C. Sarcoidosis

D. Cervical cancer

Answer: D

Q7. Which of the following is a part of normal human anatomy?

    A. Chancre

    B. Chancroid

    C. Carcinoid

    D. Choroid

Answer: D

Q8. Which of the following does not cause a macroscopic ulcer?

    A. Chancroid

    B. Lymphogranuloma venereum

    C. Donovanosis

    D. Trichomoniasis

Answer: D

Q9. All the following statements regarding *Chlamydia trachomatis* infection are true except:

    A. The organism is transmitted primarily by coitus.

    B. The majority of infected women are symptomatic.

    C. The organism may cause salpingitis.

    D. Infertility may follow acute or chronic infection.

Answer: B

Q10. A rapid diagnostic test for chlamydia has a sensitivity and specificity of 95% each. In a STD clinic, with a prevalence of chlamydial infection of 30%, the predictive value of a positive test is around 90%. In a private clinic with chlamydial prevalence of 5%, the predictive value of a positive test would be about:

    A. 90%

    B. 50%

    C. 30%

    D. 5%

Answer: B

Q11. What is the causative organism for lymphogranuloma venereum?

    A. *Haemophilus ducreyi*

    B. *Chlamydia trachomatis*

    C. *Calymmatobacterium granulomatis*

    D. *Corynebacterium donovaniae*

Answer: B

Q12. Which of the following does **not** predispose to vaginal candidiasis?

    A. HIV

    B. Eczema

    C. Pregnancy

    D. Inflammatory bowel disease

Answer: D

Q13. Clue cells are:

A. Hypervacuolated cells

B. Hyperkeratotic cells

C. Cervical cells coated with bacteria

D. Vaginal epithelial cells coated with bacteria

Answer: D

Q14. Match the disease with the corresponding relevant feature.

A. Trichomoniasis	i.	Whiff test
B. Candidiasis	ii.	Curdlike discharge
C. Bacterial vaginosis	iii.	Strawberry cervix
D. Lymphogranuloma venereum	iv.	Groove sign

Answer: A-iii, B-ii, C-i, D-iv.

Q15. Match the diseases with their respective first-line treatments in a 20-week-pregnant woman allergic to penicillin.

A. Syphilis	i.	Spectinomycin
B. Chlamydia	ii.	Erythromycin
C. Gonorrhoea	iii.	Metronidazole
D. Trichomoniasis	iv.	Azithromycin

Answer: A-iv, B-ii, C-i, D-iii

Q16. A 20-year-old woman has negative rapid plasma reagin and positive TPHA. The most likely explanation is that the patient:

A. Probably has early syphilis

B. Probably has late latent syphilis

C. Probably has been treated for syphilis in the past

D. The result is probably a biological false positive

Answer: D

Q17. Which organism is responsible for chancroid?

A. *Haemophilus ducreyi*

B. *Chlamydia trachomatis*

C. *Treponema pallidum*

D. *Mycoplasma hominis*

Answer: A

Q18. An 18-year-old who had a laparotomy for a ruptured right ectopic pregnancy has developed a 10-cm cyst on the right ovary. Her left ovary appears normal. Which of the following is the most appropriate treatment?

    A. Right ovarian cystectomy

    B. Right ovarian cyst aspiration

    C. Right salpingo-oophorectomy

    D. Right ovarian cystectomy with wedge resection

Answer: A

Q19. Which organism is responsible for donovanosis?

    A. H. ducreyi

    B. C. granulomatis

    C. G. vaginalis

    D. C. donovaniae

Answer: B

Q20. Which HPV type is mostly associated with an invasive cervical cancer?

    A. 6

    B. 11

    C. 18

    D. 35

Answer: C

Q21. A woman has RPR titre of 1:8 in early pregnancy and a history of documented successful treatment of syphilis. What would you do next?

    A. Do TPHA and FTA tests

    B. Check posttreatment RPR titres

    C. Administer IM penicillin

    D. Undertake contact tracing

Answer: B

Q22. A 26-year-old woman, 4 weeks postpartum and breastfeeding, complains of vulvovaginal irritation and a burning sensation with intercourse. Examination reveals no discharge and red and thin vaginal mucosa. Potassium hydroxide and saline preparation of vaginal secretions are negative. What is the most probable cause?

    A. Bacterial vaginosis

    B. Candida vulvovaginitis

    C. Mycoplasma vaginitis

    D. Atrophic vaginitis

Answer: D

Q23. A 40-year-old Indian woman presents with a history of intermittent small group of vesicles on her left buttock for many years. The most likely diagnosis is:

A. Lymphogranuloma venereum

B. Drug eruption

C. Recurrent HSV2

D. Dermatitis artefacta

Answer: C

Chapter 5.2.	Vaginal Discharge

Clinical Physiology

Physiological vaginal discharge is white, curdy, and odourless, and it is present in the dependent portion of the vagina. The amount of normal discharge varies from person to person. The normal vaginal discharge (secretion) is composed of vaginal and cervical cells, bacteria, water, and other chemicals. The following aerobic and anaerobic bacteria (most prevalent) may be present: *Lactobacilli, Diphtheroids, Streptococcus* species, *E. coli, Gardnerella, Bacteroides*, etc. Normal vaginal pH ranges from 3.8 to 4.5 in the reproductive age group. It is slightly higher in the postmenopausal age group. Lubrication during sexual excitement, spermatic fluid, and cervical mucus all increase the pH slightly, but the effect does not last beyond 8 hours.

Oestrogen stimulates the production of glycogen in the vaginal epithelial cells, which is metabolised to glucose and acts as a substrate for different bacteria, predominantly *Lactobacilli*. *Lactobacilli* make lactic acid, which maintains the vaginal pH and prevents bacterial colonisation to the vaginal walls. Oestrogen promotes *Lactobacilli* proliferation.

The vaginal milieu is a dynamic equilibrium of its bacterial and fungal flora that keeps changing according to age, phase of menstrual cycle, pregnancy, coitus, and antibacterial therapy.

A nonphysiological discharge is with odour, of a different colour and pH, and it adheres to the anterior and lateral walls of the vagina. Signs of lower genital tract inflammation and pruritus may be present.

Causes of increased vaginal pH:

- Bacterial vaginosis
- Trichomoniasis
- Postmenopausal age
- Within 8 hours of unprotected sexual intercourse
- Desquamative inflammatory vaginitis

Causes of decreased vaginal pH:

- Fungal infection
- Cervicitis

Clinical Features of Vaginal Discharge from Different Aetiologies

	Chlamydia	Bacterial vaginosis	Cervicitis	Candidiasis	Trichomoniasis	Gonorrhoea
Quantity	Same/↑	↑	Same/↑	Same/↑	↑	Same/↑
Consistency	Mucopurulent	Thin, whitish-grey, homogenous, frothy	Variable, depending on cause	Curdlike, does not stick to vaginal walls	Thin, foamy, homogenous	Mucopurulent
Odour	Absent	Fishy	Odourless	Yeasty	May be pungent	Absent
pH	≤ 4.5	≥ 4.5	≤ 4.5	≤ 4.5	≥ 4.5	≤ 4.5
Pruritus	Absent	Absent	Absent	Present	Present	Absent
Inflammatory changes	Absent	Absent	May be present	Dysuria, burning	Present, dysuria	Mild/absent
Red cells	May be present	Absent	May be absent	Absent	May be present	Absent
White cells	Normal/↑	Normal/occasionally ↑	May be absent	Normal/↑	May be present	Normal/↑
Lactobacilli	Present/not seen	Absent/few	Normal/↓	Moderate	Absent/few	Present/not seen
Treatment	• Azithromycin 1 g stat • Contact tracing • Test of cure in 4 weeks (it takes 3 weeks for the PCR test to become negative)	Metronidazole 2g stat, or metronidazole 400mg BD for 7 days, or clindamycin 5% vaginal cream for 7 days		• 1, 3, 7 day courses of antifungal creams or pessaries i.e. clotrimazole, miconazole, econazole • Fluconazole 150mg orally is as effective as the above treatments but it cannot be used in pregnancy	Metronidazole 2 g stat, or tinidazole 2 g stat	• Drug resistant strains ceftriaxone 250mg IM or IV or ciprofloxacin 500mg stat • Penicillin sensitive strains amoxycillin 3g probenecid 1 g orally • Penicillin allergic spectinomycin 2 g stat • Test of cure by culture at one week • Also treat for chlamydia • Contact tracing

Table 5.3. Clinical features of vaginal discharge from different aetiologies

Management of other causes of vaginal discharge:

- Nonspecific vaginitis: Povidone-iodine vaginal pessaries
- Atrophic vaginitis: Clindamycin 2% vaginal cream for 1–2 weeks

Short-Answer Questions

Question 1

A 25-year-old nonpregnant woman is complaining of a one-month history of vaginal discharge that is causing her discomfort. She has been with a new sexual partner for two months. How will you assess this patient? Discuss the differential diagnosis.

Answer:

The clinical assessment will consist of a focused history, clinical examination, lab investigations, and then, on the basis of that, I will make a differential diagnosis.

<u>History</u>:

- Type of discharge—quantity, duration, , consistency, urethral/vaginal/rectal origin
- Associated symptoms—pruritus, pain, dyspareunia, bleeding, UTIs
- Medical history—presence of conditions like diabetes, immunosuppressive diseases, STIs, use of antibiotics
- Sexual history—last sexual intercourse, previous sexual partners, type of intercourse
- Contraceptive history—oral pills, condoms, spermicides
  - IUCD may increase discharge.
- Personal history—personal hygiene, douching, clothing, synthetic/nonsynthetic, strong perfumes
- Ask about cervical smear

<u>Findings on clinical examination</u>:

- Assess the type of discharge
- Examine vulva, vagina, and cervix for signs of inflammation, erythema, ectropion, whether the discharge is sticking to the vaginal walls, site of origin, and cervical/vaginal pathology
- Take appropriate swabs from urethra, vagina, cervix, pharynx, and rectum for microscopy and culture
- MSU

On the basis of the above information, a differential diagnosis could be established according to the following algorithm:

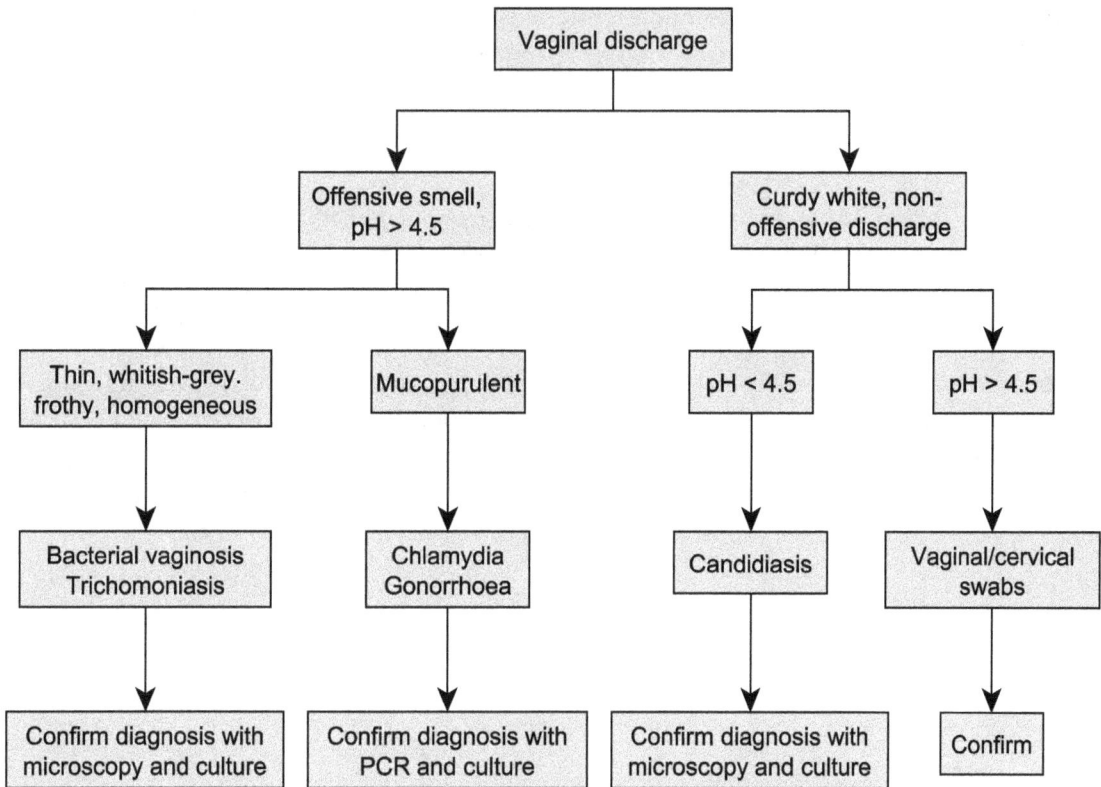

```
                            ┌─────────────────┐
                            │ Vaginal discharge │
                            └─────────────────┘
                   ┌──────────────────┴──────────────────┐
                   ▼                                      ▼
         ┌──────────────────┐               ┌──────────────────────┐
         │ Offensive smell,  │               │ Curdy white, non-     │
         │    pH > 4.5       │               │ offensive discharge   │
         └──────────────────┘               └──────────────────────┘
          ┌──────────┴──────────┐            ┌──────────┴──────────┐
          ▼                     ▼            ▼                     ▼
 ┌──────────────────┐  ┌──────────────┐  ┌──────────┐   ┌──────────────┐
 │ Thin, whitish-grey.│ │ Mucopurulent │  │ pH < 4.5 │   │   pH > 4.5   │
 │ frothy, homogeneous│ └──────────────┘  └──────────┘   └──────────────┘
 └──────────────────┘        │                │                 │
          ▼                  ▼                ▼                 ▼
 ┌──────────────────┐ ┌──────────────┐ ┌────────────┐ ┌────────────────┐
 │ Bacterial vaginosis│ │  Chlamydia   │ │ Candidiasis│ │ Vaginal/cervical│
 │  Trichomoniasis    │ │  Gonorrhoea  │ └────────────┘ │     swabs       │
 └──────────────────┘ └──────────────┘       │         └────────────────┘
          ▼                  ▼                ▼                 ▼
 ┌──────────────────┐ ┌──────────────┐ ┌────────────┐ ┌──────────┐
 │ Confirm diagnosis  │ │Confirm diagnosis│ │Confirm diagnosis│ │ Confirm │
 │ with microscopy    │ │ with PCR and   │ │with microscopy │ └──────────┘
 │ and culture        │ │    culture     │ │ and culture    │
 └──────────────────┘ └──────────────┘ └────────────┘
```

Question 2

Which laboratory tests would you do for a woman with vaginal discharge?

Answer:

The main diagnostic lab tests for treating vaginal discharge are vaginal pH testing, providing an air-dried smear of the discharge for Gram stain, and excluding gonorrhoea and chlamydia infection. If the vaginal pH and Gram stain smear are not taken, the diagnosis cannot be adequately made in a significant proportion of cases. Both urethral and endocervical samples should be taken for the diagnosis of gonorrhoea and chlamydia. Urine testing alone (PCR) misses a significant proportion of cases.

A vaginal discharge may originate from the vagina, cervix, or upper genital tract. In women under the age of 25, chlamydia should always be considered as a concomitant infection, even if the presumptive diagnosis is candidiasis.

Question 3

How will you interpret a vaginal smear slide in a case of vaginal discharge?

Answer:

The laboratory should ideally comment on white cells, red cells, vaginal epithelial cells, clue cells, lactobacilli, other bacteria, and yeasts. For urethral and endocervical smears, the presence or absence of Gram-negative intracellular diplococci (GNID) should be included. Trichomonads can only be seen in wet preparations that are made by putting some vaginal discharge in a drop of saline on a slide, covered by a cover slip.

The first thing to read on the report on Gram-stained smears is whether lactobacilli are present or not. The normal vaginal flora seen on a Gram stain comprises 95% lactobacilli. Hence, if they are not present, except for postmenopausal women not on hormone replacement therapy (HRT), significant vaginal pathology is present that warrants investigation and treatment.

The normal white cell count on vaginal smears is < 5/hpf. If the count is > 30/hpf, a severe inflammatory vaginitis is present. Clue cells with an altered bacterial flora usually indicate bacterial vaginosis. Yeasts indicate a *Candida* infection and the presence of hyphae indicates active infection. Immature epithelial cells indicate a severe vaginitis unless the woman is postmenopausal. Gram-negative intracellular diplococci should be looked for on the report of the urethral and endocervical smears.

Question 4

A 37-year-old woman presents to you with refractory (or recurrent) vaginal discharge. Discuss how you would assess and manage this woman.

Answer:

I will take a detailed gynaecological history, which will include the following:

- Duration of discharge, frequency, colour, amount, and any associated problems, such as itching, foul smell, bleeding.
- Any precipitating factors, relationship with coitus, menses.
- Use of any vaginal douching, deodorants, perfumes, or strong soaps.
- Details of past investigations and treatments (including current); for example, candidiasis can occur as a complication of treatment with metronidazole, clindamycin, or systemic antibiotics.
- Any comorbidities, such as diabetes, immunosuppressive states (HIV), chronic ailments, STIs.
- Any medical, food, or contact allergies.
- I will ensure that all the results of past investigations and treatments are available.

My examination will focus on any systemic signs of chronic ailments. I will do a detailed vulvovaginal examination, which will include the presence of any VIN, vulvar dermatitis, ulcers, excoriations, psoriasis, Lichen sclerosus and planus, and nature of the discharge. Vaginally, with a bivalve speculum, I will assess the characteristics of the discharge, such as, colour, Ph, amount, location in the vagina, smell, adherence to the vaginal walls, frothiness, and any vaginal erythema or presence of a foreign body. I will then assess the cervix, looking for any erythema, inflammation, ulcers, or IUCD strings.

I will repeat all the investigations as the diagnosis may have changed or she could have been reinfected. These investigations will include the following:

- FBE, UEC, LFT, and HbA1c
- MSU for MCS, PCR for chlamydia and gonorrhoea
- Cervical and urethral swabs for chlamydia and gonorrhoea, trichomoniasis, vaginal pH, and cytology of the air-dried Gram-stained vaginal smear; also a smear for cervical cytology

I will then treat any specific infection, based on the investigation results:

- Gonorrhoea with ceftriaxone 250 mg IM.
- Chlamydia with azithromycin 1 g stat and contact tracing.
- Trichomoniasis with metronidazole 2 g stat.
- Bacterial vaginosis with metronidazole 400 mg TDS for 7 days.
- Candidiasis with topical clotrimazole or oral fluconazole 150 mg weekly or fortnightly.
  - The presence of *Candida glabrata* indicates drug resistance, and I will treat this with boric acid, which is contraindicated in pregnancy.
- I will treat any superimposed infection with the appropriate antibiotic agent.
- Any associated dermatitis will require a steroid cream for a limited duration.
- If vaginal or cervical atrophy is present, I will prescribe topical oestradiol.

I will remove any IUCD, if present. I will refer her for treatment of any comorbidities, if found. I will advise the woman to stop all past treatments and hence avoid polypharmacy. I will also advise her regarding good perineal hygiene and advise her not to use any vaginal douching, strong perfumes, and deodorants. I will also advise against using any tight, synthetic briefs.

A prophylactic regimen will be required for recurrent infection; for example, clotrimazole 500 mg PV on days 6–11 postmenstruation. If symptoms persist despite this, enough treatment may not have been given, or the organism may be drug resistant. Antifungal resistance is increasing, and it is expected to further increase given the ready availability of antifungals over the counter.

The following is not part of the answer to this question. It is only for the reader's information:

Trichomoniasis appears to be prevalent in remote and rural areas, and is difficult to diagnose. The women infected may be asymptomatic despite having clinically evident vaginitis. Symptoms, if present, are of a vaginal discharge. The vaginal pH is elevated and could be a useful bedside diagnostic test in remote areas. Clinical examination may reveal an intense erythema of the vaginal walls and ectocervix, and colposcopic examination may reveal microscopic ulceration. It is thought that this condition may predispose to either acquisition of HIV or increased transmission if already infected with HIV. This infection has also been linked to preterm, low-birth weight infants.

When managing candida, it is helpful to clinically classify it as vulvar, vaginal, or vulvovaginal. Vulvar candidiasis is readily treated by topical or systemic antifungals and lifestyle alterations to avoid overheating of the vulva, such as not wearing underpants to bed. Sometimes an associated allergic dermatitis needs to be treated with steroids. If vaginal, establish if the infection is persistent or recurrent, and exclude diabetes mellitus.

Question 5

Discuss the clinical features of different genital ulcers.

Answer:

	Syphilis	Herpes	Chancroid	Lymphogranuloma venereum	Donovanosis
Incubation period	2–4 weeks (1–12 weeks)	2–7 days	1–14 days	3 days–6 weeks	1–4 weeks (up to 6 weeks)
Primary lesion	Papule	Vesicle	Papule or pustule	Papule, pustule, or vesicle	Papule
Number of lesions	Usually one	Multiple, may coalesce	Usually multiple, may coalesce	Usually one	Variable
Diameter (mm)	5–15	1–2	2–20	2–10	Variable
Edges	Sharply demarcated, elevated, round, or oval	Erythematous	Undermined, ragged, irregular	Elevated, round, or oval, irregular	Elevated, irregular
Depth	Superficial or deep	Superficial	Excavated	Superficial or deep	Elevated
Base	Smooth, nonpurulent	Serous, erythematous	Purulent	Variable	Red and rough ('beefy')
Induration	Firm	None	Soft	Occasionally firm	Firm
Pain	Unusual	Common	Usually very tender	Variable	Uncommon
Lymph-adenopathy	Firm, nontender, bilateral	Firm, tender, often bilateral	Tender, may suppurate, usually unilateral	Tender, may suppurated, loculated, usually unilateral	Pseudoadenopathy

Table 5.4. Causative organisms and clinical features of genital ulcers. From Holmes KK, Māndh PA, Sparling PE et al. (editors): Sexually Transmitted Diseases, 2nd ed. New York, McGraw Hill, 1990.

Multiple-Choice Questions

Q1. In a 9-year-old girl, what is the most common cause of a vaginal discharge?

A. Candidiasis

B. Atrophic vulvovaginitis

C. A foreign body

D. Vaginal trauma

Answer: B

Q2. Which of the following is **not** found in the vaginal discharge in recurrent vaginitis?

    A. IgE antibody to *Candida albicans*

    B. IgM antibody to *Chlamydia trachomatis*

    C. Spermatic fluid

    D. Spermicidal gels

Answer: B

Q3. Which of the following statements is **not** true for the pH of vaginal secretions?

    A. It is neutral or alkaline in prepubertal girls.

    B. It is around 6 in postmenopausal women.

    C. It is around 6 within 8 hours of unprotected sex.

    D. It is increased when there is *Candida glabrata* infection.

Answer: D

Q4. Match the causative organisms with the clinical features of the corresponding genital ulcers.

A. *Herpes simplex type II*	i.	Edge is sharply demarcated and elevated.
B. *Haemophilus ducreyi*	ii.	Edge is undermined, ragged, and irregular.
C. *Treponema pallidum*	iii.	Ulcer base is rough, beefy, and firm.
D. *Calymmatobacterium granulomatis*	iv.	Multiple 1–2 mm, superficial painful ulcers.

Answer: A-iv, B-ii, C-i, D-iii

Q5. Which of the following statements is true?

    A. The majority of women with chlamydia or gonorrhoea have mucopurulent cervicitis.

    B. The majority of women with chlamydia do not have mucopurulent cervicitis.

    C. For chlamydia infection, a vaginal specimen should be taken after hysterectomy.

    D. For gonorrhoea infection, a vaginal cuff specimen should be taken after hysterectomy.

Answer: B

Q6. Which of the following is least true regarding the healthy vagina of a woman of reproductive age?

    A. The pH would be in the range of 3.5–4.5.

    B. Lactobacilli metabolise glycogen to lactic acid.

    C. Parabasal cells have a small pyknotic nucleus.

    D. Oestrogen increases the ratio of superficial to parabasal cells.

Answer: C

Q7. A 6-year-old has offensive vaginal discharge that is staining her underwear. Her mother excludes sexual abuse. The most likely cause for this problem is:

    A. Chronic candida infection

    B. Oestrogen deficiency

    C. Poor perineal hygiene

    D. Chlamydia infection

Answer: C

Q8. A 6-year-old is brought by her mother with stained vaginal discharge. The most appropriate management is:

    A. Inspect vulva and do a rectal examination to exclude a foreign body

    B. Take a microbiological swab from the vagina and treat accordingly

    C. Arrange an examination under anaesthesia

    D. Arrange a pelvic ultrasound to exclude a foreign body/vaginal malignancy

Answer: C

Chapter 6
Pain

Chapter 6.1.   Pelvic Inflammatory Disease

Definition

Pelvic inflammatory disease (PID) is an infection of the upper reproductive tract in a nonpregnant woman. It consists of the infection of the uterus (endometrium, myometrium, and serosal layers), fallopian tubes, ovaries, and pelvic peritoneum, either in isolation or in various combinations. Some believe that most of the symptoms and sequelae arise from salpingitis.

Incidence

The incidence is 1–2% in young, sexually active females, usually under the age of 25. The incidence in the postmenopausal age group is about 1%.

Risk Factors

- Early age of first sexual intercourse
- Many sexual partners
- Older sexual partners
- Either current or a history of STI
- Recent uterine instrumentation

Causes

PID is mostly polymicrobial. The infection ascends from the lower reproductive tract through the mucous membrane. Lymphovascular, direct, and transperitoneal spread may also happen. The causative organisms are *Chlamydia, Gonorrhoea, Mycoplasma*, and the normal vaginal bacterial flora. In a British study, gonococcal infection was seen in 14% of PID cases (Evidence Level IV). *Chlamydia* can remain dormant in the fallopian tubes for years despite treatment and cause recurrence.

History

Symptoms are nonspecific and may be disproportionate to the actual extent of infection. Many women will be asymptomatic.

Bilateral lower abdominal and pelvic pain, which may be constant and dull, is the most common symptom. There may be current or a history of abnormal vaginal discharge, fever, nausea, and vomiting. The symptoms from a gonorrhoeal infection appear quickly and are more severe, whereas those from a chlamydial infection are of slower onset and milder.

Fitz-Hugh-Curtis syndrome develops in 5% of women due to vascular or transperitoneal spread of *Chlamydia* or gonococcus (and some other organisms) to the liver, causing perihepatitis. This condition is seen during laparoscopy in the form of violin-string adhesions between the anterior surface of the liver and the anterior abdominal wall. In the acute phase, it can cause pain in the liver area.

Recurrent disease may cause infertility in 20% of women due to tubal damage or tubal pregnancy (tenfold increase). It may also cause menstrual irregularity, dyspareunia, and chronic pelvic pain (fourfold increase).

Diagnosis

Diagnosis is clinical on the basis of a suggestive history, clinical findings, and exclusion of any pregnancy and upper reproductive tract neoplastic condition. However, clinical features lack sensitivity and specificity for diagnosis.

Clinical findings may include fever, lower abdominal tenderness with or without rebound and guarding, vaginal discharge, and cervical excitation.

High vaginal or cervical swabs are negative in nearly half the women. Urethral swab must also be taken with the cervical swab and urine PCR to exclude *Gonorrhoea* and *Chlamydia*. Positive tests strongly support a diagnosis of PID (Evidence Level IV). There may be leucocytosis and raised ESR. Lab investigations don't have good sensitivity and specificity. Ultrasound features are nonspecific. When used with power Doppler, it helps in identifying a pyosalpinx or pelvic abscess (Evidence Level III). Endometrial biopsy may show endometritis, but evidence is insufficient for its use as a routine diagnostic test (Evidence Level III). Laparoscopy helps in the direct visualisation of pelvic organs and collection of pus from Fallopian tube and POD for microbiological tests. Laparoscopy is negative in 15–30% of PID cases (Evidence Level III). It can also be used for adhesiolysis and to exclude other pathologies.

Differential Diagnosis

- Acute appendicitis
- Endometriosis
- Corpus luteum bleeding
- Pelvic adhesions
- Cystitis
- Diverticulitis and reproductive tract malignancies in postmenopausal women

Management

The aims of treatment are symptomatic relief, eradication of the infecting pathogen, reduction in the damage to pelvic organs by prompt treatment, and minimisation of the chance of recurrence.

Broad-spectrum antibiotic therapy should be started as soon as the disease is suspected and lab investigations have been completed (Evidence Level IB). Delaying treatment by 72 hours increases the risk of tubal damage threefold. Different antibiotic regimens are in use, but they must cover all of the possible organisms. A third-generation cephalosporin, doxycycline, and metronidazole are used in combination for 14 days (Evidence Level IB). The same antibiotic regimen is used in women who are HIV positive (Evidence Level III). Broad-spectrum antibiotic therapy is successful in 33–75% of women. Hospitalisation is often needed for the following:

- Pain and other systemic symptoms
- Clinically severe disease
- Tubo-ovarian abscess
- When a surgical emergency cannot be excluded

In severe cases, intravenous antibiotic therapy (cefoxitin, doxycycline, and metronidazole) should be used until 24 hours after clinical improvement is noticed. This should be followed by an oral regime (Evidence Level IB). IUCD, if present, should be removed if the disease is severe (Evidence Level IIB). The sexual partners must be treated. Patient education and follow-up are essential.

Surgical treatment, primarily by laparoscopy, may be needed in 15–20% of women. The aims are preservation of reproductive potential in younger women, drainage of an abscess, adhesiolysis, copious peritoneal lavage, or in extreme cases, unilateral adnexectomy. Ultrasound-guided pelvic-fluid aspiration is equally effective (Evidence Level III). The violin-string adhesions of Fitz-Hugh-Curtis syndrome do not need to be divided. Unresolved abscesses may be drained percutaneously under ultrasound or computed tomographic guidance.

Lack of improvement indicates the need for further investigation or surgical exploration.

Women with PID should be followed up in 3–6 months and should undergo further tests for chlamydia and gonorrhoea (Evidence Level III).

Short-Answer Questions

Question 1

You are the emergency department resident. You have been asked to see a 21-year-old, nonpregnant female with pelvic pain and vaginal discharge. How will you establish a diagnosis of PID?

Answer:

The diagnosis of PID can be established by the following approach:

Focused history:

- Pain:
  o Duration, severity, location, rhythmicity and cyclic nature, and radiation.
  o The pain of PID is in the lower abdomen, bilateral, constant, and often dull.
- Vaginal discharge:
  o Colour, quantity, odour, frothiness. Pathological discharge may be coloured, mucopurulent, odorous, frothy/foamy, and it may stick to the anterolateral vaginal walls.
- Vaginal bleeding:
  o Details of menses, any IMB/PMB.
  o IMB/PMB may or may not be present in PID.

- Cervical smear:
  - When was the last one done?
  - What was the result?
- Contraceptive history:
  - Name and type.
- Sexual history:
  - Stable relationship or multiple partners.
- History of recent uterine instrumentation, vaginal douching:
  - These are risk factors for PID.

Examination findings:

- General examination:
  - Pulse, blood pressure, temperature, and respiratory rate.
  - Is the patient well or unwell looking?
- Abdominal examination:
  - Palpation—tenderness, guarding, rebound tenderness, palpable mass.
- Bivalve speculum exam:
  - Discharge in the vagina.
  - Pus exuding from the external os.
  - Appearance of cervix:
    - It will appear inflamed in PID.
  - Take appropriate swabs from vagina, cervix, and urethra for microbiological examination.

Investigations:

- Blood and urine tests:
  - FBE, ESR, quantitative β-hCG, MSU.
- Transvaginal ultrasound scan:
  - Although the appearance of the endometrium is nonspecific, ultrasound may show a pelvic abscess, pyosalpinx, or any other pathology such as an endometrioma.

Laparoscopy is the gold standard for the diagnosis, which is often not done at the initial presentation. In early PID, laparoscopy may show normal pelvic structures, but in established PID, inflammation of the serosal layer of the uterus, salpingitis, oophoritis, pelvic peritonitis and even a pelvic abscess with adhesions may be seen.

I will start the broad-spectrum triple antimicrobial cover (ceftriaxone 250 mg IM single dose, doxycycline 100 mg oral twice daily for 14 days, and metronidazole 500 mg oral twice daily for 14 days) as soon as I suspect a diagnosis of PID.

Question 2

What treatments are available for a left-sided 7-cm tubo-ovarian abscess in a 25-year-old G1P1 woman?

Answer:

It appears from the description that the abscess is unruptured. The following treatments are available for an unruptured 7-cm tubo-ovarian abscess:

Prolonged course of broad-spectrum antibiotics: This is used when the woman is haemodynamically stable and there is no evidence of abscess rupture into the peritoneal cavity. Evidence shows that such abscesses, when less than 9 cm in size, respond well to an antibiotic regime that is continued till the abscess resolves completely. This may take up to 6 weeks or even longer. Antibiotic treatment is effective in 70% of women. Antibiotics with higher penetration into the abscess wall and pus are: clindamycin, cefotitan, cefoxitin, ertapenem, and metronidazole. If there are no signs of clinical improvement in 2–3 days after commencement of this treatment or there are signs of deterioration, a laparoscopic/laparotomic drainage of the abscess should be considered while continuing antibiotics.

Ultrasound/CT-scan-guided drainage: This treatment is suitable for unilocular and small abscesses. There is some evidence that early drainage under antibiotic cover gives a better result than antibiotics alone. The exact approach of drainage will depend upon the location of the abscess. The pus obtained must be sent for microbiological investigation.

Laparoscopic/laparotomic drainage: This treatment is not an initial option for this woman. Conservative options as mentioned above should be tried first. This method is only used when other methods have failed, there is sign of abscess rupture, or when the abscess is larger than 9 cm. The choice of drainage of the abscess by laparoscopy or laparotomy depends upon the skill of the gynaecologist. All debris and inflamed abscess wall and pus should be removed as much as possible, followed by copious peritoneal lavage. A closed-suction drain should be left in until the woman improves. Rectus sheath should be closed with a nonabsorbable suture. Tissues and pus should be sent for histological and microbiological investigation. Antibiotics should at least be continued for 2 weeks.

Combination of above treatments: If the above treatments fail, then a combination of the above treatments should be used.

Multiple-Choice Questions

Q1. Which of the following body cavities is lined by microscopic cilia?

    A. Urinary bladder
    B. Fallopian tubes
    C. Endometrial cavity
    D. Upper half of cervix

Answer: B

Q2. Which of the following is the earliest change in the development of PID in a 20-year-old woman?

A. Deciliation

B. Filling up of the fallopian tube lumen with exudate

C. Adhesion formation

D. Pelvic abscess

Answer: A

Q3. Which statement below regarding PID is false in a 20-year-old woman?

A. The majority of women with endometritis have salpingitis.

B. Bacterial vaginosis may cause endometritis.

C. The presence of plasma cells and neutrophils in the endometrium confirms the diagnosis of chlamydial endometritis.

D. It is normal for leucocytes to be present in the endometrium during the first 2 days of menses.

Answer: A

Q4. Which of the following statements below is true for PID in a 25-year-old nulliparous woman?

A. Gonococcus selectively adheres to ciliated mucus-secreting cells.

B. The damage to the fallopian tube by gonococcal infection is due to an acute complement-mediated inflammatory response.

C. The damage to the fallopian tube by chlamydial infection is due to an acute complement-mediated inflammatory response.

D. Primary chlamydial infection causes more damage to the fallopian tubes than recurrent disease.

Answer: B

Q5. Which of the following statements is true for PID?

A. The transvaginal ultrasound appearance of the uterus is very characteristic of PID.

B. The incidence of PID increases with age.

C. There is an increased incidence of Chlamydia infections in women with HLA–1.

D. The use of contraception does not change the relative risk of developing acute PID.

Answer: B

Q6. A 19-year-old girl presents with a 1-day history of lower abdominal pain. She has been in a new relationship. Her pregnancy test is negative. The WBC is 16,000, temperature is 39°C, and urinalysis is normal. Her lower abdomen is diffusely tender with rebound and voluntary guarding. Bowel sounds are heard. What is the most likely diagnosis?

A. Endometriosis

B. Ureteric stone

C. PID

D. Ovarian torsion

Answer: C

Q7. Which of the following treatment regimens will be most suitable for a 35-year-old woman with PID?

   A. Doxycycline 100 mg twice daily orally

   B. Clindamycin 450 mg 8 hourly IV and gentamicin 1mg/kg of body weight 12 hourly IV

   C. Doxycycline 100 mg twice daily orally and metronidazole 400 mg 8 hourly orally

   D. Ceftriaxone 250 mg IM, doxycycline 100 mg twice daily orally for 14 days, and metronidazole 400 mg 8 hourly orally for 14 days

Answer: D

Q8. The preferred site for obtaining a culture in a woman with acute PID during laparoscopy is:

   A. Endocervix

   B. Pouch of Douglas

   C. Fallopian tubes

   D. Endometrium

Answer: C

| Chapter 6.2. | Chronic Pelvic Pain |

Definition

Chronic pelvic pain is defined as irregular or persistent lower abdominal pain for more than six months not occurring exclusively with coitus, menstruation, or pregnancy. The pain has no particular pattern. It may happen most days of the month and may be aggravated in the premenstrual phase (Evidence Level III) or with coitus. The prevalence is about 15–20% in the premenopausal age group.

Causes

Chronic pelvic pain can happen as a result of the following disease(s). Often, there is more than one. In nearly one-third of women, no physical cause is found.

Gynaecological (20%)	Urinary tract (31%)	Gastrointestinal tract (37%)	Neurological and musculoskeletal	Psychosomatic
Endometriosis Adenomyosis PID (incompletely treated or recurrent) Pelvic adhesions Pelvic varicosities Residual ovary syndrome Retroverted uterus Pelvic congestion syndrome Fibroids (large)	Interstitial cystitis Lower urinary tract calculi	Irritable bowel syndrome (Evidence Level II) Inflammatory bowel disease Diverticulitis	Nerve entrapment (Evidence Levels III/IV) Fibromyalgia Sacroiliac arthritis Levator ani trauma (Evidence Levels I-III)	Sexual abuse Physical abuse Depression/ anxiety Personality disorder Sexual dysfunction Levator ani spasm Substance abuse Somatisation

Table 6.1. Causes of chronic pelvic pain

History

- Pain.
  - Site, severity, quality, regular or irregular, radiation, precipitating factors.
    - Burning, aching or shooting pain may indicate neuralgia.
  - Relationship to menses, coitus, urination, and defecation.
    - Pain aggravated by urination may have a lower urinary tract cause.
    - Pain aggravated by defecation may have a GIT cause.
    - Pain aggravated by menses with cyclical nature may be explained by causes of dysmenorrhoea, such as endometriosis (Evidence Levels II-IV).

     o Presence of pain anywhere else in the body.

         ▪ Sharp pain over a nerve distribution may indicate nerve entrapment (Evidence Levels III-IV).

- Menstrual history.
- Sexual history, dyspareunia, sexual dysfunction, STI
- Past medical history.
  - History of previous/recurrent PID and multiple pelvic surgery may indicate pelvic adhesions.
- Psychosocial history.
  - Life stressors, relationships, physical or sexual abuse in childhood/adult life.
- Psychiatric history.
  - Symptoms of anxiety, depression, sleep disorder (Evidence Levels I-III), substance abuse, personality disorder.
  - History of sexual abuse, especially in childhood, has been reported in 26% of women (Evidence Level III).

Investigations

- Pain diary.
  - Completing a pain diary over 2–3 months often helps in narrowing the differential diagnosis.
- Transvaginal ultrasound scan.
  - It identifies women who are less likely to have a positive finding on a diagnostic laparoscopy.
  - It accurately diagnoses an endometrioma from other adnexal masses (Evidence Level II).
- STI screen if sexually active.
  - Absence of chlamydia or gonorrhoea on swab tests does not exclude PID.
- MSU or bowel investigations.
  - Will depend upon the history and clinical findings.
- Diagnostic laparoscopy.
  - It is the only test to diagnose peritoneal endometriosis and adhesions (Evidence Levels III/IV).
  - However, in one-third to one-half of diagnostic laparoscopies, a cause is not identified (Evidence Level IV).
- Conscious pain mapping under general anaesthesia is largely experimental and not used in common clinical practice (Evidence Levels II/III).

Management

The woman should be given adequate time to completely narrate her story. She needs to feel that she has been listened to with full attention and without interruption. This helps to promote a good doctor-patient relationship and the patient's adherence to the management plan (Evidence Level I).

If the pain exacerbates premenstrually, a combined oral contraceptive pill, levonorgestrel intrauterine device, or even GnRH agonist (Evidence Levels I-IV) may help in relieving the symptoms. Dietary modification, relaxation exercises, yoga, and cessation of smoking may also help. Acupuncture and transcutaneous nerve stimulation have been observed to be helpful in some women. Physiotherapy will help if pelvic-floor abnormalities are identified.

If the pain is neuropathic, then amitriptyline, gabapentin, or pregabalin may be useful in addition to simple NSAID and narcotic analgesics. Pain from spasm of the levator muscles can be reduced by botulinum toxin injection (Evidence Levels I-III).

Specific treatment of depression and sleep disorders, which may be a consequence rather than a cause of pain, may improve women's ability to function (Evidence Levels I-III).

Symptom-based diagnostic criteria may be used to diagnose irritable bowel syndrome (IBS) with a positive predictive value of 98% (Evidence Levels II-IV) (Spiller R et al., 2007). Smooth-muscle relaxant mebeverine helps IBS pain. The efficacy of bulking agents is yet to be established (Evidence Levels I-IV) in treating IBS. Avoidance of dairy products and grains leads to sustained improvement (Evidence Level III).

If a specific cause is found, appropriate treatment should be instituted. 30% of women feel improvement in their pain symptoms after a diagnostic laparoscopy due to placebo effect. There is no evidence that division of fine adhesions helps pain, but division of dense vascular adhesions does (Evidence Level I). Laparoscopic uterosacral nerve stimulation is ineffective in treating chronic pelvic pain (Daniels J, 2009).

In the absence of any specific organic cause or improvement from other symptomatic therapies, a total hysterectomy and bilateral salpingo-oophorectomy is sometimes offered to women who have completed their families, although there is no evidence for it. Pain after hysterectomy and bilateral salpingo-oophorectomy will improve in women with dysmenorrhoea and any other gynaecological organic disease. Women should be clearly informed preoperatively that in the absence of an organic cause for pain, the pain may not improve after surgery.

There should be a low threshold for a psychiatric referral in the absence of any organic cause or improvement from treatment given.

Short-Answer Questions

Question 1

A 34-year-old woman presents to you with a twelve-year history of pelvic pain that she notices on most days, but she also notices cyclical fluctuations to the pain. She is G1P0, having terminated a pregnancy surgically when she was 19 years old. Currently, she is not in a stable relationship. She has had a diagnostic laparoscopy, which was normal.

Part a

How will you take a history?

Answer:

I will take a detailed history of her pain, which will include the following:

- Nature, location, and radiation of the pain.
  - Sharp stabbing or aching, burning pain may suggest neuropathic pain.
- Bowel habits, including alternating constipation and diarrhoea, and any bloating, as irritable bowel syndrome (IBS) can cause fluctuations in pain.
- Bladder function, as interstitial cystitis (IC) can have a cyclical pattern.
- Dyspareunia may assist with the diagnosis, and it has a negative effect on quality of life for the woman.
- Any events that occurred around the onset of pain, if she can recall.
  - Details regarding her termination of pregnancy.
- Assessment of future fertility plans.
- Woman's personal beliefs about the cause of her pain.
- Any physical or sexual abuse in her past (this may not be appropriate to assess at the first appointment).

I would also suggest that the woman keeps a detailed pain diary for two to three months, to elicit trends in the cyclical nature of the pain.

Part b

What are you looking for in your clinical examination?

Answer:

As well as potentially identifying signs that may lead to the diagnosis, a woman is at her most vulnerable state at the time of clinical examination, and often new information is revealed during this process.

- Abdominal examination
  - Superficial or focal tenderness on palpation—often due to musculoskeletal pain
    - This can be treated with local anaesthetic or physiotherapy.
  - Altered or absent sensation
- Pelvic examination
  - Presence of any discharge
  - Vaginismus
  - Hypercontractility of pelvic-floor muscles
    - This can be treated with physiotherapy.
  - Uterine or adnexal masses, nodules, or cysts
  - Uterosacral tenderness

Question 2

A 29-year-old woman presents with chronic pelvic pain for the last three years. There is no clear cause of her pain established on your history or examination. How would you investigate this woman?

Answer:

- Pain diary for 2–3 months.
- Transvaginal ultrasound scan identifies women who are less likely to have a positive finding on a diagnostic laparoscopy and accurately diagnoses an endometrioma from other adnexal masses (Evidence Level II).
- STI screen if sexually active (does not exclude PID).
- MSU or bowel investigations if any suggestion of bowel or bladder dysfunction on history.
- Diagnostic laparoscopy.
  - It is the only test to diagnose peritoneal endometriosis and adhesions (Evidence Levels III/IV).
  - However, in one-third to one-half of diagnostic laparoscopies, a cause is not identified (Evidence Level IV), and yet these procedures have small but significant risks of serious complications.
  - Evidence does not support showing laparoscopic pictures to the woman of her normal pelvis to reduce pain; it may make the woman feel unheard and that her concerns are not being taken seriously.
- MRI.
  - May show deeply infiltrating endometriosis and adenomyosis.
- Conscious pain mapping under general anaesthesia is largely experimental and not used in common clinical practice (Evidence Levels II/III).

Question 3

Discuss the treatment options for chronic pelvic pain.

Answer:

Treatment should be tailored to the patient, her predominant symptoms, and current and future fertility desires. Any underlying diseases should be treated appropriately.

- If pain is cyclical, hormonal treatment may be appropriate.
  - The combined oral contraceptive pill, taken conventionally, tricycling, or continuously.
  - GnRH agonist (can be combined with low-dose HRT safely for at least two years).
  - Levonorgestrel-containing IUCD.
- If the woman has IBS:
  - Smooth-muscle relaxant mebeverine.
  - Diet alteration (avoidance of dairy and grains may help).
  - Regular use of fibre supplementation.
  - Referral to a dietician or gastroenterologist.

- Treat neuropathic pain with amitriptyline, gabapentin, or pregabalin.
- Referral to a physiotherapist for any musculoskeletal or pelvic-floor problems.
- Dietary modification, relaxation exercises, yoga, and cessation of smoking may also help.
- Acupuncture and transcutaneous nerve stimulation have been observed to be helpful in some women.
- If the woman feels there is a psychological component to her pain, there should be a low threshold for referral to a psychologist or psychiatrist. This should be done sensitively so as not to worsen the doctor-patient relationship.
- Hysterectomy and bilateral salpingo-oophorectomy, if the woman has completed her family and she understands that the procedure may not remove the pain.

As chronic pelvic pain is often multifactorial, some of these strategies should be commenced together, with a multidisciplinary approach.

Multiple-Choice Questions

Q1. Which of the following is more likely to cause chronic pelvic pain?

    A. Pelvic congestion syndrome

    B. A small submucosal leiomyoma

    C. A small endometrial polyp

    D. Severe cervical dysplasia

Answer: A

Q2. Which of the following is more likely to cause chronic pelvic pain?

    A. Pelvic congestion syndrome

    B. Pelvic violin-string adhesions

    C. Retroverted uterus

    D. Adenomyosis

Answer: D

Q3. Which of the following statements about chronic pelvic pain is **not** correct?

    A. Chronic pelvic pain is a definite diagnosis.

    B. An estimated 50% of patients with chronic pelvic pain have multiple-symptom complaints.

    C. Laparoscopy is not the gold standard for the diagnosis of chronic pelvic pain.

    D. A pain diary often helps.

Answer: A

Q4. Which of the following is **not** a behavioural component of chronic pelvic pain syndrome?

    A. The pain is refractory to medical therapy.

    B. Signs of depression have begun.

    C. The patient's role in the family has changed.

    D. A history of sexual abuse is often present in such cases.

Answer: D

Q5. At the time of a diagnostic laparoscopy for pelvic pain, blood comes out through the Veress needle just after insertion. You remove the Veress needle. Her vital signs are stable. What will be your next step?

A. Stop surgery and observe patient for one more day in the hospital.

B. Use Hassan's cannula for pneumoperitoneum.

C. Reinsert the Veress needle at Palmer's point.

D. Perform an immediate laparotomy.

Answer: D

Q6. A 25-year-old presents with dysmenorrhoea, dyspareunia, and pelvic pain. During her gynaecological examination, which of the following will indicate the presence of endometriosis?

A. Tender nodules on the uterosacral ligament

B. Tenderness on bimanual compression of the uterus

C. Presence of an adnexal mass

D. Severe vaginismus precluding a vaginal examination

Answer: A

Q7. A 17-year-old presents with pelvic pain. During investigation, the right kidney is not seen. On vaginal examination, you feel a soft 10-cm right adnexal mass. What is the most likely cause for this mass?

A. Gartner-duct cyst

B. Ovarian mass

C. Pelvic kidney

D. Obstructed hemivagina

Answer: C

Q8. For the diagnosis of chronic pelvic pain, the duration of pain must be at least:

A. 6 months

B. 12 months

C. 18 months

D. No such defined minimum duration

Answer: A

Q9. What is the prevalence of chronic pelvic pain in the general population?

A. 1 in 6 women

B. 1 in 12 women

C. 1 in 24 women

D. 1 in 36 women

Answer: A

Chapter 6.3.   Dyspareunia

Definition

Dyspareunia is pain before, during, or after vaginal penetrative sex. It may be primary if pain starts to happen with first penetrative sex. Secondary dyspareunia happens when pain starts after a period of painless vaginal penetrative sex.

Superficial dyspareunia is when pain starts on insertion of the penis in the vagina. Deep dyspareunia is when pain starts on deep penetration of the vagina.

The causes of superficial and deep dyspareunia are quite different, and hence a thorough history and gynaecological examination are very important for the management. If no physical cause is found to explain dyspareunia, which is quite common, then psychosexual factors should be considered carefully to help explain the pain.

Causes

Superficial Dyspareunia

- Vulvodynia
- Vulvar vestibulitis
- Dermatitis, lichen sclerosus, lichen planus
- Vaginismus
- Childbirth trauma
- Psychosexual causes

Deep Dyspareunia

- Retroverted uterus
- Adenomyosis
- Endometriosis
- PID or vaginitis
- Pelvic neoplasm, irradiation
- UTI, interstitial cystitis

Vaginismus

Vaginismus is an intermittent or constant spasm of introital muscles or the pubococcygeus. Because of this spasm, any attempt at sexual penetration causes pain, which makes the sexual act painful or impossible. Mild vaginismus consists of spasm of these muscles that is relieved by reassurance during the examination. Severe vaginismus consists of spasm of these muscles that persists even after withdrawal. Women with vaginismus may have pain or fear of pain even during tampon or pessary insertion.

Like dyspareunia, vaginismus can be primary (pain starting with first intercourse) or secondary (pain starting after a period of pain-free sexual penetration). Vaginismus can be due to sexual abuse, aversion to sexual practice or partner, cultural or familial beliefs about coitus, vaginal injury, or infection.

Management

Management starts with a good history, which may indicate an organic cause. A thorough gynaecological examination, cervical smear, and swabs of the vagina and cervix will also help in finding lesions or infections. A transvaginal ultrasound examination may show a retroverted uterus, adenomyosis, endometrioma, or any pelvic neoplasm. This may also show if the uterus or ovaries are mobile and not fixed. Lastly, a laparoscopy will help in confirming any organic pelvic cause.

If no organic cause is found, then a psychosexual history should be further explored to find a precipitating cause.

If a specific organic cause is discovered, it should be treated. The treatment of dyspareunia due to psychosexual reasons should be multidisciplinary, involving appropriate counselling and proper education. Gabapentin will help in treating neuropathic pain. Amitriptyline will help vulvodynia. SSRIs may help in sexual aversion. Graduated vaginal dilators or trainers will help vaginismus. Surgery will be needed for a pelvic neoplasm or endometriosis. A change of position of coitus sometimes helps. Topical steroids will help the dermatological conditions. Local oestrogen will help atrophic vaginitis. Local anaesthetic gel will help any nonspecific painful condition.

Short-Answer Questions

Question 1

How will you take a focused history from a 25-year-old female who complains of painful sexual intercourse?

Answer:

Questions should be asked about the onset, site, and radiation of pain, including any difference in pain with the change of sexual position. The following areas in the history may suggest a precipitating cause. Questions should be asked to find out if dyspareunia is primary or secondary and superficial or deep.

- A menstrual history of dysmenorrhoea or heavy periods may suggest adenomyosis, endometriosis, or a leiomyoma.
- A gastrointestinal history of irregular bowel habits, alternating diarrhoea and constipation, may indicate irritable bowel syndrome or inflammatory bowel disease.
- Urinary history may point toward cystitis.
- Personal and sexual history may reveal sexual abuse or unpleasant sexual encounter.
- Past obstetric history may show emotional or perineal scarring from a difficult childbirth.

Question 2

What signs would you expect to elicit in the woman discussed above?

Answer:

In a majority of women, physical examination remains unequivocal. However, the following signs may be elicited:

- Woman's attitude, affect: May indicate a psychological cause.
- Abdominal palpation: Presence of mass, tenderness may indicate an extragenital cause.
- Pelvic examination: May show evidence of PID or endometriosis (tenderness, nodularity on uterosacral ligament, vaginal or cervical endometriosis). May show a retroverted uterus causing deep dyspareunia. A tender uterus may indicate adenomyosis.

Question 3

Justify your investigations for dyspareunia in the woman mentioned in the previous question.

Answer:

- Infection and STI screen: For PID.
- Transvaginal ultrasound scan: May show ovarian neoplasm/endometrioma (Evidence level IA), adenomyosis, retroverted uterus.
- Diagnostic laparoscopy: May show endometriosis, ovarian neoplasm, salpingitis, Fitz-Hugh-Curtis syndrome suggestive of past STI, adenomyosis, retroverted uterus. A negative laparoscopy will practically exclude organic causes of deep dyspareunia.

Multiple-Choice Questions

Q1. Which of the following drugs is least likely to be helpful in a 65-year-old complaining of dyspareunia?

- A. Topical oestrogen
- B. Topical steroids
- C. Topical antifungal
- D. Topical progestin

Answer: D

Q2. A 28-year-old woman had an extensive second-degree perineal laceration during childbirth 2 months ago. She is bottle feeding. She complained of dyspareunia. Which of the following drugs is least likely to be helpful in this case for treating dyspareunia?

- A. Amitriptyline
- B. Gabapentin
- C. Lignocaine gel
- D. Progesterone-only pill

Answer: D

Q3. Which of the following drugs will be most helpful in a 34-year-old woman who complains of painful intercourse without any organic cause?

A. Combined oral contraceptive pill

B. SSRI

C. Topical oestrogen

D. Topical antifungal agents

Answer: B

Q4. A 21-year-old woman had a normal vaginal delivery 6 weeks ago. She is completely breastfeeding. She complains of painful sexual intercourse. Which of the following is the most likely cause?

A. Endometriosis

B. PID

C. Prolapsed ovaries

D. Atrophic vagina

Answer: D

Q5. A 22-year-old lady, otherwise fit and healthy, complains of introital pain during sexual penetration. Which is the most likely cause?

A. Bartholin's cyst

B. Atrophic vagina

C. Vaginismus

D. Endometriosis

Answer: C

Q6. Which of the following is most likely to cause deep dyspareunia?

A. Complex endometrial hyperplasia

B. Anteverted normal-sized uterus

C. Polycystic ovary

D. Endometrioma

Answer: D

Q7. Which of the following is the most likely cause of vaginismus?

A. Sexual abuse

B. Endometriosis

C. Retroverted uterus

D. PID

Answer: A

Q8. The most common cause of dyspareunia is:

A. Vaginismus

B. Inadequate vaginal lubrication

C. PID

D. Endometriosis

Answer: B

Chapter 6.4.   Endometriosis

Definition

Endometriosis is the presence of endometrial tissue outside the uterus that induces a chronic inflammatory reaction.

Prevalence

Endometriosis is a disease of women in the reproductive age group. It is present in 40–60% of women with dysmenorrhoea, 20–30% of women with subfertility, 6% of women undergoing sterilisation, and 15% of women with chronic pelvic pain.

Most common sites of endometriosis are ovary, other pelvic organs, and pelvic peritoneum.

Causes

Many theories have been proposed to explain endometriosis. It is possible that more than one factor is operational. The proposed theories are:

i. Retrograde flow of menstrual blood. This is the most accepted theory. Retrograde flow of menstrual blood through the fimbriae causes implantation of the endometrial tissue in different parts of the pelvis. This causes a local inflammatory reaction. Any factor that stops or reduces menstrual flow helps to treat endometriosis.

ii. Genetic factors. Endometriosis is seen more commonly (7%) if a first-degree relative is affected. Monozygotic twins are highly concordant. Genetic factors may influence local response mechanisms and alter the course of the disease.

iii. Coelomic epithelium transformation. The cells of the Müllerian duct, ovaries, and peritoneum share a common origin. These cells revert to their originator primordial cells, possibly under the influence of ovarian oestrogen, and then transform into ectopic endometrial cells.

iv. Lymphovascular spread to distant sites. The endometrial cells can spread to distant sites such as lungs, brain, and joints through lymphovascular channels.

v. Iatrogenic spread. Ectopic endometrial tissue has been seen in the anterior abdominal wall following caesarean section and in episiotomy scars.

History

Symptoms may be disproportional to the extent of the disease. Women with extensive disease sometimes are asymptomatic. At other times, women with mild disease complain of a lot of pelvic pain. There is no correlation with pain and classification of endometriosis, based on guidelines from the American Society of Reproductive Medicine.

Dysmenorrhoea, deep dyspareunia, and dyschezia are the classical symptoms. Symptoms are cyclical when the disease is not too advanced, and they depend upon the anatomical sites involved.

The pain is caused by release of prostaglandins from the lesions and involvement of the nerves with deep lesions (> 5 mm). The depth of infiltration is related to the type and severity of symptoms.

Subfertility is caused by reduced coital frequency due to deep dyspareunia and the mechanical interference in the processes that lead to fertilisation.

Cyclical bleeding with menstruation from different body orifices is seen when the corresponding organs are infiltrated with endometriosis.

Examination

Abdominal palpation may be nonspecific except for some vague tenderness. On vaginal speculum examination, endometriosis could be seen in the vagina or on the cervix, if present. On digital examination, nodularity and tenderness may be felt if endometriosis is present on POD and uterosacral ligaments.

The classification systems of endometriosis are subjective and correlate poorly with pain but are of value in infertility management.

Investigations

Transvaginal ultrasound scan can show endometrioma (ectopic endometrial tissue forming cysts), which has a homogenous, slightly hypoechoic (ground-glass appearance) appearance with irregular or thick wall (Evidence Level III). Nodular endometriosis is not visible by a transvaginal ultrasound scan. Recently, techniques have been developed to visualise deep-seated infiltrating endometriosis through abdominal ultrasound scan (Menakaya U et al., 2013). It may also have a role in showing bladder and bowel endometriosis.

MRI helps in showing endometriosis, especially if it is deep seated. Surgery could be planned based on MRI findings. Available evidence does not show that it is more accurate in diagnosing endometriosis compared with laparoscopy. It is not commonly used because of cost and limited availability.

CA 125 is a glycoprotein whose serum level is raised in endometriosis, several other benign conditions, and in epithelial ovarian cancer. Its real value in endometriosis is in following the course of the disease after treatment (Evidence Level IA). It has no value as a diagnostic tool.

Micro-RNA (m-RNA) has been newly discovered bio-marker of endometriosis with a sensitivity and specificity of 90%. It is not used yet in routine clinical practice.

Anti-Müllerian hormone is used post treatment to prognosticate future fertility.

Endometriosis is diagnosed by laparoscopy (Evidence Level III), which is the gold standard. It may show endometriosis/endometrioma (chocolate cyst) on the uterosacral ligaments, POD, ovary, ovarian fossa, and fallopian tubes. Endometriosis affecting the bowel or bladder may need colonoscopy or cystoscopy. The most common colour is dark blue to black but it can be of any colour, depending upon the blood supply, haemorrhage, and fibrosis.

Differential Diagnosis

The symptoms of endometriosis have considerable overlap with the following conditions:

- Chronic pelvic pain
- Pelvic inflammatory disease
- Irritable bowel syndrome

- Inflammatory bowel disease
- Interstitial cystitis
- Ovarian cysts

A focused history and examination will help in arriving at the correct diagnosis.

Management

Medical

Medical treatment is used to alleviate pain. It does not help subfertility, nor is it curative. There is no evidence that ovarian suppression improves endometriosis-associated infertility (Evidence Level IA). Symptoms recur following cessation of treatment.

NSAIDs

NSAIDs are useful in women not wanting daily hormonal pills; however, the evidence is inconclusive about its (specifically Naproxen's) effectiveness in treating pain of endometriosis.

Combined Oral Contraceptive Pills

The hormonal preparations described below are all equally effective (Evidence Level IA).

These are useful in women not wishing to conceive in the near future. They act by reducing menstrual blood loss and decidualisation of ectopic endometrial tissue. Increasingly, low-dose pills are being used without any high-level supportive evidence. These pills can be taken over a long time without many side effects. Tricycling is more effective in controlling the symptoms.

Progestins

Medroxyprogesterone acetate has been used to alleviate pain. It acts by abolishing menstruation.

Danazol

Danazol is a 17-α-ethinyl testosterone derivative that acts by suppressing pituitary gonadotropins. The side effects are hot flushes, acne, loss of libido, and weight gain. The median time of recurrence of symptoms after cessation of hormonal therapy was 6.1 months (Evidence level III).

Gestrinone

Gestrinone is a 19-nortestosterone derivative with progestogenic and antiprogestogenic actions. It is as effective as danazol and GnRH analogues, with fewer side effects.

Dienogest

It is a nortestosterone derivative with antiandrogenic activity of approximately one third of that of cyproterone acetate. It has a strong progestogenic effect. It acts by reducing the endogenous production of oestriol. It also has immunological and antiangiogenic effects, which inhibits cell proliferation. After 3 months of treatment, a statistically significant difference compared to placebo and a clinically meaningful reduction of pain compared to baseline has been shown. Dose: 2 mg daily.

Levonorgestrel-Containing Intrauterine Devices

The levonorgestrel-containing IUCD acts by suppressing both normal and ectopic endometrium. It is especially useful in treating rectovaginal endometriosis and recurrence of the disease. It reduces pain symptoms and the effects last for up to 3 years (Evidence Level IA).

GnRH Analogues

This causes hypogonadotropic hypogonadism and consequently reduces the size and activity of ectopic endometrial tissue (Evidence Level III). It is also used before surgery to reduce the extent of disease and postsurgical recurrence. Its prolonged use causes osteoporosis and severe menopausal symptoms. Add-back oestrogen protects against osteoporosis at the lumbar spine during treatment and for up to 6 months after treatment (Evidence Level IA). The median time of recurrence of symptoms after cessation of hormonal therapy was 5.2 months (Evidence Level III).

Aromatase Inhibitors

Aromatase enzyme has been found in endometriotic tissues, suggesting oestrogen production by these tissues. GnRH analogues only inhibit ovarian oestrogenic production. Aromatase inhibitors have the potential of inhibiting oestrogen production from the endometriotic tissues and consequently inhibiting disease expansion. Significant bone-density loss is an important side effect.

Surgical

Surgery for advanced disease should only be done by experienced gynaecologists.

The role of surgery in improving pregnancy rate for moderate to severe disease is uncertain (Evidence Level III). It is effective in treating pain as well as subfertility for mild to moderate disease. For early-stage disease, laparoscopic excision of endometriosis or laser/diathermy ablation are equally effective. Ablation reduces pain compared with diagnostic laparoscopy (Evidence Level IA). For an endometrioma, excision is better than drainage combined with ablation of the cyst wall, in terms of symptom control and recurrence (Evidence Level IA). However, it may lead to decreased ovarian reserve. Laparoscopic uterine nerve ablation alone is not effective in reducing pain (Evidence Level IB). Laparoscopic adhesiolysis may help in restoring ovarian-tubal anatomy. Bilateral oophorectomy, with or without a hysterectomy, will create a hypo-oestrogenic state and will help in medical ablation of the endometriosis. Hysterectomy alone without oophorectomy will eliminate retrograde menstruation and hence is also a useful treatment, when ovarian preservation is required. Evidence of benefit is insufficient to justify the use of preoperative or postoperative hormonal treatment, especially pregnancy rate (Evidence Level IA). Tubal flushing with oil-soluble media and intrauterine insemination improve pregnancy rates in infertility associated with endometriosis (Evidence Level IB).

HRT after TAHBSO

There is some role for a combined hormone replacement therapy (HRT) in young women who have undergone bilateral oophorectomy for endometriosis and are being incapacitated with vasomotor menopausal symptoms. There is, however, a small increase in the recurrence of endometriosis symptoms. The ideal regimen of HRT after bilateral oophorectomy is unclear, but adding a progestogen will suppress activation of the disease by oestrogen (Evidence Level IV). HRT should only be started after a 6-month period following surgery to reduce the recurrence of the disease.

Endometriosis in pregnancy:

Women with endometriosis have a higher risk of miscarriage, placental abruption, placenta previa (4 times increased risk), fetal growth restriction and caesarean section.

Short-Answer Questions

Question 1

How will you manage subfertility due to endometriosis in a 28-year-old woman who is asymptomatic and is otherwise well? She has regular menstrual cycles. Her tubes are patent, and her husband's semen count is normal.

Answer: It appears from the above description that she is ovulating regularly. If not, a midluteal progesterone test can be done to ascertain ovulatory status. For mild disease, the chance of spontaneous conception in her age group will be around 35–40%.

Medical treatment, especially hormones, have no role in increasing fertility. In fact, it causes more harm in terms of lost time and side effects. Laparoscopic ablation by diathermy or laser of endometriotic nodules in mild to moderate disease improves conception rate (Evidence Level IA). The role of surgery in increasing conception rate for moderate to severe endometriosis is uncertain (Evidence Level III). Laparotomy for dense pelvic adhesion and endometrioma also increases conception rate. Removal of the lining of the endometrioma has a better prognosis for fertility than just draining the endometrioma (Evidence Level IA). Every attempt should be made to preserve as much ovary as possible. Ovarian hyperstimulation with gonadotropins with intrauterine insemination results in a higher conception rate than intrauterine insemination alone (Evidence Level IB). Surgical treatment of advanced disease should be done by highly skilled operators. Flushing of fallopian tubes with lipid-based agents improves conception rates in young women with endometriosis-related subfertility (Evidence Level IB).

Question 2

A 43-year-old woman complains of right-sided pelvic pain for 2 years. She had an abdominal hysterectomy and left salpingo-oophorectomy 3 years ago for endometriosis. How will you manage this?

Answer:

History: A focused history will indicate possible sources of the pain. For example, if the pain is cyclical with dyspareunia and dyschezia, it may indicate endometriosis. Dysuria may indicate cystitis. The pain of renal or ureteric colic will be of sudden onset, very severe, and will radiate from the loin to the groin. Altered bowel habits with alternate constipation and diarrhoea will indicate bowel-related pain.

Examination: An acute abdomen will indicate possibly a torted right ovarian cyst or a ruptured appendicitis. Painful loin will indicate a renal origin of the pain. A vaginal examination may reveal vaginal endometriosis. On digital vaginal examination, painful nodules or lumps could be felt in the POD, suggestive of endometriosis.

Investigations:

- MSU to exclude cystitis.
- Transvaginal ultrasound scan to exclude any endometrioma. It will not show mild disease.
- Abdominal ultrasound scan to exclude nongynaecological cause of pain, such as appendicitis, ureteric stones, or even a bladder calculus/neoplasm.
- MRI, when available, could be used for deep-seated endometriosis, to map its extent.

Treatment: Symptomatic treatment for pain should be given, depending upon the severity of the pain. Laparoscopy is both diagnostic and therapeutic for endometriosis. Ablation of mild disease with adhesiolysis is very effective in treating pain. Endometrioma should be excised as far as possible with at least an attempt for some ovarian conservation. For advanced endometriosis, a skilled operator and laparotomy may be needed. The patient should be adequately counselled about unintended intraoperative trauma to abdominal viscera, such as bowel, bladder, ureter, nerves, and vessels, and even the need for a colostomy. Patients with known advanced endometriosis should have a bowel preparation preoperatively. Medical treatment following surgery is highly effective in prolonging the pain-free interval and delaying the recurrence of the disease. The details of the medical treatment are discussed in the main body of the chapter. Serial CA 125 will help in monitoring the disease posttreatment.

Question 3

Discuss the risk of malignant transformation of endometriosis.

Answer:

Overall, the risk of malignant transformation of endometriosis is low. Malignant transformation of ovarian endometriosis is more common than nonovarian endometriosis. The reason for this is poorly understood. Malignant transformation of the rectovaginal fascia endometriosis is more common than all the other nonovarian endometriosis. Risk factors include unopposed oestrogen and tamoxifen use. Hence, women with a history of endometriosis requiring HRT must have combined HRT. Endometriomas larger than 9 cm have a higher incidence of malignant transformation. The incidence of malignant transformation is also higher in women greater than 45 years of age (Johnson N et al., 2013). Overall, there is no definite data to indicate that the early surgical treatment of endometriotic implants is associated with a reduced risk of malignancy (Glanc P et al., 2017).

The risk of ovarian cancer in women with endometriosis is four times higher. A possible explanation is loss of heterozygosity and mutations in suppressor genes (p53). Cervical endometriosis is reported to cause abnormal cervical cytology.

Malignant transformation of endometriosis to endometrioid adenocarcinoma is the most common, followed by sarcoma and other Müllerian tumours. The prognosis is favourable.

Multiple-Choice Questions

Q1. Which of the following is **not** true for endometriosis?

    A. Pelvic lymph nodes are involved in 30% of cases.

    B. The rectosigmoid colon is involved in 10–15% of advanced disease.

    C. Viable endometrial glands and stroma can be identified in 25% of cases.

    D. Abnormal bleeding is noted by 15–20% of women with endometriosis.

Answer: C

Q2. Which of the following is least common in endometriosis?

    A. Bowel obstruction

    B. Hydronephrosis

    C. Massive ascites

    D. Haemothorax

Answer: C

Q3. Which of the following is **not** correct for endometriosis?

    A. It is seen in men on exogenous oestrogen.

    B. It has been reported in prepubertal girls.

    C. An estimated 5% of symptomatic disease presents after menopause.

    D. The risk of malignant transformation is about 30%.

Answer: D

Q4. Which of the following statements is **not** correct for endometriosis?

    A. The rectovaginal septum is the most common extragonadal location for malignant transformation of endometriosis.

    B. The risk of developing ovarian cancer is increased fourfold.

    C. Cervical endometriosis can cause abnormal cervical cytology.

    D. Sarcoma is the most common malignancy arising from the endometriotic nodules.

Answer: D

Q5. Which of the following is the most common site of endometriosis?

    A. Fallopian tube

    B. Ovary

    C. Uterosacral ligament

    D. Broad ligament

Answer: B

Q6. Which of the following is **not** a cardinal histological feature of endometriosis?

    A. Ectopic endometrial glands

    B. Ectopic endometrial stroma

    C. Haemorrhage into adjoining tissue

    D. Lack of inflammatory features

Answer: D

Q7. Which of the following is **not** true for endometriosis?

    A. The recurrence rate following medical therapy is 5–15% in the first years.

    B. The recurrence rate following medical therapy is 15–40% in 5 years.

    C. The recurrence rate following danazol therapy is 15–30% in 2 years.

    D. Medical treatment improves the conception rate for mild disease.

Answer: D

Q8. Which of the following is **not** true for medical therapy of endometriosis?

    A. The primary aim with hormonal treatment is amenorrhoea.

    B. The recurrence of the disease is proportional to the extent of the disease.

    C. Medical therapy is very effective in treating pain if the patient is taking medication.

    D. Optimal regression is seen in lesions that are less than 2 cm in diameter.

Answer: C

Q9. Which of the following is the most effective surgical treatment for endometriosis?

    A. Drainage of endometrioma

    B. Laparoscopic uterine-nerve ablation

    C. Total hysterectomy

    D. Ablation/excision of endometriosis

Answer: D

Q10. Following the uneventful removal of a small endometrioma from the ovary, which of the following should be done to prevent adhesion formation around the ovary?

    A. Close the ovarian incision with running 4-0 chromic catgut suture

    B. Microsurgically close with 6-0 Prolene suture

    C. Microsurgically double layered closure with 6-0 Dexon suture

    D. Leave it open to heal by itself

Answer: D

Q11. How can the presence of endometriosis in the pelvis of a woman with Müllerian agenesis be explained?

    A. It is due to menstrual outflow obstruction.

    B. It is due to retrograde menstrual flow.

    C. It is due to coelomic metaplasia.

    D. It's not possible because there are no ovaries.

Answer: C

Q12. A 25-year-old presents with dysmenorrhoea, dyspareunia, and pelvic pain. Which of the following will indicate the presence of endometriosis?

    A. Tender nodules on the uterosacral ligaments

    B. Tenderness on bimanual uterine compression

    C. The presence of an adnexal mass

    D. Severe vaginismus precluding a bimanual examination

Answer: A

Chapter 7
Disorders of Fertility

Polycystic Ovarian Syndrome

Definition

Polycystic ovarian syndrome (PCOS) is an ovarian disorder characterised by anovulation causing menstrual dysfunction and hyperandrogenism with a spectrum of manifestations. It is seen in 6–7% of the premenopausal population.

Pathophysiology

PCOS has a genetic predisposition, and more than one gene may be involved. It is postulated that girls are born with polycystic ovaries, and on being subjected to "stressors," they develop polycystic ovarian syndrome at different stages of reproductive life. The common stressors are obesity and psychosocial influences.

Hormonal Changes

Due to increased GnRH pulse amplitude or increased pituitary sensitivity to GnRH, LH is secreted constantly in increased quantity in 2/3 of women with this condition. Increased LH secretion causes increased androgen production from ovarian theca cells. About half of women with PCOS will also have increased adrenal androgen (DHEAS) production.

Hirsutism develops if the androgens get converted into the active metabolite DHT (dihydrotestosterone) by the enzyme 5α-reductase. 3α-diol-G is a measure of the 5α-reductase activity.

Women with PCOS also have increased levels of nonbound oestradiol and oestrone. High levels of androgens and insulin reduce SHBG and hence, more oestradiol remains in the nonbound biologically active state. Increased oestrone is due to increased peripheral conversion of androgens by the adipocytes. The increased oestradiol not only causes endometrial hyperplasia, but it also causes increased GnRH pulsatility, which causes persistent elevated levels of LH and, consequently, anovulation.

In about 1/5 of women with PCOS, due to increased GnRH pulsatility, prolactin secretion also increases slightly.

Role of Insulin Resistance

Insulin resistance is defined as a metabolic state in which the normal level of insulin produces a subnormal effect on glucose metabolism. Obesity, body fat distribution, and muscle mass affect insulin resistance. The exact mode of development of insulin resistance is not properly understood. In obese patients, it is thought to be due to changes in the different proteins produced by the adipocytes, and in nonobese patients, it may be due to adipocyte or β-cell dysfunction.

Insulin resistance is defined as a metabolic state in which the normal level of insulin produces subnormal effect on glucose metabolism. Obesity, body fat distribution, and muscle mass affect insulin resistance. The exact mode of development of insulin resistance is not properly understood. In obese patients, it is thought to be due to changes in the different proteins produced by the adipocytes, and in nonobese patients, it may be due to adipocyte or β-cell dysfunction.

Insulin resistance leads to hyperinsulinaemia, which causes hyperandrogenism by reducing the synthesis of SHBG by hepatocytes. Hyperandrogenism may cause anovulation by inhibiting ovarian granulosa cells.

History

The symptoms of PCOS are largely due to anovulation and hyperandrogenism. Pain is not a feature of PCOS.

- Anovulation: oligomenorrhoea, heavy withdrawal bleeding.
- Hyperandrogenism: acne, oily skin, abnormal hair growth around central regions of the body, acanthosis nigricans, alopecia.
- Obesity: not all women with PCOS are obese. Symptoms of PCOS are worse in obese women due to insulin resistance.

Examination

Signs of PCOS may be obesity and different manifestations of hyperandrogenism, as mentioned above. Hirsutism is objectively assessed by the Ferriman-Gallwey scoring system. Presence of virilism indicates an androgen-secreting neoplasm.

Investigations

The haematological investigations are directed toward establishing hyperandrogenism and its potential source. These include LH, free and total testosterone, SHBG and free-androgen index/free testosterone, and DHEAS to exclude adrenal androgenesis. Increased fasting insulin level will reflect insulin resistance. TFT and prolactin levels should be checked to exclude other causes of menstrual irregularity.

To assess the long-term sequelae of PCOS, a glucose tolerance test and lipid profile should also be done.

A transvaginal scan may show polycystic appearance of the ovaries, which is described as 10 or more peripherally arranged follicles up to 8 mm in diameter, ovarian volume > 10 cm^3, and prominent stroma.

Diagnosis

Diagnosis is established by the presence of any 2 of the following 3 features:

i. Polycystic appearance of the ovaries: About 20% of normal women without PCOS have polycystic ovaries without any relevant symptoms. These women are at increased risk of developing PCOS in the future.

ii. Clinical and biochemical markers of hyperandrogenism.

iii. Anovulation/menstrual irregularity.

Management

The treatment of PCOS will start with the management of obesity, if present, and cosmetic treatment for hirsutism if required.

Importance of managing obesity: A small amount of weight loss can lead to ovulation. It also helps in reducing maternal and fetal morbidities. The risk of antenatal problems is reduced by preconception weight management.

Weight management is achieved by lifestyle modification in terms of diet and exercise. Drug treatment and bariatric surgery should be considered in morbidly obese women.

Pharmacological treatment of PCOS: This will differ according to the desired goal. The 3 common desired goals are as follows:

i.   <u>To achieve ovulation</u>: In a woman with PCOS, ovulation is induced by the use of oral antioestrogens (clomiphene or tamoxifen), gonadotropins, and more recently, aromatase inhibitors. Insulin-sensitising agents (metformin) potentiates the effects of clomiphene by decreasing insulin resistance and consequent hypoandrogenism. Following the failure of medical treatment, ovulation could be effected surgically by laparoscopic ovarian drilling. This is as effective as using gonadotropins and also rectifies biochemical abnormalities, such as high LH and androgen levels.

ii. <u>To treat hirsutism</u>: Hirsutism is treated by combined oral contraceptive pill or cyproterone containing oral contraceptive pills. Use of nonandrogenic progestins such as desogestrel, norgestimate, and drospirenone in the combined oral contraceptive pill is an advantage. Specific peripheral androgen-blocking agents can also be used in combination with the combined oral contraceptive pills mentioned before. These agents include spironolactone and flutamide. Because of the risk of feminisation of a male fetus and menstrual irregularity, they should always be used with a combined oral contraceptive agent. Eflornithine cream inhibits hair growth and shows noticeable reduction of hair growth within weeks. On cessation of therapy, hair growth returns. Eflornithine cream can also result in acne by obstructing the sebaceous glands.

iii. <u>To treat oligomenorrhoea</u>: This is treated by controlling hyperandrogenism and anovulation. In a woman not desiring conception, a combined oral contraceptive pill or a cyclical progestogen should be used. Metformin also helps to make the menstrual cycle regular.

Long-Term Consequences

PCOS is an incurable disease with varied metabolic ramifications. Obesity itself and insulin resistance can lead to diabetes mellitus and cardiovascular disease. In a relatively young woman, because of increased oestradiol levels, endometrial hyperplasia leading to endometrial carcinoma may result. Obesity with hyperandrogenism leads to abnormal lipid profile.

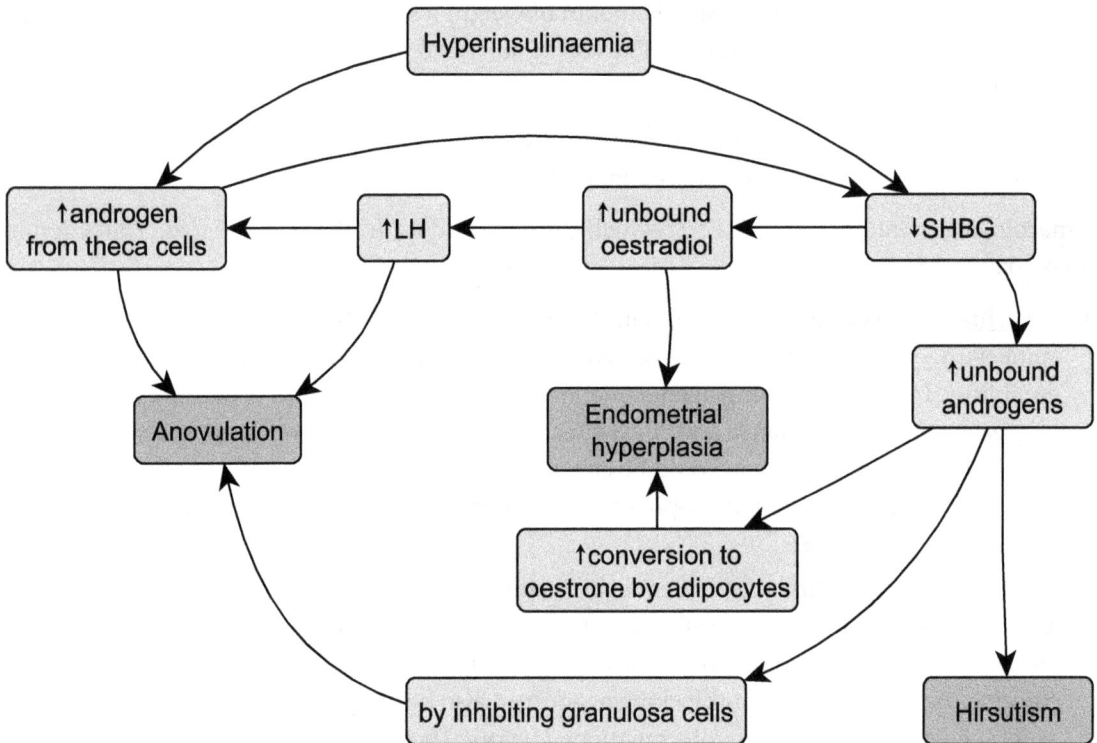

Figure 7.1. Schematic representation of the pathogenesis of anovulation, hyperandrogenism, and endometrial hyperplasia

Short-Answer Questions

Question 1

Discuss the approach to investigation of hirsutism in a 25-year-old female.

Answer:

A focused history of abnormal hair growth should be obtained, which should include duration of abnormal hair growth, slow/rapid growth, and age of onset. Any associated features, such as obesity, oligomenorrhoea, infertility, and the presence of acanthosis nigricans, should be investigated. History of drug use, such as danazol, anabolic steroids, phenytoin, and corticosteroids, should be obtained.

Clinical examination may show hypertrichosis (abnormal hair growth in peripheral areas), acanthosis nigricans (a marker of insulin resistance), or virilism (due to androgen-producing neoplasm). In PCOS, the abnormal hair growth is mostly in the central areas of the body.

The basic investigations will be aimed at finding the site and severity of hyperandrogenism. These will include LH, testosterone, SHBG, and free-androgen index. In women with anovulation or oligomenorrhoea, serum FSH and oestradiol levels should be checked to exclude hypogonadotropic hypogonadism or premature ovarian failure. TSH should be checked in hyperandrogenic patients. A transvaginal ultrasound scan is done to look for polycystic ovaries or ovarian neoplasm.

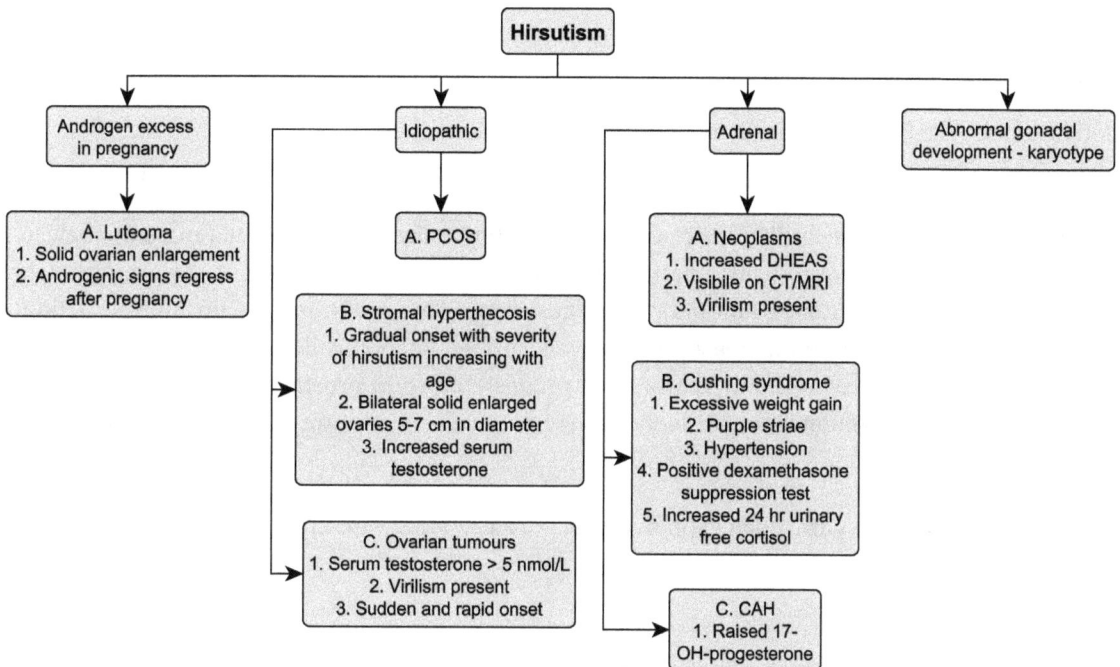

Figure 7.2. Clinical features and investigations for hirsutism

Question 2

Discuss the use of metformin in PCOS.

Answer:

Metformin is a biguanide oral antidiabetic agent that acts by:

i. Reducing hepatic glucose production and thereby reducing hyperinsulinaemia

ii. Reducing hyperinsulinaemia by sensitising peripheral tissues to the action of insulin

In PCOS, the use of metformin is primarily to induce ovulation. The evidence is limited for its use in treating other symptoms of PCOS.

Metformin induces ovulation with or without the simultaneous use of clomiphene by reducing hyperinsulinaemia, gonadotropins, and androgens. A Cochrane review showed an OR of 3.88 for promoting ovulation. In a meta-analysis, pregnancy rates did not differ a great deal between the placebo group and the metformin group (Lord et al., 2003, *BMJ*).

Dose of metformin = 1500 mg/day.

The side effects are mainly GIT-related.

It has also been suggested that oocyte quality improves following treatment with metformin, but the evidence is not strong.

Question 3

Part a

Briefly describe the biochemical events that lead to ovulation.

Answer:

The serum LH level rises steadily in the second half of the follicular phase of the menstrual cycle, as a result of stimulation from follicular oestrogen. The LH causes luteinisation of the granulosa cells, which start to secrete increasing amounts of progesterone. This progesterone, through its action on the pituitary, causes a marked increase in LH levels, a phenomenon called LH surge. The LH surge stimulates meiosis of the oocyte and synthesis of progesterone and prostaglandins in the developing follicle. Progesterone stimulates the proteolytic enzymes, causing rupture of the follicular wall.

Part b

In a 28-year-old woman with polycystic ovary syndrome, briefly describe why ovulation does not occur.

Answer:

In the given context, ovulation does not occur because of the following reasons:

A) Increased LH secretion from the pituitary in response to the increased GnRH pulse amplitude or increased pituitary sensitivity to GnRH causes increased androgen production from the ovarian theca cells. This directly inhibits ovulation.

B) A decreased level of sex hormone–binding globulin as a result of increased androgen and hyperinsulinaemia causes increased levels of unbound, biologically active androgens in the blood. This causes apoptosis of the granulosa cells, and hence, progesterone is not secreted, and the LH surge does not occur.

C) The increased nonbound oestradiol as a result of decreased sex hormone–binding globulin causes increased GnRH pulsatility, which causes persistent elevated levels of LH and, consequently, anovulation.

Part c

List the consequences of persistent anovulation in the above woman.

Answer:

The clinical consequences of persistent anovulation in this woman are the following:

   i. Infertility

   ii. Menstrual bleeding problems, ranging from amenorrhea to dysfunctional uterine bleeding

   iii. Hirsutism, alopecia, and acne

   iv. An increased risk of endometrial cancer and perhaps breast cancer

   v. An increased risk of cardiovascular disease

   vi. An increased risk of diabetes mellitus in patients with insulin resistance

Part d

List the mode of action of insulin-sensitising drugs in PCOS.

Answer:

The mode of action of an insulin-sensitising drug in the context of PCOS is primarily to induce ovulation. Evidence for the action of this drug on other aspects of PCOS is limited. The most commonly used insulin-sensitising drug is metformin, a biguanide. The modes of action are as follows:

   i. It reduces hepatic glucose production and thereby hyperinsulinaemia. The reduced insulin level leads to reduction of LH and androgen levels, which promotes ovulation.

   ii. It also reduces hyperinsulinaemia by sensitising peripheral tissues to the action of insulin.

Multiple-Choice Questions

Q1. Which of the following statements regarding PCOS is true?

   A. The presence of polycystic ovaries is essential for the diagnosis.

   B. An estimated 20% of normal asymptomatic women will have polycystic ovaries.

   C. A normal ovarian volume is 12 cm^3.

   D. Polycystic ovaries are always bilateral.

Answer: B

Q2. Which of the following statements is true?

   A. The main ovarian androgen is androstenedione.

   B. The main ovarian androgen is DHAS.

   C. The main adrenal androgen is testosterone.

   D. Granulosa cells produce androgens.

Answer: A

Q3. Regarding anovulation in PCOS, which of the following statements is **not** true?

    A. Increased LH secretion leads to anovulation.

    B. Increased androgen secretion leads to anovulation.

    C. Increased nonbound androgen leads to anovulation.

    D. Increased insulin secretion directly leads to anovulation.

Answer: D

Q4. Which of the following is **not** a consequence of persistent anovulation in the context of PCOS?

    A. Dysfunctional uterine bleeding

    B. Alopecia

    C. Increased risk of endometrial cancer

    D. Increased risk of ovarian cancer

Answer: D

Q5. Which of the following statements is true for hirsutism due to PCOS?

    A. The distribution of abnormal hair does not follow any pattern.

    B. Spironolactone reduces androgen synthesis.

    C. Hirsutism is produced due to the action of dihydrotestosterone (DHT) on the pilosebaceous unit.

    D. 10% of women with PCOS will have increased levels of DHEAS.

Answer: C

Q6. Which of the following is **not** a sign of PCOS?

    A. Hirsutism

    B. Virilism

    C. Infertility

    D. Increased ovarian stroma

Answer: B

Q7. Which of the following is a sign of PCOS?

    A. Hypertrichosis

    B. Presence of excessive vellus hair

    C. Presence of excessive terminal hair

    D. Temporal balding

Answer: C

Q8. Which of the following is caused by spironolactone?

    A. Menstrual irregularity

    B. Masculinisation of a female fetus

    C. Inactivated 5-α-reductase

    D. Does not affect serum potassium level

Answer: A

Q9. Which of the following is **not** true regarding the mode of action of a combined oral contraceptive pill in PCOS?

    A. Suppress LH secretion

    B. Suppress ovarian androgen secretion

    C. Increase sex hormone–binding globulin synthesis

    D. Increase gluconeogenesis

Answer: D

Q10. Which of the following is **not** true in the context of PCOS treatment by metformin?

    A. Promotes gluconeogenesis

    B. Promotes peripheral tissue sensitisation to insulin

    C. Reduces hyperandrogenism

    D. Decreases LH secretion

Answer: D

Q11. Which of the following does **not** increase in PCOS?

    A. Oestrone

    B. TSH

    C. 17-hydroxyprogesterone

    D. DHEAS

Answer: B

Q12. Which of the following is a **not** a sequela of PCOS?

    A. Breast cancer

    B. Endometrial cancer

    C. Coronary artery disease

    D. Diabetes mellitus

Answer: A

Q13. Which of the following is **not** increased in PCOS?

    A. DHEAS

    B. LH

    C. Prolactin

    D. TSH

Answer: D

Q14. A 23-year-old obese woman has developed hirsutism and deepening of the voice over the past one year. Her menses are irregular and infrequent. Examination shows severe facial hair, clitoromegaly, and a slightly bulky uterus. Her serum testosterone is 17 nmol/L and DHEAS of 9.8 μmol/L. What will be your next investigation?

A. Serum androstenedione

B. Serum 17-hydroxyprogesterone

C. Selective venous catheterisation

D. Transvaginal ultrasound of the ovaries

Answer: D

Q15. The significance of the ultrasound finding of polycystic ovaries in the prepubertal sister of a woman with PCOS is that:

A. She will develop PCOS.

B. It is a marker of insulin resistance.

C. There is partial 21-hydroxylase deficiency in the family.

D. She will have an earlier menopause.

Answer: B

Q16. Which of the following is **not** associated with an increase in non-androgen-dependent hair (hypertrichosis)?

A. Ranitidine

B. Diazoxide

C. Cyclosporin

D. Phenytoin

Answer: A

Q17. In a lady born with a relative deficiency of 17-α-hydroxylase, you would expect to see:

A. Hirsutism

B. Absent vagina

C. Hypertension

D. Salt-losing syndrome

Answer: C

Q18. A 22-year-old female, 150 cm tall and 49 kg in weight, has had severe hirsutism for 7 years and oligomenorrhoea since menarche. Her sister, who suffers from mild hirsutism, uses combined oral contraceptive pills. She has mild clitoromegaly but is otherwise normal. Investigations are as follows: LH 19 IU/L, FSH 6 IU/L, Testosterone 3.0 nmol/L, DHEAS 21.0 µmol/L and 17-hydroxyprogesterone 16 nmol/L.

The most likely diagnosis is:

   A. PCOS

   B. Ovarian hyperthecosis

   C. Late-onset congenital adrenal hyperplasia

   D. Androgen-secreting tumour of the adrenal gland

Answer: C

Q19. A 26-year-old female presents with acute virilisation and has a normal pelvic examination. Her investigations are as follows: LH 2 IU/L, FSH 3 IU/L, 17-hydroxyprogesterone 2.9 nmol/L, testosterone 8.9 nmol/L, and DHEAS 5.3 µmol/L. Which of the following is the most probable diagnosis?

   A. Cushing's syndrome

   B. PCOS

   C. Adrenal adenoma

   D. Sertoli-Leydig cell tumour

Answer: D

Q20. Which of the following statements regarding late-onset 21-hydroxylase deficiency is least correct?

   A. The 21-hydroxylase gene mutation is on chromosome 6.

   B. Late-onset 21-hydroxylase deficiency accounts for approximately 5% of hirsutism.

   C. DHEAS levels are usually elevated.

   D. Definitive diagnosis is done with a dexamethasone suppression test.

Answer: D

Q21. A 40-year-old woman presents with a rapid onset of virilisation. She has a normal pelvis. Her serum testosterone is 12.3 nmol/L, and DHEAS is 25.4 µmol/L. What is the most likely diagnosis?

   A. Late-onset congenital adrenal hyperplasia

   B. Adrenal cortical adenoma

   C. PCOS with insulin resistance

   D. Cushing's syndrome

Answer: B

Q22. A 23-year-old woman has periods 3–4 times a year. Her periods are very heavy and prolonged. She has noticeable facial hair. Her BMI is 33. An endometrial biopsy would most likely show:

A. Subnuclear vacuoles

B. Supranuclear vacuoles

C. Crowding of straight tubular glands

D. Stromal oedema with perivascular decidualisation

Answer: C

Q23. Which of the following statements regarding hyperandrogenic chronic anovulation (HCA) and PCOS is most correct?

A. Approximately 5% of normal ovulatory women have an ultrasound appearance of PCO, and approximately 75% of women with HCA have an ultrasound appearance of PCO.

B. Approximately 20% of normal ovulatory women have an ultrasound appearance of PCO, and approximately 75% of women with HCA have an ultrasound appearance of PCO.

C. Approximately 5% of normal ovulatory women have an ultrasound appearance of PCO, and approximately 90% of women with HCA have an ultrasound appearance of PCO.

D. Approximately 20% of normal ovulatory women have an ultrasound appearance of PCO, and approximately 90% of women with HCA have an ultrasound appearance of PCO.

Answer: B

Q24. A 20-year-old has severe acne that is unresponsive to conventional treatment. Which of the following tests will you do before prescribing isotretinoin?

A. Lipid profile

B. Liver function tests

C. Kidney function tests

D. Pregnancy test

Answer: D

Q25. Which of the following statements is **not** correct in the context of PCOS treatment by metformin?

A. It causes weight loss.

B. It improves the rate of conception.

C. It reduces hepatic glucose production.

D. It reduces androgen level.

Answer: A

Q26. A blood assay of which of the following steroids is the most direct measure of adrenal androgen activity?

 A. Cortisol

 B. Androstenedione

 C. Dehydroepiandrosterone sulphate

 D. Testosterone

Answer: C

Q27. In a 16-year-old girl with unresponsive acne, which of the following tests should be done before prescribing isotretinoin?

 A. Full blood count

 B. Liver function tests

 C. Lipid profile

 D. β-HCG in urine

Answer: D

Q28. Which of the following reduces sex hormone–binding globulin concentration?

 A. Pregnancy

 B. Weight loss

 C. Hyperinsulinaemia

 D. Oestrogen

Answer: C

Chapter 7.2.   Infertility

Definitions

Asthenospermia	Reduced or absent sperm motility.
Azoospermia	No sperm in semen.
Conception	The stage of pregnancy when implantation has occurred. In this book, it is used interchangeably with fertilisation.
Fecundability	Probability of conceiving within a single menstrual cycle. Incidence is 20% and decreases with the increasing duration of infertility.
Fecundity	Probability of achieving a live birth within a single cycle.
Infertility	Inability to conceive after 1 year of unprotected intercourse. Incidence is 10–15% of the normal population and increases with the age of the female.
Oocyte	Egg surrounded by zona pellucida and cumulus cells.
Primary infertility	Infertility with no prior conception.
Salpingitis isthmica nodosa	Diverticulum of the inner layer of the fallopian tube passing through the muscularis layer.
Secondary infertility	Infertility with prior conception, irrespective of the fate of that conceptus.
Subfertility	Decreased capacity for pregnancy.
Zona pellucida	A translucent, acellular, porous layer of mucopolysaccharide secreted by the oocyte.
Zygote	The single-cell diploid stage of the fertilised ovum.

Table 7.1. Chapter 7.2. Definitions

Chapter 7.2.1.   Infertility

Clinical Physiology of Conception

For implantation of the blastocyst in the endometrium, the following must occur in a timely and synchronised fashion:

- Ascent of sperm through the cervix, uterus, and the fallopian tube ("tube")
- Ovulation
- Ovum (egg) transport through the tube
- Fertilisation (conception)

The reproductive efficiency in humans is only 20% (fecundability). The ovum is released from the ovary in the metaphase II stage of meiosis, with the zona pellucida and a few layers of granulosa cells around it. This happens around day 14 of a 28-day cycle. The fimbrial end of the tube picks up the oocyte from the ovary. Entry of the egg into the tube is facilitated by the contraction of the muscle layer of the tube. Further transport of the oocyte inside the tube is achieved by the muscle layer and cilia of the tube. Within 2–3 minutes of ovulation, the oocyte is in the ampulla of the tube, where fertilisation occurs. If not fertilised, the egg starts to disintegrate within 24 hours once it is inside the ampulla.

To maximise the chance of fertilisation, the spermatozoa ("sperm") should already be present in that area of the tube. Although the sperm lives for up to 7 days, the ability to fertilise an egg only lasts up to about 72 hours. The sperm is attracted to the egg by a process known as chemotaxis, which involves the binding of progesterone to a surface receptor on the sperm. This results in increased sperm motility. During its journey from the cervical mucus to the tube, the sperm undergoes capacitation and an acrosomal reaction that involves enzymatic changes in the sperm head, which increases its ability to penetrate the cumulus cells and zona pellucida. Capacitation can also occur in vitro.

The journey of the sperm from the cervical mucus to the tube takes only a few minutes. The cervix serves as a reservoir of sperm for up to 72 hours. A few hundred sperms reach the oocyte, but only one is able to penetrate the cumulus, zona pellucida, and cell membrane of the egg. The zona pellucida precludes more than one sperm from entering the oocyte. Once inside the egg, the sperm head forms the male pronucleus.

The egg completes its second meiotic division once the sperm head is inside it, and its nucleus forms the female pronucleus. The male and female pronuclei, which contain the haploid sets of chromosomes, then lose their nuclear membrane, and the chromosomes from each nucleus align along the developing spindle. A diploid zygote is formed, completing the process of fertilisation.

A significant proportion of zygotes fail to further divide due to a variety of factors, such as failure of spindle formation and appropriate chromosomal arrangement, gene defects, environmental factors, and the effects of any teratogenic agents.

Multiple pregnancy may result if the dividing cell mass completely separates into two or more distinct cell masses. This process can only occur up to the stage of blastula (a ball of cells surrounding a central cavity) formation, since all the cells of the blastula (blastomeres) are totipotent.

In humans, the fertilised egg spends about 80 hours in the tube, 90% of which is in the ampulla. The fertilised egg arrives at the uterus anywhere from the 32-cell stage to the blastula stage. Implantation of the blastocyst occurs approximately 3 days after the embryo enters the uterus. The blastocyst produces human chorionic gonadotropin (hCG), which acts on the corpus luteum to maintain the synthesis of oestradiol (E2) and progesterone. This prevents the onset of menstruation and allows a pregnancy to continue.

Factors Affecting Fertility

i.   Age: Female and male fertility decline with age, although the latter declines much more slowly.

ii. Coital frequency: Fecundability rises sharply with coital frequency. Coitus every 2–3 days maximises the chance of conception.

iii. Timing of intercourse: The maximum chance of conception occurs if the intercourse happens a day before ovulation. Couples should be encouraged to have daily intercourse for 3 days midcycle.

iv. Alcohol intake: Drinking 1–2 units of alcohol once or twice a week does not affect the fetus. Ideally, women trying to conceive should not drink alcohol at all. Binge drinking is detrimental to the developing fetus. Drinking 3–4 units of alcohol per day does not affect semen quality.

v.   Smoking and caffeine: Smoking, both active and passive, adversely affects female fertility and semen quality. Caffeinated drinks decrease conception rate.

vi. BMI: Women with a BMI > 30 and < 19 take longer to conceive, most likely because of anovulation. Restoration of a normal body weight helps in ovulation. Men with BMI > 30 are likely to have decreased fertility.

vii. Occupation: Men with increased scrotal temperatures from working very close to heated areas, such as close to industrial boilers and furnaces, will have reduced semen parameters. Exposure to radiation may cause azoospermia, which is reversible. Exposure to other chemicals, such as pesticides and paints, may lead to oligospermia.

viii. Drugs: NSAIDs inhibit ovulation. Immunosuppressive agents may affect conception. Chemotherapy can cause ovarian failure. Thyroxine, antidepressants, and drugs used for asthma have been reported to cause anovulation. Marijuana and cocaine may be detrimental to ovulation and tubal motility.

History

Ideally, both the woman and her male partner should be interviewed together. The history should explore all the areas mentioned in the "Factors Affecting Fertility" section. In addition, it should also include the following:

- Previous reproductive, obstetric, or gynaecological history
- Evidence of ovulation in the history
  - Is the menses regular every 28–35 days?
  - Is there a rise in the basal body temperature in the luteal phase of the cycle?
  - Is there midcycle pain (mittelschmerz) suggestive of ovulation?
  - Does cervical mucus become clear and stretchy (spinnbarkeit) at midcycle?

- o Does she experience molimina (breast tenderness, dysmenorrhoea, and bloating) on a monthly basis?
- History of previous infection, such as STI and PID
- Sexual history: frequency and timing of coitus, dyspareunia, vaginal dryness
- Past medical history: endometriosis, PCOS, hyperprolactinaemia, hypothyroidism, Cushing's syndrome, antiphospholipid syndrome
- Genetic: Turner's syndrome
- Past surgical history: ruptured appendix, tubal surgery
- Family history: premature menopause, hereditary disorders
- Social history: stress, nutrition, exercise

In men, the focused history should also include:

- Whether he has fathered a child before
- History of mumps, genital trauma, undescended testicles, cystic fibrosis, bladder-neck surgery, vasectomy reversal
- History of premature ejaculation, hypospadias, ability to have successful intercourse

Examination

Examination of the Woman

- General examination, including:
  - o BMI
  - o Acne
  - o Hirsutism
- Breast examination
  - o Galactorrhoea
  - o Bitemporal hemianopia
- Any thyroid swelling
- Abdomen
  - o Abnormal mass
  - o Surgical scars
- Vaginal examination
  - o Any vaginal/cervical abnormality
  - o Any abnormal discharge
  - o Uterine size, shape, and tenderness
  - o Abnormal adnexal mass
  - o Any nodularity in the POD or on the uterosacral ligaments

Examination of the Man

As long as the semen count is normal and a male partner is able to achieve successful intercourse with the deposition of semen into the vagina, examination of the male partner is not necessary. When an examination is indicated, it should include the following:

- BMI
- Gynaecomastia
- Testicular volume and consistency
- Varicocele
- Any penile abnormality

Causes

In a World Health Organisation study of 8,500 infertile couples, the distribution of causes of infertility was as follows:

- Female factor—37%
- Male factor—8%
- Male and female factors combined—35%
- Unexplained—20%

The causes of female infertility were broadly divided as follows:

- Ovulatory disorders—25%
- Pelvic (including endometriosis)—25%
- Tubal disorders—22%
- Hyperprolactinaemia—7%

Investigations

1. Evidence of ovulation
   - Apart from the factors mentioned in the history, a midluteal serum progesterone (day 21 in a 28-day cycle) > 25 nmol/L indicates ovulation.
2. Biochemical markers of PCOS
   - If there are features of androgenisation and anovulation on history and examination.
   - FSH, LH, SHBG, serum testosterone and free testosterone.
3. Serum thyroxine and prolactin
   - If there are suggestive features on history and examination.
4. Blood group, antibody screen, serum rubella and hepatitis antibodies, VDRL, HIV, FBE, and iron studies
5. Chlamydia and gonorrhoea screening
   - If relevant features in the history.
   - Thomas et al. (2000) have suggested that if chlamydia IgG antibody titre is greater than 1:32, it is suggestive of tubal damage in 35% of women.

6. Cervical cytology

  • If not done in the last 12 months.

7. In women older than 35 years, tests for ovarian reserve (number of nongrowing primordial follicles) are also recommended, which are:

  • Serum FSH on day 2 or 3; if > 15 mU/mL, it indicates decreased ovarian reserve.
  • Serum oestradiol on day 2 or 3; if > 70 pg/mL, it indicates decreased ovarian reserve.
  • Anti-Müllerian hormone (AMH):
    ○ It is produced by granulosa cells.
    ○ Maximum production occurs in the preantral and small antral stages (< 4 mm in diameter) of follicular development.
    ○ Low serum AMH levels indicate decreased ovarian reserve.
    ○ With aging and consequent decreasing ovarian reserve, AMH level falls.
    ○ As opposed to FSH and oestradiol levels, it can be done at any time in the cycle as its level remains stable throughout the cycle.
    ○ When combined with antral follicle count, it gives the best strategy for IVF treatment—natural or stimulated IVF.
    ○ AMH levels can also help to identify those women who are at risk of ovarian hyperstimulation following the use of ovulation-inducing drugs.

8. Tubal patency tests

  • These are tests to establish a normal endometrial cavity and tubal patency, either unilateral or bilateral.
  • They must be performed within a week of finishing menses to avoid harm to the developing embryo.
  • These tests should be done under antibiotic cover.
  • A history of salpingitis is a relative contraindication.
  • These tests can be done either by sonohysterography, hysterosalpingography, or a combination of hysteroscopy, laparoscopy, and chromotubation.

9. Semen analysis

  • It is the most important test to evaluate male infertility. It reflects sperm production that happened 72 days before.
  • The sample is collected after 3 days of abstinence. Frequent ejaculation can lower the seminal volume and even the sperm count in some men.
  • The entire specimen should be collected because the initial part contains the highest density of sperm.
  • The specimen should be transported to the lab at body temperature (sperm are very temperature-sensitive) and should be examined within 1–2 hours of collection. Sperm motility declines 2 hours after ejaculation.

- The following parameters are looked at:

Volume	1.5—5 mL
pH	> 7.2
Sperm count	> 20 million/mL
Percent motility	> 50%
Forward progression	> 2%
Normal morphology	> 15%
Round cells	< 5 million/mL
White blood cells	< 1 million/mL

- o White blood cells in the seminal fluid may indicate prostatitis or epididymitis. The presence of excessive round cells indicates defective spermatogenesis.
- A suboptimal sperm analysis should be repeated after 3 months.

10. Transvaginal pelvic ultrasound scan

- This gives most of the relevant information about the cervix, cervical canal, endometrial cavity, phase of the endometrium, endometrial polyps, submucosal or intramural fibroids, state of the myometrium, adenomyosis, ovaries, polycystic ovaries, and any abnormal adnexal mass.
- When combined with sonohysterography using a sono-opaque dye, it also provides information about tubal patency.

11. Other tests

- There is no evidence that the following actually contribute to infertility:
  - o Antisperm antibodies in men and women
  - o Luteal-phase deficiency
  - o Subclinical genital infection in normally ovulating women
  - o Subclinical endocrine abnormality in normally ovulating women

Management

The 3 types of anovulatory dysfunction are shown in the following table:

Type of anovulation	FSH, LH, E$_2$	Symptoms	Associated diseases	Treatment
Hypogonadotropic hypogonadism (common)	Low FSH Low LH Low E$_2$	Amenorrhoea Anovulation	Sheehan's syndrome, Anorexia nervosa	Ovulation induction or ART
Normogonadotrophic hypogonadism (most common)	Normal FSH Normal LH Normal E$_2$	Secondary amenorrhoea, Irregular anovulation	PCOS, Adrenal and ovarian tumours	Ovulation induction or ART
Hyper gonadotrophic hypogonadism (least common)	High FSH High LH Low E$_2$	Amenorrhoea, Menopausal symptoms	Ovarian failure, Turner's syndrome	ART with donor oocyte

Table 7.2. Anovulatory dysfunction

The following ovulation-inducing management options and agents are in use:

Weight Modulation

Higher and lower body mass indices both cause anovulation and subfertility. With a higher BMI, loss of only 5–10% body weight restores ovulation in 55–100% of women in 6 months. Women with BMI less than 19 should be advised to gain weight and reduce exercise in order to ovulate.

Clomiphene Citrate

Clomiphene is a selective oestrogen-receptor modulator with antioestrogenic and weak oestrogenic action. It competitively inhibits the negative feedback of oestrogen on the hypothalamus, thereby increasing GnRH secretion from the hypothalamus. Consequently, FSH and LH secretion from the pituitary are increased, which leads to increased oocyte maturation with increased E$_2$ synthesis. This drug is administered orally for 5 days, starting on day 2, 3, or 4 of the menstrual cycle. The starting dose is 50 mg daily, which can be incrementally increased up to 250 mg in successive cycles if ovulation does not occur. Ovulation occurs about 7 days after the ingestion of the 5th clomiphene tablet.

Ovulation is confirmed by measuring the serum progesterone level 2 weeks after the last tablet (or one week after ovulation).

If ovulation occurs, the same dosage of clomiphene should be continued for 3–6 cycles. A new course of clomiphene should only be started once a pregnancy has been excluded. In the absence of ovulation, even on the maximum dose of clomiphene, 5000 IU of hCG is injected a week after the last clomiphene tablet. This further increases the chance of ovulation.

An estimated 80% of women on clomiphene will ovulate, although only 40% will get pregnant. Success is highest in the first few months of treatment. In hypothalamic pituitary failure (hypogonadotropic hypogonadism), with very low level of oestradiol, clomiphene is not successful in ovulation induction.

Side Effects

- Lack of libido, vaginal dryness, and dyspareunia because of the antioestrogenic effect
- Vasomotor symptoms (10%), abdominal pain, bloating, urticaria, and alopecia
- 5% increase in the incidence of twin pregnancy
- 5% increase in fetal malformation if the drug is administered in the first 6 weeks of pregnancy
- Ovarian hyperstimulation

Metformin

Metformin is an insulin sensitiser and an adjunctive therapy for ovulation induction. It decreases the insulin level by decreasing hepatic glucose production. It also directly stimulates the ovary, leading to ovulation.

The dose is 1,500 mg/day. This is slowly increased due to side effects.

On its own, it leads to ovulation in 60% of women. When combined with clomiphene in clomiphene-resistant women, 25% of women will ovulate.

This drug is described in more detail in the PCOS chapter.

Side Effects

- Nausea and vomiting
- Lactic acidosis

Aromatase Inhibitors (Letrozole)

Letrozole is used when clomiphene ovulation induction has been unsuccessful. It acts by inhibiting E_2 inhibitors' synthesis with a negative feedback, causing an increased LH:FSH ratio. Ovarian androgens are also increased, increasing FSH sensitivity.

Dose: 2.5 to 5 mg, oral, daily for 5 days, starting day 3, 4, or 5 of the menstrual cycle.

Comparison of Clomiphene and Letrozole

	Clomiphene	Letrozole
Thick cervical mucus	Common	Less common
Thin endometrium	Common	Less common
E_2 level at ovulation	Normal	Lower
Pregnancy rates	Comparable or worse	Comparable or better
Follicular production	More than letrozole	Less than clomiphene
Half-life	5 days	50 hours
Multiple gestation	Higher	Lower
Clinical experience	Widely used	Limited

Table 7.3. Comparison of clomiphene and letrozole

Gonadotropins (FSH and HMG)

They are used in the following cases:

- Clomiphene or letrozole failure
- E_2 level is low ($<$ 30 pg/mL)
- Lack of withdrawal bleed after progestin administration

This treatment is expensive and requires close E_2 and sonographic (follicular) monitoring. The rate of multiple pregnancy is 15%.

Laparoscopic Drilling

Laparoscopic drilling is used in anovulatory PCOS women when other treatments have been unsuccessful. Ovarian drilling is done using a monopolar laparoscopic diathermy needle to destroy the cells. Up to 3–7 holes are made in each ovary. It promotes ovarian healing and ovulation. It has similar cumulative pregnancy rates as 3 to 6 cycles of ovulation-inducing drugs. The rate of multiple pregnancy is considerably lower compared with other groups.

Its drawback is the expense. It is a surgical procedure and has all of the inherent anaesthetic and surgical risks and complications, including adhesion formation and premature menopause if done too aggressively.

Other Drugs

- Tamoxifen (SERM)
- Bromocriptine (dopamine agonist)
- GnRH

ART will be discussed separately.

Management of Pelvic Causes of Infertility

Uterus and Cervix

Congenital uterine abnormalities rarely cause infertility. Women with intrauterine adhesions as a solitary finding get pregnant in 75% of cases after hysteroscopic adhesiolysis. Some submucous myomas may interfere with sperm transport and implantation. Larger myomas can occlude the interstitial part of the tube. A cervical myoma can also impede sperm transport. A myomectomy does improve conception rates, but the quality of evidence is poor for pregnancy rate, improved live birth rate, and decreased miscarriage rate.

Endometriosis

Endometriosis is present in 15–60% of infertile women. If the endometriosis is minimal to mild, the chance of achieving a spontaneous pregnancy in the next 9 months is about 30–40%. Medical treatment for endometriosis will cause ovarian suppression and delayed conception (Evidence Level IA). It has no benefit over no treatment at all. Laparoscopic ablation of endometriosis may improve fertility in mild to moderate endometriosis (Evidence Level IA). Laparotomy or laparoscopy for severe disease also improves fertility. A cystectomy for endometrioma gives better results than drainage and electrocautery (Evidence Level IA). There is no benefit from postoperative treatment with danazol or GnRH agonists, but preoperative treatment does have benefits. Pregnancy rates after IVF for endometriosis are about 20% per cycle of treatment.

Management of Tubal Causes of Infertility

The incidence of infertility from tubal causes is on the rise due to the rising incidence of salpingitis. Tubal obstruction is more common at the distal end. Hydrosalpinges big enough to be seen on ultrasound should be excised to improve the IVF success. The surgical outcome following tubal reconstructive surgery depends upon the following:

- Extent of adhesions
- Nature of adhesions
- Diameter of hydrosalpinx (> 2 cm)
- Appearance of the endosalpinx
- Thickness of the tubal wall

The following methods are used to establish tubal patency:

	Hysterosalpingogram (HSG) – X-ray	Sonohysterography – ultrasound	Hysteroscopy, laparoscopy and chromotubation
Cost	Cheap	Cheap	Expensive because of surgery and anaesthesia
Simplicity	Simple and easy to do	Simple and easy to do	Invasive; able to do laparoscopically
Timing of procedure	Proliferative phase	Proliferative phase	Proliferative phase
Place	Needs radiological setup	Possible in outpatient clinic	Operating theatre
Dye	Radio-opaque dye	Sono-opaque dye	Methylene blue
Results	Better in diagnosing tubal patency than obstruction; for diagnosing tubal obstruction: sensitivity 65%, specificity 83%	Good statistical comparability and concordance with other methods	Gold standard; confirms HSG-diagnosed obstruction in only 38% of cases; confirms HSG-diagnosed patency in 94% of cases
Advantages	• Can detect uterine cavity abnormalities, site of tubal occlusion • No GA required • Two-fold increase in pregnancy rates using oil-based dye	• Can detect uterine and myometrial abnormalities, such as adenomyosis • Easy to access the whole pelvis including ovaries, corpus luteum, and endometrium • No GA required	• Allows view of whole pelvis • Adhesiolysis, salpingolysis, ovarian drilling can be performed simultaneously
Disadvantages	Assessment of pelvic structures, pathology, and treatment not possible	Can't diagnose mild endometriosis and filmy adhesions; treatment not possible	Inherent risks and costs of a surgical procedure; site of tubal occlusion not always easy to identify
Risks of dye	Anaphylaxis	Anaphylaxis Granuloma formation	Anaphylaxis
Risks of procedure	Failure Cervical trauma Radiation exposure	Failure Cervical trauma (No radiation)	Usual anaesthetic and laparoscopic risks

Table 7.4. Comparison of methodologies for investigation of tubal patency

Chapter 7.2.2.   Ovarian Hyperstimulation Syndrome (OHSS)

OHSS is a systemic disease resulting from vasoactive chemicals released from hyperstimulated ovaries. These chemicals (vascular endothelial growth factor) increase capillary permeability, and hence, leakage of fluid from the vascular compartment to third spaces occurs. This causes intravascular dehydration and increased blood viscosity.

Severe Complications

- DVT
- Renal and hepatic dysfunction
- Acute respiratory distress syndrome (ARDS)
- Death

Epidemiology

Although the disease can happen with the use of any ovulation-inducing drug, 33% of IVF cycles are affected by a mild form of the disease. An estimated 3–8% of IVF cycles are affected by severe disease. The incidence is increased in women who are lean and younger (< 35 years) and in women with PCOS, multiple pregnancies, and prior OHSS. High E_2 levels and multiple developing follicles are also risk factors (Evidence Level IV).

History

The common symptoms are abdominal distension, pain, nausea, and vomiting, on a background of ovarian stimulation.

Classification

The classification by Mathur (2005) is as follows:

Mild OHSS	Moderate OHSS	Severe OHSS	Critical OHSS
• Abdominal bloating and pain • Ovarian diameter < 8 cm	• Moderate abdominal pain • Nausea and vomiting • Ascites • Ovarian diameter 8–12 cm	• Ascites, obvious clinically • Hydrothorax • Oliguria • Haematocrit > 45% • Hypoproteinaemia • Ovarian diameter > 12 cm	• Tense ascites • Large hydrothorax • Haematocrit > 55% • WCC > 25 x 10^9/mL • Oliguria/anuria • DVT • ARDS

Table 7.5. Classification by Mathur of OHSS

Management

Outpatients

Women with mild and sometimes moderate disease can be managed in an outpatient setting.

1. Blood investigations: FBE (especially haematocrit), UEC, LFT, and coagulation screen. Repeat every 2–3 days.
2. Ultrasound scan for ovarian size and morphology, and ascites.
3. Daily weight and abdominal girth measurement.
4. Analgesia: Paracetamol and/or codeine is appropriate. NSAIDs are contraindicated because of renal toxicity.
5. Oral fluid intake: Drink to thirst, not excessively.
6. Avoid excessive exercise and coitus because of the risks of trauma or ovarian torsion.
7. Progesterone luteal support could be continued but not hCG.
8. Review every 2–3 days. In the absence of pregnancy, the condition resolves by the time of the next period.

Inpatients

Women with moderate disease that is not improving on outpatient management and all women with severe or critical disease should be managed as an inpatient. The inpatient management is largely supportive with an aim to provide symptomatic relief under the care of a multidisciplinary team, including an intensivist.

In addition to the management in the outpatient setting, blood tests should be repeated daily, and ultrasound scans should be performed twice-weekly. Haemoconcentration is reflected by raised haemoglobin and haematocrit levels.

Parenteral opiates can be used for additional analgesic requirements, along with antiemetics such as prochlorperazine, metoclopramide, and cyclizine. Regular clinical assessments of hydration status, the cardiorespiratory system, presence of ascites, and a palpable abdominal mass should be performed.

Tight fluid balance should be measured, as urine output less than 1000 mL/24hrs or a persistently positive fluid balance indicates a nonresolving condition. Patients should drink as per thirst. Avoid diuretics as they deplete intravascular volume. Colloid volume expansion may be required.

A chest X-ray is indicated if there is shortness of breath and clinical suspicion of a hydrothorax or pulmonary embolism.

Ascites should be tapped under ultrasound guidance when excessive abdominal distension causes distress. Increasing abdominal pain, oliguria, weight gain, and shortness of breath reflect worsening OHSS.

Thromboprophylaxis should be given to all inpatients until at least discharge, or even longer.

Surgery is only necessary if ovarian torsion cannot be excluded.

Pregnancy can continue normally. In critically ill women, a termination of pregnancy may be needed. There is no evidence of increased congenital malformations or other pregnancy complications with OHSS (Evidence Level IIA).

Prevention

- Monitoring oestrogen levels, follicle numbers, and size
- Delaying hCG injection or cancelling IVF cycle, if above are present
- Using progesterone rather than hCG for luteal support

Chapter 7.2.3.   Assisted Reproductive Technology

Assisted reproductive technology (ART) consists of techniques that are used to increase fecundability by artificial methods of enhancing the chances of fertilisation. These techniques include the following:

- In vitro fertilization (IVF)
- Intracytoplasmic sperm injection (ICSI)
- Gamete intrafallopian transfer (GIFT)
- Zygote intrafallopian transfer (ZIFT)
- Cryopreserved embryo transfers
- Use of donor eggs

GIFT and ZIFT are now rarely used because of the successes of IVF and ICSI. IVF and ICSI have the following steps:

- Ovarian stimulation with FSH HMG, follicle tracking, and serum oestradiol level assessment
- Prevention of premature LH surge and ovulation
- Oocyte maturation using hCG
- Oocyte harvesting (retrieval)
- Fertilisation by IVF/ICSI
- Embryo culture
- Endometrial preparation for implantation using progestins
- Fresh embryo transfer

Chapter 7.2.4.   Hyperprolactinaemia

Prolactin is a polypeptide, monomeric hormone secreted from the anterior pituitary lactotrophs with a half-life of 20 minutes.

Hyperprolactinaemia is defined as a serum prolactin level in excess of 25 ng/mL with galactorrhoea or amenorrhoea or both. It is present in 15% of anovulatory women and 20% of women with amenorrhoea.

Galactorrhoea is watery or milky secretions from the breast of a woman who is not lactating. About 60% of women with galactorrhoea will have a hyperprolactinaemia.

Clinical Physiology of Prolactin

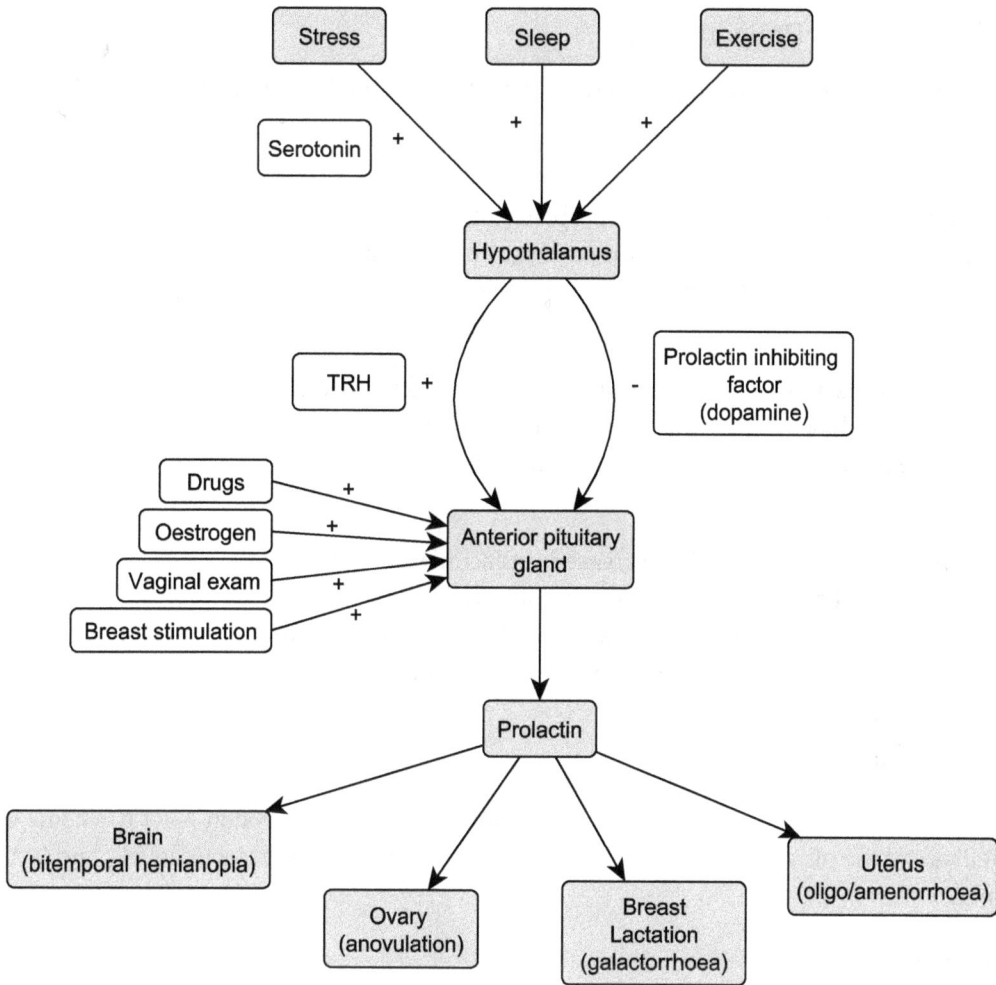

Figure 7.3. Clinical physiology of prolactin

Diurnal Variation of Prolactin Secretion

The prolactin level varies during the day and menstrual cycle. The maximum level is during sleep and after lunch. The best time to collect prolactin estimation is midmorning. The prolactin level is maximum at midcycle.

Factors That Increase Prolactin Level

- Sleep (serotonin-mediated), stress, exercise, breast and skin stimulation, gynaecological examination.
- Pregnancy:
  o Placental oestrogen causes the hyperplasia of pituitary lactotrophs and hence increased secretion. However, the increased oestrogen also blocks the prolactin receptor in the breast tissue, and hence, lactation does not occur despite a high level of prolactin.
- Drugs:
  o Tranquilisers, narcotics, tricyclic antidepressants, antihypertensive (methyldopa); all of these either block the synthesis or action of dopamine.
  o COC pills cause oestrogenic stimulation of lactotrophs.
- Disease:
  o Chronic renal failure due to decreased prolactin excretion.
  o Hypothyroidism due to decreased inhibition of TRH.
  o Craniopharyngioma: disrupts connection between hypothalamus and pituitary.
  o Pituitary: adenoma, hyperplasia, empty sella syndrome.
  o Cushing's disease.

Functions of Prolactin

Prolactin promotes breast tissue hyperplasia and lactation once the oestrogen level has come down after the delivery of the placenta. Suckling of the breast further increases prolactin levels, and lactation is maintained.

Adverse Effects

- Anovulation due to the reduction in the frequency and amplitude of LH pulsatility
- Retards follicular development
- Decreases sensitivity of corpus luteum to LH, consequently there is decreased synthesis of progesterone
- Directly inhibits ovarian secretion of E_2 and progesterone

Investigations

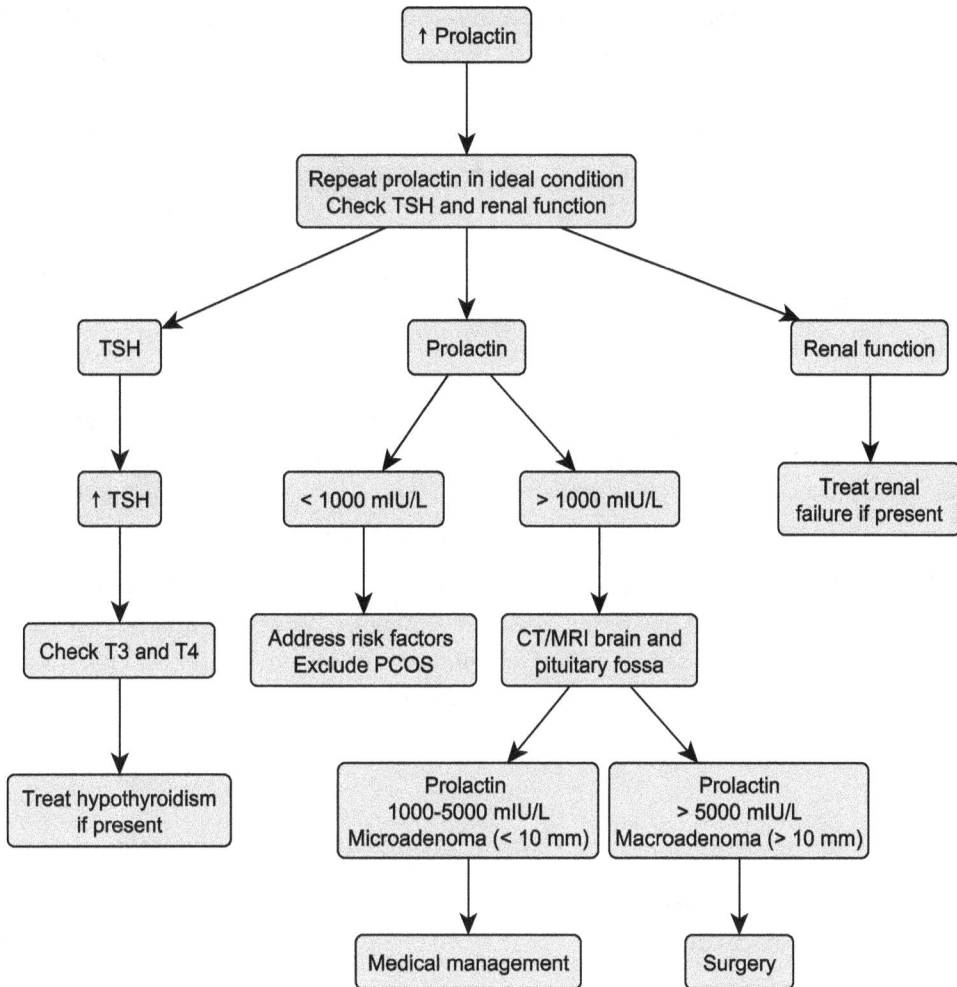

Figure 7.4. Diagnostic algorithm for hyperprolactinaemia

Management

Take a focused history of the presenting problems, factors affecting prolactin secretion, any chronic illnesses, and use of any relevant drugs. Ask whether the blood test for the prolactin level was done soon after a gynaecological or breast examination. Establish the woman's expectation of treatment. Explore if the woman wants to conceive, or if her main aim is symptomatic improvement.

Expectant

Asymptomatic women with hyperprolactinaemia and microadenoma who do not wish to conceive may be followed without any medical treatment by measuring serum prolactin levels once a year.

Medical

Asymptomatic women with hyperprolactinaemia and microadenoma with low oestradiol levels and who do not want to conceive may be treated by the combined oral contraceptive pill. Since side effects, cost, and compliance are all better for the COC pill compared with bromocriptine/cabergoline, the former is the preferred treatment.

If these women desire to conceive, then dopamine receptor agonists, such as bromocriptine, pergolide, and cabergoline, should be used.

Bromocriptine: It inhibits prolactin secretion. It may need to be taken orally 3 to 5 times daily. The most common side effect is orthostatic hypotension (incidence 15%). Other side effects such as nausea, vomiting, and nasal stuffiness may occur in about half of women. With daily vaginal administration (2.5 mg daily), the side effects are nonexistent. Prolactin levels decrease in a few days, and reduction in tumour size takes about 6 weeks. Macroadenomas are reduced in size in 80–90% of women. In 10% of women with microadenomas, despite bromocriptine administration, the prolactin level does not reduce. This is possibly because of an altered sensitivity of lactotrophs to bromocriptine. The treatment should be continued for one year, unless pregnancy ensues in that time.

Cabergoline: It is a long-acting dopamine receptor agonist that directly inhibits pituitary lactotrophs. The dose is 0.5 mg twice weekly. It has fewer side effects than bromocriptine and is more effective. It reduces prolactin level in 83% of women, induces ovulation in 72%, and stops galactorrhoea in 90%. It is the drug of choice these days, and treatment should be continued at least for 6 months after the prolactin level has returned to normal.

Surgery

Transsphenoidal microsurgical resection of prolactinoma is the mainstay of surgical treatment.

- Recurrence rate for microadenoma   21%
- Recurrence rate for macroadenoma   19%
- Long-term cure rate for microadenoma   58%
- Long-term cure rate for macroadenoma   26%

The indication for surgery is failed medical treatment for a macroadenoma. It is preferable to treat macroadenomas medically first to reduce the size before attempting surgery.

Radiotherapy

Radiotherapy is rarely used—only when all other treatments have failed.

Chapter 7.2.5.   Unexplained Infertility

When a woman is unable to conceive despite patent fallopian tube(s), ovulation, a normal semen count of the male partner, and successful and timely coitus, the condition is classified as "unexplained." In practice, this is the largest group of infertility patients.

Such women benefit from intrauterine insemination following ovarian stimulation.

There is no evidence to substantiate that luteal-phase deficiency, antisperm antibodies in males and females, subclinical genital infection, or subclinical endocrinopathies, such as hyperprolactinemia hypothyroidism, or hyperthyroidism, cause infertility.

Chapter 7.2.6.   Male Infertility

The classification of male causes of infertility is as follows:

- Testicular disease (30–40%)
- Primary hypogonadism (hypergonadotropic hypogonadism)
  - Disorders of sperm, number, morphology, and motility
  - Congenital and developmental disorders, e.g., Klinefelter's syndrome (XXY) or cryptorchidism
  - Acquired disorders, e.g., varicocele, testicular cancer, and radiation
- Secondary hypogonadism (hypergonadotropic hypogonadism—LH, FSH, and GnRH deficiency)
  - Congenital disorders, e.g., Kallmann syndrome, haemochromatosis
  - Acquired disorders, e.g., pituitary neoplasms, craniopharyngioma
  - Systemic disorders, e.g., malnutrition, marijuana use, chronic illnesses, and obesity
- Disorders of sperm transport (10–20%)
  - For example, absent or obstructed vas deferens

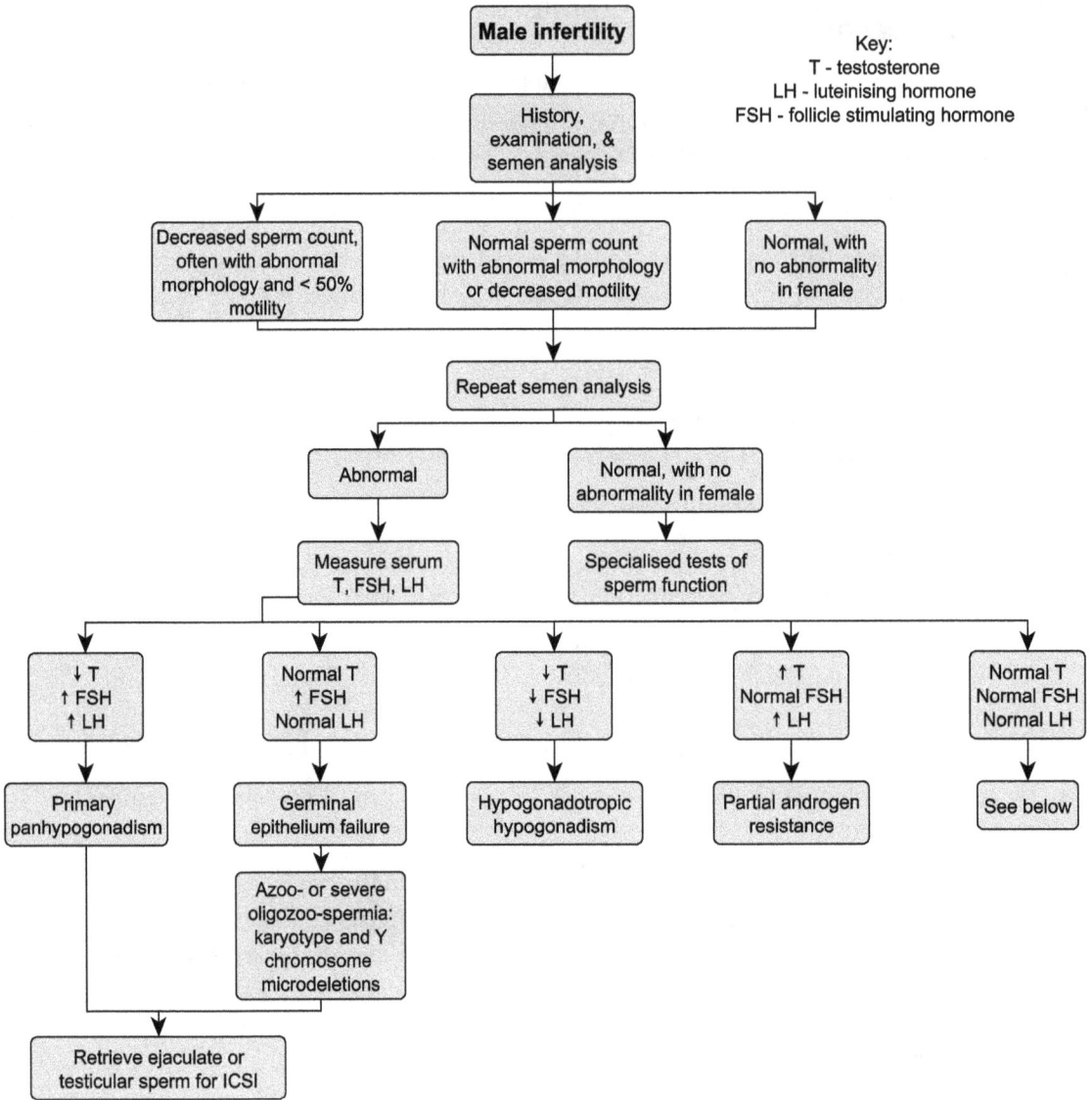

Figure 7.5. Approach to diagnosis of male infertility, modified from uptodate.com.
If normal T, LH, and FSH, then detailed semen analysis and treatment of abnormalities is required

Chapter 7.2.7.   Surrogacy

Surrogacy is a way of creating a family in which a woman (surrogate) carries a pregnancy for a related or unrelated couple, with the express intention of giving up all parental rights to the commissioning (intended) parent(s).

Definitions

Commercial surrogacy	The surrogate is rewarded financially or otherwise over and above her medical and allied expenses for undertaking the pregnancy.
Altruistic surrogacy	The surrogate is only compensated for medical and allied expenses for undertaking the pregnancy.
Gestational surrogate	Same as surrogate. A gestational surrogate has no genetic bond to the embryo.

Table 7.6. Chapter 7.2.7. Definitions

Indications

- A woman's inability to conceive
- A woman's or fetus's health would be endangered if she were to fall pregnant
- A couple of the same sex wishing to have a child

Medical and Psychological Evaluation

The gestational surrogate and the commissioning parent(s) should undergo a thorough medical and psychological evaluation. The surrogate should be screened for the following:

- HIV, viral hepatitis, syphilis, gonorrhoea, chlamydia, varicella, rubella, and CMV
- Use of tobacco, alcohol, and recreational drugs
- Her moral and ethical views regarding surrogacy
- Emotional state

The surrogate's partner should also be screened for STIs and CMV.

The commissioning parent(s) should also be screened for the same infectious diseases as the surrogate.

Prerequisites for Surrogate

- Young
- In good general health, with no chronic or communicable diseases
- Good past obstetric history: previous full-term pregnancy and delivery

Contractual Issues

The lawyers of the surrogate and commissioning parent(s) should draft legally binding contracts for both parties. The contract should specifically cover the following areas:

- To what extent could the commissioning parent(s) influence the conduct of the surrogate and her partner that may affect the pregnancy?
- Can the surrogate continue the pregnancy if the commissioning parent(s) want(s) her to terminate it?
- Will the surrogate be asked to breastfeed or provide her breast milk?
- In the event of sudden death of the commissioning parent(s), what will be the responsibility of the surrogate, and what will happen to the newborn?

IVF

The commissioning parent(s) could provide the egg and sperm, if able to. Otherwise, egg or sperm could be procured from registered donors. Both the surrogate and the commissioning mother (if providing the egg) are made to synchronise their menstrual cycles. The egg is harvested from the commissioning mother, fertilised in vitro, and transferred into the uterus of the surrogate at the appropriate time. Frozen embryos could also be used.

Consequences of Surrogacy

- The live-birth rate of the surrogate is comparable to age-matched controls undergoing IVF.
- The developmental milestones of the child are comparable to children born in a conventional situation.
- Surrogates do not suffer from any short-term or long-term consequences, either medically or emotionally, as a result of participating in surrogacy.

Short-Answer Questions

Question 1

How does cancer affect a woman's fertility?

Answer:

Cancer prevalence increases with age. The rate of survival from cancer treatment is improving, but the incidence of cancer is not reducing.

A woman's chance of developing temporary or permanent ovarian failure is related to her age, diagnosis, and specific treatment methods for the cancer.

With increasing age, ovarian reserve decreases. In addition, if a woman undergoes chemotherapy, it adversely affects cell division and DNA function within the developing follicle. Even if the menstrual period returns after a period of amenorrhoea, follicle numbers are reduced, and the markers of ovarian reserve start to become abnormal.

Alkylating agents (cyclophosphamide, protein) are particularly toxic to the ovary.

Radiotherapy to the pelvis can damage pelvic structures irreparably, especially the endometrium and myometrium. Cranial radiation can affect pituitary function.

Question 2

Discuss the methods for fertility preservation in a woman who is about to start cancer treatment.

Answer:

The following options for fertility preservation during chemotherapy and radiotherapy are available, although many are largely experimental.

i.   GnRH analogues: They have been shown to protect the ovary during chemotherapy in animal models. The mechanism of this effect is poorly understood; however, it could be mediated by either ovarian blood-flow reduction or AMH activity. Immunomodulators are also being trialled for this purpose.

ii. Embryo-freezing: Cryopreservation of embryos prior to treatment offers the best chance of a successful pregnancy. The pregnancy rate for each transferred embryo is 25–30% for a woman under 37 years of age. The problems of this method are the following:

   • It will delay start of cancer treatment.
   • Ovarian stimulation may have harmful effects on hormonally sensitive tumours, e.g., breast, endometrium.
   • Many women with cancer do not respond well to ovarian stimulation.
   • Lack of a partner or a stable relationship.

iii. Oocyte freezing: Instead of embryo freezing, mature oocytes could be frozen after ovarian stimulation. This is suitable for women who don't have a male partner or are not in a stable relationship. Initial experience with this technique does not show an increase in complications such as miscarriage or congenital abnormality. The drawback of this technique is the time needed for ovarian stimulation, which may delay the start of chemotherapy and radiotherapy.

iv. Ovarian tissue freezing and grafting: It is now possible to cryopreserve the whole or part of an ovary prior to chemotherapy and radiotherapy. There is no need for ovarian stimulation. The ovary is removed laparoscopically. Drawbacks are the following:

   • The ovarian tissue removed may harbour malignant cells, particularly in acute leukaemia, and hence can lead to relapse of the cancer after grafting of the ovarian tissue.
   • The follicular development in the grafted tissue does not always follow typical cyclical patterns.

Question 3

How does infertility affect cancer?

Answer:

Infertile women are at significantly increased risk of developing ovarian and uterine cancers, especially when nulliparous. Multiple cycles of high doses of clomiphene have been shown to increase uterine cancer risk.

Question 4

Critically appraise the ovarian reserve markers.

Answer:

Ovarian reserve implies the quantity of primordial follicles in an ovary at a given point in time. Different markers have been discovered that represent ovarian reserve and are used in IVF.

<u>Serum FSH</u>: Measurement of serum FSH on day 2 or 3 of the cycle has been used as a marker of ovarian reserve. As the oocyte pool decreases with advancing age, higher levels of pituitary stimulation are needed for follicular development. Hence, a higher serum FSH level represents lower ovarian reserve. However, FSH level varies from month to month and within the same month, and it also varies due to the pulsatile release from the pituitary. No cut-off level for poor outcome is agreed.

<u>Inhibin B</u>: It is produced from small antral follicles in response to FSH stimulation and hence is dependent on FSH levels.

<u>Anti-Müllerian hormone (AMH)</u>: It is secreted mainly by the preantral follicles and is a marker of the size of the antral follicular pool. A lower value indicates a small antral pool, whereas a higher value indicates PCOS. Its advantage is that there is no inter/intracyclic variation, and hence it can be measured at any stage of the cycle. Additionally, short-term use of the COC pill has no effect on its level. It is not a predictor of pregnancy outcome.

It also induces the regression of the Müllerian duct in a male fetus, where it is synthesised by the Sertoli cells.

<u>Antral follicular count (AFC)</u>: The number of small antral follicles (2–10 mm) also reflects ovarian reserve. Its drawback is its dependency on the sonographer. Studies have not shown any benefit over AMH. A combination of AMH and AFC offers better prediction of oocyte yield.

<u>Oocyte quality</u>: Oocyte numbers correlate with oocyte quality in older women. This is based on the fact that with increasing age, the number of oocytes decreases, whereas the incidence of karyotypic abnormalities increases. However, a young IVF patient with low oocyte count may still show good oocyte quality.

There is a higher incidence of aneuploidy in IVF embryos, but none of the above markers reflect that. They are also poor predictors of pregnancy outcomes.

Question 5

How will you assess and manage a 30-year-old man with azoospermia?

Answer:

Assessment:

- Repeat semen analysis in 3 months
- Focused history
  - Medical disorders
  - Mumps
  - Cystic fibrosis
  - Drugs, including recreational drugs
  - Testicular trauma
- Examination
  - Penile and testicular abnormalities
  - Presence of vas deferens
  - Features of Klinefelter's syndrome
- Investigations
  - Serum FSH, LH, and testosterone
  - Depending upon the result, further tests will be required—for example:
    - Testicular biopsy if obstruction likely
    - Karyotype if high FSH

Treatment:

- Counselling
- Treat the cause—for example:
  - If hyperprolactinemia, treat with dopamine agonist
  - Surgery if vas deferens obstructed
- Artificial insemination with donor sperm
- Adoption
- ICSI

Question 6

How does age affect male fertility?

Answer:

Increasing age affects male fertility adversely. After the age of about 40 years, the following changes occur:

- Disordered spermatogenesis
- Reduced sperm testosterone
- Reduced sexual desire and activity
- Changed testicular morphology
- Deterioration of sperm quality volume, morphology, and motility
- Fragmentation of sperm DNA

The adverse effect of age on male fertility is much less than on female fertility, but if both male and female are of advanced age, fecundity is substantially reduced.

Question 7

How does age affect female fertility?

Answer:

Increasing age affects female fertility adversely. After the age of about 35 years, apart from decreasing oocyte numbers, the following changes in the oocyte quality occur:

- Disordered spindle formation
- Disordered chromosome segregation
- Disordered mitochondrial function
- Disordered function of the cytoskeleton
- Disordered fertilisation and implantation
- Disordered cell division of the zygote

There is increased evidence of miscarriage (51%), ectopic pregnancy, and stillbirth in older women. Obstetric complications due to increased maternal age are the following:

- GDM
- Placenta praevia
- Placental abruption
- Hypertension
- Caesarean section

All these adverse effects could be avoided by a donor egg.

Question 8

Discuss the effects of obesity on gynaecological pathophysiology.

Answer:

The disease of obesity (BMI > 30 kg/m^2) is on the rise in the developing world. The risks of increased mortality and morbidity from hypertension, CAD, dyslipidaemia, type 2 diabetes, stroke, gallstones, osteoarthritis, sleep apnoea, and cancers of the endometrium, breast, and colon are increasing. They are further increased with morbid obesity or when obesity begins in the adolescent years.

The increased adipose tissue aromatises androgens to oestrogens. Obese women also have lower levels of sex hormone–binding globulin (SHBG), which allows a greater fraction of androgen to circulate in the blood "unbound" and hence be active. Additionally, because of low SHBG, more androgens are converted to oestrone. As a result of this, the following diseases develop:

- Hirsutism due to increased unbound androgen.
- PCOS, because obesity causes increased insulin resistance, and hyperinsulinaemia leads to PCOS.
- Menstrual abnormalities and anovulation due to the interactions of increased androgens and oestrogens with other hormones and IGF-1 causing abnormal feedback to the GnRH pulse generator.
- Higher incidence of endometrial cancer is due to increased amount of oestrogens.

Obesity also increases intra-abdominal pressure and damages the pelvic floor, causing an increased incidence of stress incontinence or exacerbation of the condition if it is preexisting. A dose-response relationship between BMI and stress incontinence exists.

Postoperatively, there is a higher incidence of complications in obese patients, such as DVT, pulmonary embolism, problems in wound healing, and necrotising fasciitis.

Question 9

A couple, both 28 years old, have been trying to conceive for over 2 years. A diagnosis of unexplained infertility is made. What will be your advice to the couple? Which factors will affect the result of the treatments?

Answer:

My advice will be as follows:

Counselling:

- Importance of timely intercourse, a day prior to the expected ovulation.
- Up to 3% of couples with unexplained infertility will conceive in each cycle.
- Up to 60% of couples with unexplained infertility of less than 3 years will conceive within 3 years.

Behavioural modification:

- Reduce smoking, alcohol, and caffeine intake, and stop recreational drugs.
- Reduce or increase weight depending on the BMI. Ideal BMI for conception is 22–27 kg/m^2.

Proposed treatment plan:

- Folate and iodine supplementation, if not already being taken.
- Do Pap smear if due.
- Check rubella immunity.
- Intrauterine insemination, with or without ovulation induction. The pregnancy rate is 46% without ovulation induction and 10% with ovulation induction.
- Ovulation induction with clomiphene, or with gonadotropins if that is unsuccessful.

	Clomiphene	Gonadotropins
Pregnancy rate	4–6% each cycle	8–10% each cycle
Multiple pregnancy rate	8%	20–25%
Cost	Cheap	Expensive
Incidence of OHSS	< 1%	1–5%

- IVF/ICSI pregnancy rate is 30%.
- Donor sperm if nothing works.

Factors affecting the result of treatment:

- Age—better result with younger age
- Previous pregnancies—better result with previous pregnancies
- Duration of infertility—better results when the diagnosis of unexplained infertility was made within 3 years
- Absence of comorbidities, such as obesity and diabetes
- Lifestyle factors—smoking, alcohol, caffeine, and recreational drugs

Question 10

You have found bilateral hydrosalpinges (left = 3 cm, right = 2 cm) during a laparoscopy for pelvic pain in a 25-year-old nulliparous woman.

Part a

What will you do intra-operatively?

Answer:

Look for causes of pelvic pain, such as salpingitis, adhesions, and endometriosis, and deal with them. Bilateral salpingectomy could only be done if prior consent had been obtained. The role of salpingostomy is unclear.

Part b

At a 3-week postoperative visit, what will you tell her?

Answer:

- I will explain the intra-operative findings and inquire about the pelvic pain.
- The hydrosalpinges are most likely from prior infection (chlamydia, gonorrhoea), endometriosis, ruptured appendix, or other pelvic surgery.
- It is very unlikely that a spontaneous conception will occur.
- Incidence of a tubal pregnancy will be higher if a conception does occur.
- She will need an STI screen and contact tracing if the STI screen is positive.
- Laparoscopic bilateral salpingectomy followed by IVF is the most realistic option for her to achieve a conception.
- IVF without salpingectomy has lower pregnancy rates, possibly due to the leakage of fluid from the hydrosalpinx into the endometrial cavity, adversely affecting implantation of the blastocyst.

Part c

What are the surgical risks of laparoscopic bilateral salpingectomy?

Answer:

- Risks of bleeding:
  - Veress needle going into major iliac vessels
  - Lateral trocars damaging superficial inferior epigastric vessels or inferior epigastric artery (1: 1000)
  - Trauma to paratubal venous plexus
  - Port site
- Infection
- Visceral trauma during initial trocar placement or intra-operatively
- Gas embolism
- Conversion to laparotomy (0.2–1%)
- Risk of death (1: 12000)

Multiple-Choice Questions

Q1. Fallopian tube motility is adversely affected by which of the following syndromes?

    A. Turner's

    B. Marfan's

    C. Kartagener's

    D. Noonan's

Answer: C

Q2. For ovulation induction, clomiphene works best in which of the following?

    A. Hypogonadotropic hypogonadism

    B. Normogonadotrophic hypogonadism

    C. Hypergonadotrophic hypogonadism

    D. All of the above

Answer: B

Q3. Which of the following statements about ovarian hyperstimulation syndrome (OHSS) is incorrect?

    A. Late-onset OHSS is more likely to be severe.

    B. Late-onset OHSS lasts for less time than early-onset OHSS.

    C. OHSS within 9 days after hCG administration reflects excessive ovarian response.

    D. OHSS after 9 days of hCG administration reflects endogenous hCG stimulation
       from an early pregnancy.

Answer: B

Q4. Which of the following seminal fluid parameters better correlates to fertilising ability of the spermatozoa?

    A. Volume

    B. Morphology

    C. Absolute number

    D. Motility

Answer: B

Q5. The highest probability of conception following treatment is when:

    A. Anovulation is the only abnormality.

    B. Tubal disease is the only abnormality.

    C. Sperm abnormality is the only abnormality.

    D. The woman is 40 years of age.

Answer: A

Q6. Which of the following is false for infertility treatment?

A. Perinatal mortality is not increased.

B. Spontaneous abortion rate is increased.

C. Incidence of ectopic pregnancy is increased.

D. Incidence of multiple pregnancy is increased.

Answer: B

Q7. What do increased serum FSH and LH levels indicate?

A. Pituitary tumour

B. Pituitary failure

C. Ovarian tumour

D. Ovarian failure

Answer: D

Q8. Increased BBT correlates with increased serum level of which of the following?

A. Oestradiol

B. Progesterone

C. FSH

D. LH

Answer: B

Q9. For conception to occur, which is the best time for sexual intercourse is?

A. When LH surge occurs

B. 1 day before LH surge

C. 2 days before LH surge

D. 1 day after LH surge

Answer: A (LH surge occurs 1 day before ovulation)

Q10. Which of the following is the most plausible explanation for decreased oocyte quality with aging?

A. Age-related deterioration of granulosa cells

B. Increased meiotic nondisjunction

C. Effect of environmental factors, such as smoking, pollution, and increasing BMI

D. Damage to germ cells from comorbidities that happen with aging

Answer: B

Q11. By what percentage does vaginal douching reduce the chance of conception?

A. 10%

B. 20%

C. 30%

D. 40%

Answer: C

Q12. Which of the following statements regarding basal body temperature (BBT) is correct?

   A. A rise in BBT indicates that ovulation will occur.

   B. A rise in BBT is a precise indication of ovulation.

   C. BBT can be recorded any time of the day or night.

   D. BBT is recorded just after waking up in the morning, and the thermometer is placed sublingually.

Answer: D

Q13. A 45-year-old lady presents with secondary infertility after having 2 vaginal births, 16 and 20 years ago. She had amenorrhoea for 7 months. Her pregnancy test is negative. Which of the following tests should be done first?

   A. Serum FSH/LH levels

   B. Endometrial biopsy

   C. Tubal patency test

   D. Midluteal progesterone

Answer: A (Need to exclude menopause)

Q14. A 25-year-old is diagnosed with a bicornuate uterus during the investigation for infertility. Which of the following abnormalities needs to be excluded further?

   A. Skeletal

   B. Renal

   C. Gastrointestinal

   D. Cardiac

Answer: B

Q15. Artificial insemination with the husband semen is **not** indicated in which of the following conditions?

   A. Unexplained infertility

   B. Impotence

   C. Azoospermia

   D. Oligospermia

Answer: C

Q16. Which of the following conditions has the highest risk of Asherman's syndrome after a D&C?

   A. Termination of pregnancy

   B. Postpartum haemorrhage

   C. Endometrial hyperplasia

   D. Atrophic endometrium

Answer: C (A greater surface area of endometrium is curetted)

Q17. A 33-year-old lady had a miscarriage at 13 weeks' gestation nearly 6 months ago. She has had amenorrhoea since then. There was no withdrawal bleeding following a progesterone challenge test with a prior course of oestradiol. What is the cause of her amenorrhoea?

A. Ovarian failure

B. Pituitary failure

C. Asherman's syndrome

D. Anovulation

Answer: C (A failed oestrogen and progesterone challenge test indicates end-organ failure, i.e. Asherman's syndrome.)

Q18. Which of the following is the most frequent cause of slightly elevated prolactin?

A. Stress

B. Sleep

C. Coitus

D. Exercise

Answer: A

Q19. Which of the following drugs will raise serum prolactin levels?

A. Antioestrogens

B. Gonadotropins

C. Phenothiazines

D. Prostaglandins

Answer: C

Q20. Semen analysis shows the absence of sperm but the presence of fructose. What is the most likely cause for this presentation?

A. Mumps orchitis in the past

B. Prostatic infection

C. Block in the efferent duct system

D. Sample collected after too-frequent ejaculations

Answer: C

Q21. The most common Müllerian abnormality is:

A. Unicornuate uterus

B. Bicornuate uterus

C. Septate uterus

D. Müllerian agenesis

Answer: C

Q22. Which of the following could be used to treat abdominal distension and discomfort in a 23-year-old with OHSS?

    A. Mefenamic acid

    B. Ethacrynic acid

    C. Tranexamic acid

    D. Abdominal paracentesis

Answer: D

Q23. A rising serum FSH to promote development of developing follicles in the perimenopausal years is because of:

    A. Depleting oocyte numbers

    B. Depleting oocyte quality

    C. Depleting ovarian blood supply

    D. Decreasing ovarian size

Answer: A

Q24. The earliest histological evidence of ovulation is:

    A. Predecidual reaction

    B. Decrease in glycogen in the endometrial cells

    C. Subnucleolar vacuolations

    D. Pseudostratification

Answer: C

Q25. A woman presents with amenorrhoea, 4 months after an evacuation of retained products of conception for an incomplete miscarriage at a 9 weeks' gestation. Her serum FSH is 8 IU/L. What is the most likely explanation?

    A. Ovarian failure

    B. Pituitary failure

    C. Asherman's syndrome

    D. Product of conception still retained in the uterus

Answer: C

Q26. A 20-year-old presents with a history of lower abdominal pain for almost 2 days, 3 weeks before her period finishes. She has a 28-day cycle, and her period lasts for up to a week. The most probable cause of her pain is:

    A. Spinnbarkeit

    B. Mittelschmerz

    C. Couvelaire uterus

    D. Molimina

Answer: B

Q27. Which of the following analgesics should be used in a healthy 22-year-old with mittelschmerz who does **not** want to ovulate?

A. Paracetamol

B. NSAIDs

C. Narcotic

D. A combination of all of the above

Answer: B

Q28. A hysterosalpingogram should be performed on which of the following days of a 28-day menstrual cycle?

A. Day 4

B. Day 8

C. Day 12

D. Day 16

Answer: B

Q29. A hysteroscopy is **not** used for the investigation of which of the following conditions?

A. Subfertility

B. A woman passing large clots during her periods

C. Asherman's syndrome

D. Recurrent stillbirth

Answer: D

Q30. Which of the following applications of reproductive technology is least justified on ethical grounds?

A. Tubal reanastomosis in a 41-year-old female

B. Donor insemination of an unmarried woman

C. Surrogate motherhood for a married professional woman who does not want to stop the treatment of mild endometriosis

D. IVF in a 27-year-old woman with blocked fallopian tubes whose father has Huntington's chorea

Answer: C

Q31. A 32-year-old woman with 4 years of infertility had a recent laparoscopy that showed moderate pelvic endometriosis without adhesions. Medical treatment for endometriosis has been recommended. You advise her that:

A. The pregnancy rate after medical therapy is not related to the initial stage of the disease

B. Danazol is most effective when administered as a single daily dose

C. The degree of ovarian suppression achieved by GnRH agonists is greater than that achieved by danazol

D. Newer drugs for endometriosis have better pregnancy rates than surgery

Answer: C

Q32. Following ovulation, the survival of the unfertilised human egg is approximately:

A. 12–24 hours

B. 24–48 hours

C. 2–3 days

D. 4–5 days

Answer: A

Q33. Which of the following tests would be helpful in investigating azoospermia in a 33-year-old man?

A. Serum prolactin

B. Serum FSH

C. Karyotype

D. Cystic fibrosis genetic studies

Answer: C

Q34. The incidence of ovarian hyperstimulation syndrome after clomiphene ovulation induction is:

A. < 1%

B. 5–10%

C. 15–20%

D. 25–30%

Answer: A

Q35. A 22-year-old nulliparous woman with oligomenorrhoea and idiopathic hyperprolactinaemia is on bromocriptine 2.5 mg BD. She wants to fall pregnant. She experiences orthostatic symptoms and moderate nausea. A pregnancy test is negative. Serum TSH and MRI brain are normal. The most appropriate step in her management is to:

A. Continue with bromocriptine, and she will become tolerant to it.

B. Stop bromocriptine.

C. Halve the dose till she becomes tolerant.

D. Increase the dose.

Answer: C

Q36. The chance of pregnancy in a healthy 20-year-old nulliparous woman from a single act of coitus one day before ovulation is about:

A. 1%

B. 5%

C. 20%

D. 30%

Answer: C

Q37. A man with X-linked recessive disorder marries a normal homozygous woman. They have two children. The probability that both the children will have the disorder is:

  A. 0

  B. 1 in 8

  C. 1 in 4

  D. 1 in 2

Answer: A

Q38. The human zygote reaches the uterus in approximately:

  A. 36 hours after ovulation

  B. 5 days after ovulation

  C. 7 days after ovulation

  D. 9 days after ovulation

Answer: B

Q39. Crossing over of chromosomes takes place during:

  A. metaphase 1

  B. mitotic prophase

  C. meiotic prophase 1

  D. meiotic prophase 2

Answer: C

Q40. Which of the following is most common?

  A. Tay-Sachs disease

  B. Phenylketonuria

  C. Duchenne dystrophy

  D. Cystic fibrosis

Answer: D

Q41. In which of the following conditions will medical treatment enhance pregnancy rates compared with no treatment?

  A. Anorexia nervosa

  B. Hyperprolactinaemia in an ovulating woman

  C. Antibodies to sperm in the woman

  D. Ovarian failure due to resistant ovarian failure

Answer: A

Q42. The reporting requirements for randomised trials are contained in the:

  A. NICE standard

  B. CONSORT statement

  C. COCHRANE database

  D. QUOROM checklist

Answer: B

Q43. A 26-year-old with hypothalamic amenorrhea wants to get pregnant. In this context, ovulation induction with GnRH is effective if:

A. The drug is administered as a continuous infusion for 14 days

B. The drug is administered in a pulsatile fashion

C. hCG is used to trigger ovulation

D. HMG is administered simultaneously

Answer: B

Q44. Which of the following genetic conditions is not associated with a particular ethnic group?

A. Tay-Sachs disease

B. Sickle cell disease

C. Alpha thalassaemia

D. Von Willebrand disease

Answer: D

Q45. Which of the following statements is correct regarding the use of clomiphene for primary infertility?

A. The risk of teratogenicity is 2%.

B. The risk of ovarian cancer increases by 5%.

C. The risk of multiple pregnancy is 5–10%.

D. The risk of ovarian hyperstimulation is 15%.

Answer: C

Q46. In women receiving clomiphene citrate for induction of ovulation, the frequency of complications is:

A. < 1%

B. 5–10%

C. 15–20%

D. 25–30%

Answer: B

Chapter **8**
Contraception

Chapter 8.1.   Combined Oral Contraceptive Pill

Clinical Physiology

The combined oral contraceptive pills (COC) have synthetic oestrogen and progestin components.

Progestins

The following types of progestins have been used so far:

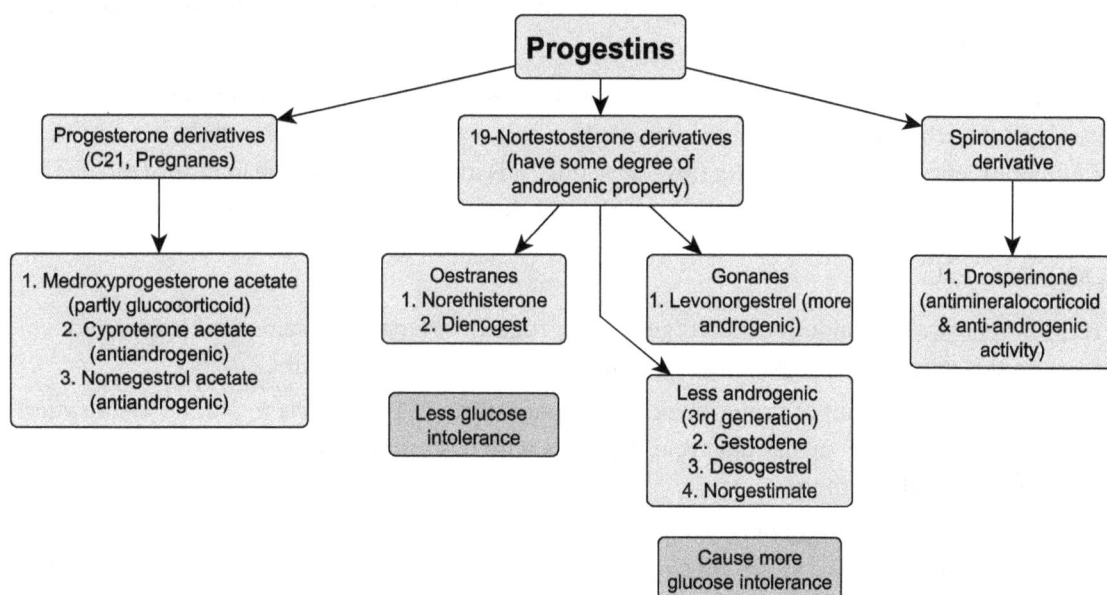

Figure 8.1. Types of progestins used in hormonal contraception

In terms of contraceptive efficacy, there is no difference between the different types of progestins. However, compared with oestranes, gonanes have significantly higher progestogenic effect; hence a smaller amount is required in the COC. The progestins differ in their side effect profile and also in their affinities for oestrogen, androgens, and progesterone receptors. Some attach to receptors directly, such as levonorgestrel, whereas others need bioactivation, such as desogestrel, which is almost completely converted to its active, metabolite etonogestrel, in the liver.

Oestrogens

The following types of oestrogens have been used in the COC:

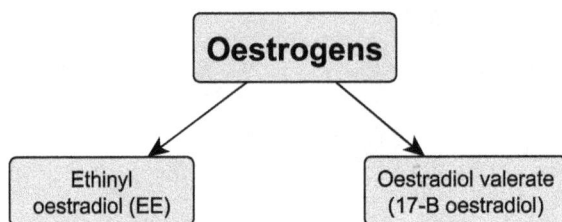

Figure 8.2. Types of oestrogens used in hormonal contraception

Oestradiol valerate is the prodrug for 17-β oestradiol which is identical to oestradiol produced by the ovary. Ethinyl oestradiol is about 100 times more potent than conjugated equine oestrogen or oestrone sulphate and 1.7 times more potent than mestranol.

The synthetic oestrogens and progestins in COC have an ethinyl group at position 17, which makes them more potent when taken orally. This is because the ethinyl group slows down their breakdown in the liver.

The amount of oestrogens and progestins in COC has reduced significantly over the years to reduce the side effects, while maintaining its contraceptive efficacy. Most of the commonly used COC have 30–35 μg of EE, the lowest being 20 μg (low-dose pill). It is unclear whether the low-dose pill has fewer side effects compared with the normal-dose pill, but is known to have poorer cycle control.

Types of COC

1. Monophasic: The amount of oestrogens and progestins remain the same for 21 days. No steroid is given for the next 7 days, when the withdrawal bleed occurs.

2. Biphasic: The amount of progestins changes once during 21-day cycle to minimise side effects and mimic a natural menstrual cycle. The pills with oestradiol valerate have a higher chance of no withdrawal bleeding.

3. Multiphasic: The amount of oestrogens and progestins changes 2–4 times during a pill cycle. This regimen enables a lower dose of steroid administration to the woman and hence fewer side effects.

Recently, some new COC have been developed where the steroids (oestradiol and nomegestrol) are given for 24 days with no active pills for 2 days. This is supposed to reduce side effects in the steroid-free period, such as pelvic pain, headache, and bloating.

Lengthening the steroid-free period to more than 7 days detracts from COC's contraceptive efficacy.

Mode of Action

The oestrogen component of the COC prevents ovulation mainly by inhibiting the release of GnRH from the hypothalamus. It also inhibits gonadotropin secretion from the pituitary gland. Pituitary suppression is better achieved in 35–50 μg pills.

The progestin component of the COC makes the cervical mucus thicker and more viscous, thereby obstructing sperm migration. They also reduce uterine and tubal contractility, which reduces migration of both sperm and ova. Progestins also reduce the glycogen content of the endometrial cells, thereby making them less responsive to implantation.

No study has shown any significant difference in the contraceptive efficacy of different formulations of the COC. The pregnancy rate is 0.3% at 1 year with perfect use.

Benefits

- Decreased dysmenorrhoea severity and blood loss.
- Decrease in functional ovarian cysts and benign ovarian tumours.
- Decrease in benign breast disease.
- Decrease in the incidence of PID and acne.
- Decrease in the incidence of endometrial and ovarian cancer by 50%. This effect lasts for up to 15 years after stopping the COC.
- Possible protective effect against rheumatoid arthritis, duodenal ulcers, and thyroid problems.

Side Effects

Most common:

- Nausea (CNS effect), breast tenderness, and fluid retention (mild) caused by increased aldosterone synthesis and decreased sodium and fluid excretion. These effects are oestrogenic in origin.

Less common:

- Melasma.
- Mood changes and depression could be oestrogenic or progestogenic in origin.
- Androgenic effects include weight gain and acne. These are progestogenic side effects.
  - Weight gain is due to the anabolic effects of progestins.
  - Progestins increase sebum production. whereas oestrogens decrease it. Hence, women with acne should be prescribed a COC with a low progestin-oestrogen ratio.
- Failure of withdrawal bleed due to progestins suppressing endometrial proliferation.
- Breakthrough bleeding due to insufficient oestrogen, an excess of progestins. or both. It is treated by increasing oestrogen content or by prescribing a more potent oestrogen.

- Effect on protein metabolism:
  - Synthetic oestrogens increase hepatic production of globulins and clotting factors V, VIII, X. and fibrinogen.
  - Increased synthesis of angiotensinogen leads to hypertension.
  - Progestins, however, decrease the synthesis of sex hormone–binding globulin (SHBG).
  - The incidence of venous and arterial thrombosis is increased due to increased production of globulins and clotting factors, as mentioned above, and is oestrogen-dose dependent.

- Effect on carbohydrate metabolism:
  - Impaired glucose metabolism is a progestogenic side effect and is dose dependent

- Effect on lipid metabolism:
  - Oestrogen increases HDL, total cholesterol, and triglycerides. It decreases LDL.
  - Progestins decreases HDL, total cholesterol, and triglycerides but increases LDL.

- Effect on myocardial infarction:
  - COC increases the incidence of myocardial infarction, especially in the presence of smoking and hypertension.

- Effect on cerebrovascular accidents:
  - The risk is increased, especially in the presence of smoking and hypertension.

- Effect on cancers:
  - The risk of breast cancer is increased while the COC is taken, but this decreases to the background risk ten years after the COC has been discontinued.
  - The incidence of liver cancer, cervical intraepithelial neoplasia, and cervical cancer increases.

Interaction with Other Drugs

COC interacts with some other drugs by increasing their efficacy, e.g., aspirin, warfarin, diazepam, metoprolol, and antiretroviral drugs. Hence, lower doses of these drugs may be effective when COC is being used concurrently.

COC also interacts with some drugs that are hepatic enzyme inducers, and hence, their own efficacy gets reduced (e.g., phenytoin, phenobarbital, carbamazepine, rifampicin, and griseofulvin). Hence, with the concomitant use of these drugs, the dose of COC must be increased, or alternative contraceptive methods should also be used.

Contraindications

Absolute:

- History of cardiovascular disease, such as:
  - Thromboembolism
  - Thrombophlebitis
  - Cerebrovascular accident
  - Congestive cardiac failure
  - Uncontrolled hypertension

- Presence of systemic diseases that may affect the vascular system:
    - Systemic lupus erythematosus
    - Diabetes mellitus with end-artery involvement

- Undiagnosed uterine bleeding.
- Elevated serum triglycerides.
- Use in pregnancy may masculinise the external genitalia of a female fetus.
- Presence of active liver disease.
- Smoking in over-35-year age group.

Relative:

- Heavy smoking in less-than-35-year age group.
- Migraine.
- Depression.
- Prolactin-secreting macroadenoma.

How to Start the COC?

The COC should only be started after proper counselling and excluding any contraindications. Usually a 30–35 μg monophasic pill is chosen in an otherwise normal woman. Progestins with lower androgenic effect should be selected. The use of multiphasic pills allows a reduced progestin component and is not the COC of first choice in an uncomplicated young woman.

In adolescents, once the regular ovulatory cycles have started, a COC can be prescribed.

After spontaneous or induced abortion of less than 12 weeks' gestation, a COC can be started immediately.

For deliveries of babies after 28 weeks in a woman who is not breastfeeding, a COC can be started 2–3 weeks after delivery.

In women who are completely breastfeeding without the use of any artificial feeds, a COC should not be started. A COC could be started where artificial feeding has been commenced, even periodically.

Missed Pills

If an active pill has been delayed for more than 12 hours, if the woman is suffering from diarrhoea or vomiting, or if she is on drugs that interfere with the pill, the pill may fail as a contraception. In such situations, the woman should be advised to use some alternative contraception until 7 active pills have been ingested after the risk has resolved.

Chapter 8.2. Oestrogen-Only Contraception

In Australasia, oestrogen-alone contraception is available in the form of vaginal rings. These are 54 mm, quite soft and malleable plastic rings. They are impregnated with ethinyl oestradiol, which is released at a constant rate and is absorbed by vaginal mucosa with systemic effects.

It prevents ovulation by inhibiting the gonadotropins. The contraceptive effect lasts up to five weeks from the insertion of one ring. Contraceptive efficacy and systemic effects are similar to COC. In some other countries, these vaginal rings also contain desogestrel. The menstrual cycle control is also good despite low levels of serum ethinyl oestradiol.

The ring is inserted into the vagina by the woman, and she removes it after three weeks. Withdrawal bleeding occurs in the following week. A new ring is reinserted into the vagina after a week's break. Spontaneous expulsion of the ring is very rare.

Chapter 8.3. Progestin-Only Contraception

Progestin-only contraception has been used for a long time in the following forms:

- Oral pills
- Intramuscular injections
- Intrauterine contraceptive devices
- Implants

Progestin-Only Contraception Oral Pill

These oral pills contain one of the following progestins:

- Norethindrone: 0.35 mg/pill
- Norgestrel: 0.03 mg/pill
- Levonorgestrel: 0.075 mg/pill
- Lynestrenol: 0.5 mg/pill
- Desogestrel: 0.075 mg/pill

The progestin component in this pill is about 25% of that in the COC pill, and hence it is referred to as the "minipill."

The mode of action is the same as that described for progestins in the COC. The gonadotropins are not consistently inhibited. The impermeability of the cervical mucus to sperm caused by these pills lasts up to 22 hours after the ingestion of the pill. Hence these pills must always be taken at a constant time every day. Because of its inability to inhibit ovulation consistently, these pills are not as effective in controlling tubal pregnancy as intrauterine pregnancy.

The failure rate is 1.1 to 9.6 per 100 women in the first year.

Minipills are less effective than COC.

Clinical Use

These pills are used in women who breastfeed. These pills do not interfere with prolactin secretion and action and so do not suppress lactation. Hence, they can be safely used by lactating women who intend to use additional contraception. Together with lactational amenorrhoea, minipills provide very effective contraception.

The minipill may also be used in women who cannot take the COC because of side effects or contraindications.

How to Start the Minipill?

In the presence of menses, this pill should be started on the first day of menses. Additional contraception should be taken for the first seven days because very few women may ovulate around day 7–9. The pill should be taken at the same time every day, or at most three hours after the expected time of ingestion. If the pill is ingested after three hours of the expected time, additional contraception should be taken for 48 hours. In case of diarrhoea or vomiting or forgetting to take pills, the pill should be started as soon as possible, and additional contraception should be taken for seven days.

Side Effects

- Irregular vaginal bleeding due to inconsistency of ovulation suppression.
- Functional ovarian cysts are more common.
- Levonorgestrel-containing pills may cause acne.

Injectable Progestins

The most common injectable contraceptive progestin is depot medroxyprogesterone acetate (DMPA). It is the only C-21 progestin that is used for contraception with a rate of pregnancy with perfect use of 0.3%.

Mode of Action

- Inhibits ovulations by preventing the midcycle FSH peak
- Makes the endometrium thin and glycogen-depleted, thus making it unfavourable for implantation
- Thickens the cervical mucus

Dose

A common dose is 150 mg deep intramuscular injection every 3 months. The injection site should not be massaged to allow slow, sustained absorption. It should be administered within 7 days of the LMP to allow it to be effective from the very first cycle.

An alternative is 104 mg subcutaneously every 3 months. This is absorbed more slowly than the intramuscular preparation.

Pharmacokinetics

The contraceptive blood level of > 0.2 mg/mL is reached within 24 hours. It remains detectable in the blood for 7–9 months after the injection and hence the delay in return to fertility. Return to ovarian follicular activity precedes that of luteal activity. Following DMPA administration, the FSH level remains in the midfollicular range (4–7mIU/mL). Oestradiol and progesterone levels remain completely suppressed.

Advantages

- 3-monthly dosing schedule.
- More effective than COC.
- No lactation impairment.
- Does not promote thrombosis.
- Does not affect overall breast cancer risk in humans.
- Risks of ovarian and endometrial cancer decrease.
- Improves PMS.

Disadvantages

- Irregular uterine bleeding.
- Delayed ovulation after cessation of administration.
- Weight gain around 3 kg per year.
- Bone loss after prolonged use, which is partly reversible.

Contraindications

A history of CVS disease, thromboembolism, breast cancer, or liver disease.

Subdermal Progestin Implant

The most common subdermal progestin implant used in Australasia is the etonogestrel implant. It is a 4-cm-long, 2-mm-wide plastic cylindrical structure.

Mode of Action

- Ovulation suppression
- Thickening of cervical mucus
- Interferes with the implantation of the blastocyst

Insertion

The subdermal progestin implant is usually inserted in the biceps groove of the nondominant upper arm within 5 days of the LMP, after infiltrating local anaesthetic.

Pharmacokinetics

Etonogestrel is the active metabolite of desogestrel, which has progestational activity but only weak androgenic effects. The contraceptive level is reached after 8 hours of administration, reaching the peak level at about 4 days and slowly declining. The contraceptive efficacy lasts up to 3 years and hence should be removed with a small incision just before or at 3 years. Following removal, the hormones become undetectable in the blood within a week; hence fertility return is immediate.

Advantages

- Very effective contraception
- No decrease in bone density
- Immediate return to fertility

Disadvantages

- Irregular uterine bleeding in 20% of women
- Weight gain
- Depression

Chapter 8.4. Intrauterine Contraceptive Devices

The single biggest advantage of intrauterine contraceptive devices (IUCD) and progestin implants is that they remove totally the user error factors, and hence, contraceptive efficacy is enhanced. There are 2 types of IUCD in use:

- Levonorgestrel-containing IUCD
- Copper-containing IUCD

These are both small, T-shaped, plastic devices with monofilament strings attached to the lower end of the vertical arm. The levonorgestrel (52 mg) is in the vertical arm, whereas copper is in both the vertical and horizontal arms.

They are the most cost-effective in terms of long-term contraception and are equal to tubal occlusion in terms of efficacy.

Advantages

- Long term—lasts 5 years
- Reversible
- Very highly effective
- Minimal systemic side effects
- Suitable for mentally handicapped women
- Suitable for women who forget to take pills
- Useful when oestrogen is contraindicated
- No effect on lactation
- Cheapest and most cost-effective over a 5-year period

Advantages Specific to the Levonorgestrel-Containing IUCD

- Reduces menstrual blood loss and dysmenorrhoea
- Treats endometriosis and endometrial hyperplasia
- Can be used as progestin replacement in hormone replacement therapy

Mechanism of Action

1. The levonorgestrel-containing IUCD releases 20 µg of levonorgestrel into the endometrial cavity every day.

- Spermicidal and hence prevents spermatic migration to the fallopian tubes
- Thickens cervical mucus
- Inhibits ovulation

2. The copper-containing IUCD's contraceptive efficacy and duration are proportional to the amount of copper in the IUCD and the size of the IUCD.

- Spermicidal due to a foreign-body inflammatory reaction
- Copper aids in the inflammatory reaction
- Prevents spermatic migration to the fallopian tubes

Time of Insertion

The levonorgestrel-containing IUCD can be inserted at any time in the menstrual cycle, but inserting it during menses excludes any possibility of a pregnancy. It should be inserted 3 weeks after a vaginal birth and immediately after a termination of pregnancy.

Time of Removal

An IUCD can be removed at any time within 5 years or at 5 years, which is the normal duration of action of these IUCDs. Some copper-containing IUCDs can last up to 7 years. Return of fertility is prompt.

Failure Rate

52 mg levonorgestrel-containing IUCD: 0.2% in the first year of use

13.5 mg levonorgestrel-containing IUCD: 0.4% in the first year of use

380A copper-containing IUCD: 0.8% in the first year of use

Side Effects

- Heavy, prolonged menses or intermenstrual bleeding with copper-containing IUCD. These patterns of bleeding are significantly reduced with the levonorgestrel-containing IUCD. Excessive bleeding in the first few months of insertion could be treated with reassurance, iron supplementation, and prostaglandin synthetase inhibitors.
- Expulsion of IUCD (incidence 2–10%) happens usually when inserted immediately postpartum or immediately after a termination of pregnancy/miscarriage.

- Uterine perforation (incidence 0.1%) happens exclusively during insertion. If the woman cannot feel the strings of the IUCD in the vagina, its presence in the uterus must be confirmed by pelvic ultrasound examination. If the IUCD is discovered in the peritoneal cavity, it should be removed laparoscopically to reduce the chance of complications such as bowel perforation or obstruction. IUCDs that are only partially perforating the myometrium as a result of insertion can completely perforate the uterine wall within a few months as a result of the strong uterine contractions.

- Effect on pregnancy:
  - There is no evidence of increased fetal malformation from either of the IUCDs.
  - The IUCDs are always extra-amniotic.
  - The incidence of miscarriage in the presence of an IUCD is about 55%.
  - An IUCD should be removed if the string is visible in a woman desirous of continuing the pregnancy.
  - IUCDs do not increase the risk of sepsis in the pregnancy.
  - Both types of IUCD reduce the risk of ectopic pregnancy; however, the risk of a pregnancy being ectopic is increased if a woman becomes pregnant.
  - There is also an increased risk of preterm delivery if the pregnancy is continued in the presence of an IUCD.

- Infection:
  - The risk of pelvic infection nearly 3 weeks after IUCD insertion is unchanged from the baseline risk.
  - Administration of an antibiotic at the time of insertion is not indicated, provided the method of insertion is sterile.
  - There may be increased chances of actinomycosis colonisation in plastic-containing IUCDs. In an asymptomatic woman with actinomycosis colonisation, removal of the IUCD is not required. The condition can be treated with antibiotics.

Contraindications

- Possibility of an existing pregnancy/GTD with persistently elevated β-HCG
- Presence of infection—PID, endometritis, or bacterial vaginosis
- Possibility of a genital tract malignancy
- Presence of undiagnosed genital tract bleeding
- Uterine malformations—bicornuate uterus, septate uterus, uterus didelphys
- Women not in a stable relationship
- Wilson's disease for copper-containing IUCD
- Young age or nulliparity

Chapter 8.5. Emergency Contraception

This is also known as postcoital contraception or the morning-after pill.

The different methods are:

- Yuzpe method
  - High-dose (100 µg) ethinyl oestradiol and 0.5 mg levonorgestrel.
  - Pill needs to be taken within 72 hours of sexual intercourse.
  - This method has largely been superseded due to its side effects, such as nausea.
  - Failure rate is 3.2%.

- High-dose progestin
  - Levonorgestrel: two 0.75 mg tablets, taken 12 hours apart, or a single 1.5-mg dose.
  - Improved compliance and fewer side effects.
  - Should be taken within 72 hours of sexual intercourse.
  - Failure rate is 1.1%.

- Mifepristone
  - 10 mg.
  - Can be used up to 120 hours after sexual intercourse.
  - Failure rate is 1%.

- IUCD
  - Both copper- and levonorgestrel-containing IUCDs can be used.
  - Should be used within 120 hours of sexual intercourse.
  - Failure rate is 1%.

In the event of failed emergency contraception, the drugs do not exert any adverse effects on the developing embryo.

Mode of Action

- Inhibition of ovulation
- Making the endometrium unsuitable for implantation
- Interfering with luteal function

Follow-up of Emergency Contraception

The woman should be advised to have a pregnancy test if her subsequent period is delayed. Levonorgestrel does not provide contraception for the rest of the cycle. It may be better to start the woman on long-term contraception.

Short-Answer Questions

Question 1

A 16-year-old wants to use contraception. How will you counsel her?

Answer:

I will conduct the consultation in a sensitive and nonjudgmental way. The girl should be preferably seen alone. I will speak clearly without any medical jargon, so that I am easily understood.

The consultation will start with a detailed history, such as menstrual history, any previous pregnancies, history of sexually transmitted infections, sexual history, and whether she is in a stable relationship. I will also seek information from the girl about whether she wants contraception to prevent getting pregnant or for other reasons, such as menstrual problems or the prevention of an STI.

I will then take a full medical history, including a history of any previous medical or surgical conditions such as DVT or ruptured appendix, and whether she was on any medicines, especially antiepileptic or anticoagulant drugs. I will also ask about alcohol intake, smoking, and any allergies. I will then ask about a family history of any diseases, such as hormone-dependent malignancies and thrombophilias.

I will take her verbal consent to perform a complete physical examination followed by a gynaecological examination. For the latter, I will ensure privacy and seek the presence of a chaperone. I will use a bivalve speculum to examine the vagina and cervix, and I will take high vaginal and cervical swabs for *Gonorrhoea* and *Chlamydia* respectively. I will then do a bimanual examination to ensure the normality of the uterus and absence of any adnexal pathology. Having established the normality of the pelvis and excluded any contraindication to contraceptive methods, I will briefly discuss each method, such as COC, depot medroxyprogesterone acetate, IUCD, subdermal etonogestrel implant, and the oestrogen vaginal ring.

Combined oral contraceptive pill is not only a very effective form of contraception if taken regularly, but it also treats dysmenorrhoea, menorrhagia, endometriosis, and irregular menstrual cycles, and it prevents some of the STIs. Provided there is no contraindication, the first-choice dosages of the pills would be either 20 µg or 30 µg monophasic pills with a nonandrogenic progestin. The side effects of nausea, headache, and sometimes breast tenderness will be explained. There is not much difference in terms of side effects between a low-dose monophasic and a multiphasic pill.

Depot medroxyprogesterone acetate injection should not be preferred because of its osteoporotic effects with long-term use. IUCDs are not used in a 16-year-old nulliparous girl because of the very small risk of infection in the first 3 weeks after insertion. Subdermal implants and depot medroxyprogesterone acetate both cause irregular vaginal bleeding, which could be very annoying. Teenagers are relatively poor users of barrier methods of contraception. Emergency contraception is not a substitute for regular contraception.

I will discuss the pros and cons of the different contraceptive methods as above and give her some reading material to take home. I will then consult her a second time to make a final choice of contraception on the basis of a thorough understanding of all of her options.

Question 2

Define breakthrough bleeding (BTB). Discuss its risk factors, types, and management.

Answer:

BTB is unscheduled bleeding from the genital tract when the woman is on a combined oral contraceptive pill. BTB does not decrease the pill's efficacy.

Risk factors:

- Insufficient oestrogen or high-dose progestin in COC
- Irregular pill taking
- Smoking
- Low-dose oral pills

Types:

- Early
- Delayed

Early BTB: It is the more common of the two types. The incidence ranges from 10–30% in the first 3 months of use. The incidence decreases after continuous use. This is due to unscheduled endometrial breakdown as it adjusts from its normal thickness to a lesser thickness due to the pill use.

Delayed BTB: This happens after several months or years of use. It is due to progestin-induced decidualisation of the endometrium, which is more fragile and hence breaks down easily, causing unscheduled bleeding.

Management:

- Reassurance and encouragement to continue with the pill regularly.
- Cessation of smoking.
- Switch to a normal-dose COC.
- If BTB happens just before the end of the pill cycle, stop the pill and start a new cycle after 7 days.
- Irrespective of where the BTB occurs in the pill cycle, a course of conjugated oestrogen 1.25 mg or oestradiol 2 mg daily for 7 days controls the bleeding.
- Continued BTB despite the above management needs further investigation for abnormal bleeding from the genital tract.

Question 3

Name the drugs that affect the efficacy of the combined oral contraceptive pill.

Answer:

The following drugs, which affect liver metabolism, could affect the COC's efficacy: rifampicin, phenobarbital, phenytoin, carbamazepine, griseofulvin, and ethosuximide.

Drugs that affect the absorption of the pills from the gastrointestinal tract will affect the efficacy of the COC, such as laxatives and colonic washout preparations.

Question 4

Discuss the effect of the COC on venous thromboembolism (VTE).

Answer:

Oestrogens increase the synthesis of clotting factors V, VIII, X, XII, and fibrinogen, and hence all COCs increase the risk of VTE. Fourth-generation progestins such as drospirenone increase clotting by a mild diuretic effect. Low-dose oral contraceptives do not increase the risk of myocardial infarction in healthy, nonsmoking women, but high-dose contraceptives do. The risk of VTE increases with smoking, but the risk of arterial thrombosis does not increase with smoking. The venous system has a lower blood-flow velocity with relatively low platelet and high fibrinogen counts. The arterial system, on the other hand, has a high blood-flow velocity with high platelet and low fibrinogen counts—hence the differential response to thrombosis. The risk of arterial thrombosis is proportional to the dose of oestrogen.

Hypertension is also a risk factor for stroke in contraceptive users.

Question 5

List the risk factors for VTE with simultaneous use of COC.

Answer:

- Personal or family history of VTE
- Inherited or acquired thrombophilia
- Puerperium
- Smoking
- Obesity
- Major surgery or trauma
- Immobilisation or long flights

Question 6

List 2 pharmacological effects of drospirenone and the clinical use of those pharmacological effects.

Answer:

1. Antiandrogenic effect
   - Decreased hirsutism
   - Decreased acne
2. Diuretic effect
   - Decreased bloating
   - Decreased breast tenderness
   - No effect on weight

Question 7

List the failure rate of different contraceptives.

Answer:

COC	0.1 to 1	/100 woman years
POP	1 to 3	/100 woman years
Depot medroxyprogesterone acetate	0.1 to 2	/100 woman years
Copper IUCD	1 to 2	/100 woman years
Levonorgestrel IUCD	0.5	/100 woman years
Male condom	2 to 5	/100 woman years
Female diaphragm	1 to 15	/100 woman years
Natural family planning	2 to 3	/100 woman years
Vasectomy	0.02	/100 woman years
Female sterilisation	0.13	/100 woman years

Table 8.1. Failure rates of various contraceptives

Question 8

Discuss the contraceptive efficacy of breastfeeding.

Answer:

Women who breastfeed have a delay in resumption of ovulation postpartum due to prolactin-induced inhibition of pulsatile gonadotropin-releasing-hormone release from the hypothalamus. The degree to which breastfeeding suppresses ovulation is affected by the intensity of the breastfeeding, the basal nutritional status of the mother, and the body mass index of the mother.

The presence of following conditions will increase the contraceptive efficacy of breastfeeding in the following cases:

- The woman is less than six months postpartum.
- She is breastfeeding exclusively (i.e., not providing food or other liquid to the infant).
- She has persistent amenorrhea.

Under such circumstances, the chance of a pregnancy is less than 1%.

Question 9

A 22-year-old healthy woman who is not in a stable relationship wants to discuss her contraceptive options after undergoing a termination of pregnancy. What will you discuss?

Answer:

I will conduct my consultation in a supportive and nonjudgmental way, ensuring privacy. I will discuss the advantages and disadvantages of the following contraceptive options.

Barrier method:

Advantages: Available when needed, provides immediate contraception, can be started immediately, cheap, does not have to be taken daily, no systemic side effects, protective against certain STIs.

Disadvantages: Low efficacy, can result in failure if improperly used, woman has to depend on male partner for its timely use, allergic reaction. Does not protect against HPV infection.

Write the advantages and disadvantages of all the contraception options described in the text.

Question 10

A 20-year-old woman wishes to take the combined oral contraceptive pill for contraception. She has only heard that it can cause lots of side effects and is unaware of any benefits other than contraception. List any benefits of the combined oral contraceptive pill (other than contraception) that you could tell her about.

Answer:

- Periods
  - Regular (treatment for irregular)
  - In control of period (for times travelling, etc.)
  - Lighter periods (therefore useful in treatment of menorrhagia)
  - Less anaemia
  - Helps with dysmenorrhoea

- Symptoms
  - Helps with PMS
  - Reduces acne (by increasing SHBG)
  - Reduces hirsutism (PCOS)

- Benign pathology
  - Fewer symptomatic fibroids and incidence of fibroids
  - Fewer functional ovarian cysts
  - Fewer benign breast lumps and benign breast disease
  - Increases SHBG (therefore useful in reducing hirsutism)
  - Reduced risk of PID
  - Reduced incidence and severity of endometriosis
  - Inhibits ovarian cysts
  - Reduces fibrocystic disease of breast

- Cancer
  - Reduced risk of endometrial cancer and hyperplasia
  - Reduced risk of ovarian cancer

Multiple-Choice Questions

Q1. The clinical pregnancy rate after a single midcycle coitus without the use of contraception is:

    A. 4%.

    B. 8%.

    C. 12%.

    D. 16%.

Answer: B

Q2. Which of the following is incorrect?

    A. Oestrogen decrease sebum production

    B. Oestrogen increases SHBG

    C. Oestrogen increases the synthesis of clotting factor X

    D. Oestrogen increases LDL levels

Answer: D

Q3. Which of the following statements regarding breakthrough bleeding is incorrect?

    A. It is usually due to insufficient oestrogen.

    B. It is usually due to too much progestin.

    C. Both A and B are true.

    D. It is treated by a lesser oestrogenic oral contraceptive.

Answer: D

Q4. In some women, a withdrawal bleed does not occur at the end of a cycle of combined oral pill. This is because of:

    A. Too much oestrogen.

    B. Not enough progestin.

    C. Progestin causing suppression of endometrial growth.

    D. Both A and B.

Answer: C

Q5. Progestin in the COC causes a/an:

    A. Decrease in HDL.

    B. Decrease in LDL.

    C. Increase in total cholesterol.

    D. Increase in triglycerides.

Answer: A

Q6. Which of the following neoplasms has been associated with the use of the COC?

A. Ovarian cancer

B. Endometrial cancer

C. Breast cancer

D. Hepatic adenoma

Answer: D

Q7. Which of the following is the most correct regarding the mode of action of the copper-containing IUCD?

A. Decreases tubal motility

B. Causes a spermicidal Inflammatory response in the endometrium

C. Makes the endometrium unsuitable for implantation

D. Thickens cervical mucus

Answer: B

Q8. A woman finds herself pregnant with an IUCD in place. If possible, she would like to continue with the pregnancy. Which of the following is the best course of action?

A. Don't remove the IUCD, and continue with the pregnancy.

B. Remove the IUCD, and continue with the pregnancy.

C. Remove the IUCD, and terminate the pregnancy.

D. Give antibiotics, and continue with the pregnancy.

Answer: B

Q9. Progestins decrease the synthesis of which of the following?

A. Clotting factor V

B. Clotting factor VIII

C. Clotting factor X

D. SHBG

Answer: D

Q10. How much levonorgestrel is released daily by a levonorgestrel-containing IUCD (Mirena)?

A. 10 µg

B. 20 µg

C. 30 µg

D. 40 µg

Answer: B

Q11. Which of the following is part of the mechanism of ovulation suppression during lactation?

A. Increased prolactin secretion

B. Decreased GnRH lactation

C. Decreased LH secretion

D. All of the above

Answer: D

Q12. For how long can a sperm survive inside the female genital tract?

    A. 2–4 hours

    B. 12–14 hours

    C. 1–3 days

    D. 5–7 days

Answer: D

Q13. What percentage of pregnancies will be ectopic in women with an IUCD inserted?

    A. 5%

    B. 15%

    C. 25%

    D. 35%

Answer: A

Q14. Select the most suitable contraception options from the list given on the right for the following group of patients.

A	A healthy 17-year-old	i.	Levonorgestrel IUCD
B	A multiparous 25-year-old with heavy periods	ii.	Combined contraceptive pill
C	A lactating woman	iii.	Progesterone-only pill
D	A 35-year-old, history of endometriosis, family complete	iv.	Depo-Provera injection
E	A 30-year-old multiparous lady with Wilson's disease	v.	Any of the above but not a copper-containing IUCD

Answer: A-ii, B-i, C-iii, D-iv, E-v

Q15. Should pregnancy occur after use of the Yuzpe postcoital contraception regimen (100 μg of ethinyl oestradiol and 500 μg of levonorgestrel repeated at 12 hours), the particular concern about the resulting pregnancy is that:

    A. Miscarriage rate is increased.

    B. An ectopic pregnancy is more common.

    C. The male fetus is more likely to have hypospadias.

    D. The incidence of a molar pregnancy is increased.

Answer: B

Q16. The failure rate among typical users of which method of contraception is less than 1%?

    A. Combined oral contraceptive pill

    B. Depot medroxyprogesterone acetate

    C. Minipills

    D. Condoms

Answer: B

Q17. Which of the following is incorrect?

A. Norethisterone and norethynodrel are first-generation progestogens and were used in the first oral contraceptives.

B. Levonorgestrel is a second-generation progestogen and more potent than norethisterone.

C. Triphasic oral contraceptive pills with second-generation progestogens are associated with less favourable lipid profile than monophasic preparations with the same progestogens.

D. Desogestrel, gestodene, and norgestimate are third-generation progestins and are less androgenic than levonorgestrel.

Answer: C

Q18. Which of the following is **not** an advantage of depot medroxyprogesterone acetate?

A. No significant effect on coagulation system

B. No significant effect on blood pressure

C. Low incidence of menstrual irregularity

D. No suppression of lactation

Answer: C

Q19. The Pearl Index is the:

A. Percentage of women becoming pregnant while using a particular contraceptive method.

B. Percentage of women not becoming pregnant while using a particular contraceptive method.

C. Number of pregnancies per 100 woman-years' use of a particular contraceptive method.

D. Number of pregnancies per 1000 woman-years' use of a particular contraceptive method.

Answer: C

Q20. A 17-year-old on combined oral contraceptive pill for 1 year without any problems complains of vaginal spotting. She should:

A. Have a different pill with higher oestrogen content.

B. Have a different pill with higher progestin content.

C. Get checked for STI.

D. Be prescribed additional cyclical oestrogen for 2 months.

Answer: A

Q21. Oral contraceptives are associated with a decreased risk of each of the following except:

A. Cervical cancer.

B. Endometrial cancer.

C. Endometriosis.

D. PID.

Answer: A

Q22. What is the contraceptive option for a woman with epilepsy on phenytoin?

    A. Combined oral contraceptive pill with 35 µg of ethinyl oestradiol

    B. Combined oral contraceptive pill with 50 µg of ethinyl oestradiol

    C. Combined oral contraceptive pill with 80 µg of ethinyl oestradiol

    D. Progestogen-only pill with 35 µg of levonorgestrel

Answer: B

Q23. The failure rate among typical users of which method of contraception is less than 1%?

    A. Combined oral contraceptives

    B. Progestogen-only contraceptive

    C. Depot medroxyprogesterone acetate

    D. Condoms

Answer: C

Q24. Which of the following is not true for depot medroxyprogesterone acetate?

    A. It causes amenorrhoea in approximately 50% of women at 1 year.

    B. It causes amenorrhoea in approximately 95% of women at 2 years.

    C. It results in a modest reduction in bone-mineral density.

    D. It provides good contraception in women with epilepsy.

Answer: B

Q25. Which of the following statements about oestrogen is **not** correct?

    A. Oestriol synthesis in pregnancy is increased by aromatisation in the fetal adrenal.

    B. Oestrogen is a positive inotrope.

    C. Oestrogen causes vasodilatation.

    D. Oestrogen increases the effect of nitric oxide on vascular smooth muscle.

Answer: A

Q26. Which of the following has the highest one-year continuation rate?

    A. Withdrawal

    B. Depot medroxyprogesterone acetate

    C. Minipill

    D. Levonorgestrel-containing IUCD

Answer: D

Q27. Which of the following statements regarding actinomycosis is false?

    A. It is associated with toxic shock syndrome.

    B. It can be recognised with cervical cytology.

    C. It occurs with Lippes loop IUCD.

    D. It is best treated by IM penicillin.

Answer: A

Chapter 9
Menopause

Chapter 9.1. Menopause

Definition

Menopause is cessation of menstruation for a continuous period of at least 12 months in a woman aged 40 years or over, due to complete loss of follicular function.

Clinical Physiology of Menopause

At birth, an ovary has nearly a million oocytes. At puberty, nearly 400,000 are present, of which only 400 progress to ovulation during the reproductive lifetime. At about 37–38 years of age, only 25,000 oocytes are left. The loss of follicles is due to apoptosis. From this age onward, the rate of loss of follicles accelerates. The accelerated loss of follicles is due to aging of the follicles and reduced secretion of inhibin by the granulosa cells. Inhibin exerts a negative-feedback effect on FSH secretion by the anterior pituitary. The reduced secretion of inhibin allows a rise in FSH, which is a marker of reduced follicular activity. This is continuous throughout the premenopausal age and beyond.

The rise in LH level starts a few years after the FSH level has started to rise and plateaus just after menopause has been reached. The transition from perimenopause to menopause is completed when the follicular function in the ovaries is totally lost. In the Western world, the median age of menopause is 51 years. The age of menopause is genetically determined (whereas age of menarche depends upon nutritional status and general health).

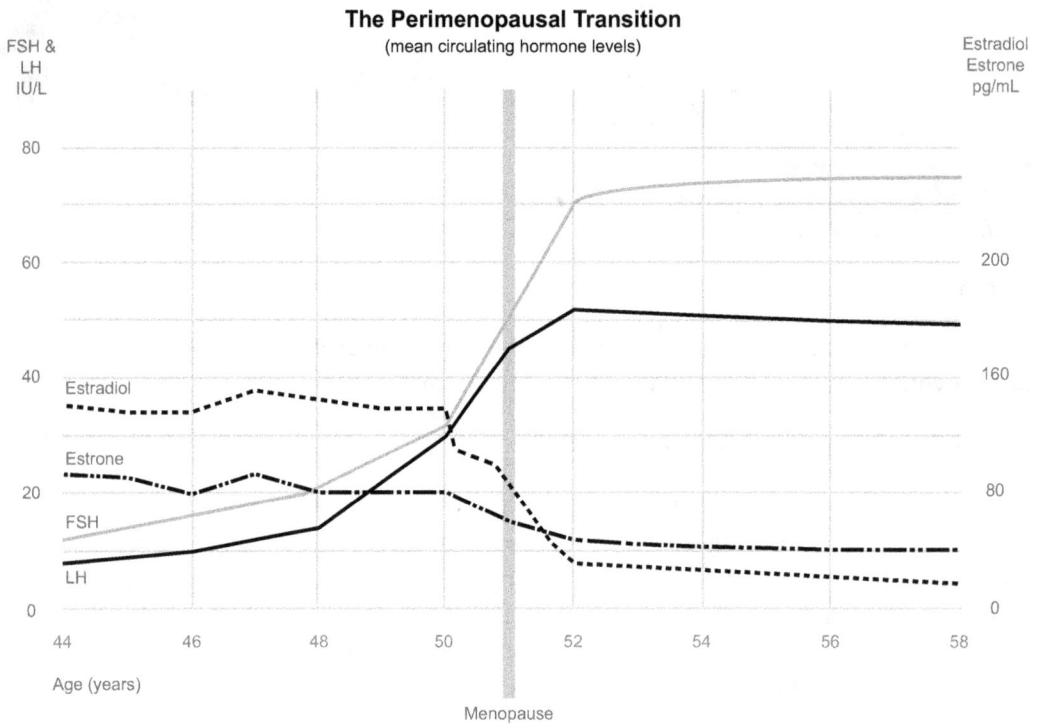

Figure 9.1. Transition of hormone levels before and after menopause. (Adapted from Rannevik G et al., 1995)

Climacteric, also known as perimenopause, is a period that spans from the end of the reproductive years to the postmenopausal years.

The following factors are associated with an early menopause:

- Smoking—dose dependent
- Familial history
- Slimmer women
- Irregular menses in women under 40 years of age
- Chemotherapy and radiotherapy

The following factors are associated with a later onset of menopause:

- Increasing parity
- Increased alcohol consumption

Genital Atrophy

Because of oestrogen deprivation after menopause, the urogenital tissues undergo the following changes:

- Thinning of the epithelium
- Reduced vascularity
- Reduced muscle bulk
- Increased fat content
- Increased neutrophils
- Altered vaginal flora

Apart from clinical examination, a vaginal smear for cytology will show characteristic atrophic changes such as the following:

- Failure of maturation of epithelial cells
- A relative excess of parabasal epithelial cells

History

Symptoms of menopause are primarily due to oestrogen depletion rather than the absolute level; hence, many women are symptomatic even with normal FSH and oestradiol levels. Symptoms start a few years before the menopause is reached. The symptoms of menopause can be broadly divided into the following groups:

- Vasomotor: hot flushes, night sweats, palpitations, headaches
- Genitourinary: vaginal dryness, dyspareunia, dysuria, recurrent UTI, decreased libido
- Psychological: depression (increased incidence if past history of depression/PMS), anxiety, insomnia, irritability, memory loss, poor concentration, lack of motivation
- Locomotor: arthralgia, myalgia, formication, tiredness

Hot flushes are the most prominent and common symptom, which is felt by nearly 70% of women, and only 20% seek help. It starts in the head and neck area and spreads to the whole body, raising the body temperature by 1°C. Approximately 25% of women will keep feeling hot flushes even after 5 years. It coincides with the paroxysmal increase in the intensity and frequency of GnRH pulsatility. This increased pulsatility is due to the action of serotonin and noradrenaline at the hypothalamus, resulting into disordered thermoregulation.

Hot flushes can cause sleep deprivation and irritability. Sleep efficiency is lower, and the latency to rapid eye movement sleep is prolonged.

Genitourinary Problems

Vagina: dryness, thinning, and atrophy of vaginal walls in 13.1% of women; pale, absent rugae; visible capillaries with a pH of 6–7.5 (< 4.5 in reproductive years)

Urethra: atrophy of epithelium, recurrent UTI, stress and urge incontinence

Sexual dysfunction: decreased vascularity of vagina and vulva, decreased lubrication, and possibly neuropathy

Cardiovascular Disease

Because of the altered HDL: LDL ratio after menopause due to a decreased serum-oestradiol level, the incidence of cardiovascular disease increases, but it does not reach the incidence in men. The Heart and Oestrogen/Progestin Replacement Study (HERS) showed no benefit from hormone replacement therapy in terms of cardiovascular diseases and a substantial rise in venous thromboembolism. The Women's Health Initiative (WHI) study showed that after 5 years of hormone replacement therapy (HRT), the risks of breast cancer, cardiovascular, and cerebrovascular disease increased, although the incidence of fractures and colorectal cancer decreased.

Osteoporosis

In women, bone mass is at its maximum toward the end of the third decade. It remains more or less constant until menopause, when it starts to decline. It is the trabecular bone that is responsive to oestrogen. Oestrogen promotes osteoblastic activity and reduces osteoclastic activity. Vertebrae, femoral neck, and radius have high trabecular bone content, and hence osteoporotic fractures happen in these bones. At least 2 mg oestradiol is essential to increase bone mass.

Diagnosis

Menopause is diagnosed clinically by the cessation of menstruation due to total loss of follicular function, with or without the symptoms. Serum FSH, LH, and oestradiol levels could be checked if in doubt. Serum FSH and LH are higher, and oestradiol level is lower in menopause. Climacteric is diagnosed clinically on the basis of the symptoms described above.

Differential Diagnoses

- Hyperthyroidism
- Hyperprolactinaemia
- Pheochromocytoma
- Carcinoid
- Panic disorder
- Diabetes
- Side effects of drugs, such as antioestrogens and SERMs

Management

Not all menopausal women need treatment. Treatment should be individualised according to the woman's main symptoms. The lowest dose of oestrogen/progestin that ameliorates the symptoms should be administered after a detailed discussion of the pros and cons and the effectiveness of any alternative therapy (Evidence Level IB). The lowest dose varies from woman to woman. The need for continuing the therapy should be reviewed every year. There is little evidence to support the routine use of HRT, also known as menopausal hormone therapy (MHT), for prophylaxis of long-term menopausal sequelae.

The treatment can start even in the perimenopausal years if the woman's symptoms seem to affect her quality of life. The treatment should continue as long as the symptomatic relief is required or the benefits of the hormonal therapy outweigh its risks. The hormone therapy should be slowly stopped. Up to 40% of women will have recurrence of symptoms after cessation of treatment. A thorough clinical examination should be undertaken. HRT should not be prescribed to women with multiple risk factors for VTE (Evidence Level IV). A baseline mammography and lipid profile should be checked. Blood pressure and lipid profile checks should be done periodically. Yearly breast examination and two-yearly mammograms should be offered.

Oestrogen Use

Oestrogen alone should only be used if the uterus and cervix have been removed. It is very effective for vasomotor (more effective than placebo; Evidence Level I) and genitourinary symptoms and for the prevention of osteoporosis. It also reduces the incidence of colorectal cancer by 33%.

The much-publicised risk of oestrogen therapy for menopause is the increased risk of breast cancer to the magnitude of 8/10,000 women per year. There is also a slight increase in the risks of coronary heart disease (RR 1.24) and thromboembolic phenomena. The side effects of this therapy are breast tenderness, abdominal bloating, and hypertension. Many of these side effects ameliorate after prolonged use or by changing the dose or type of oestrogen.

The route of administration depends upon the principal symptom(s) and any comorbidity such as a past history of thromboembolic phenomena. Oral administration is the most commonly used route. It causes a higher level of oestrone than oestradiol. Oral oestrogens undergo a significant "first-pass" effect in the liver, which causes a 30% reduction in their bioactivity. Due to the first-pass effect, some beneficial changes happen, such as an increase in HDL and a decrease in fibrinogen and plasminogen activator inhibitor. An increase in coagulation factors also happens due to the same effect, which is a harmful consequence of oestrogen therapy.

Oral synthetic oestrogens are much more potent than natural ones. Serum oestradiol level, following oral administration, fluctuates between women and based on the time of the day. The oral route of administration is more suited for women with vasomotor symptoms and osteoporosis. For women with genitourinary symptoms, vaginal administration is more appropriate, which is done in the form of vaginal tablets, pessaries, rings, and creams. A very small amount of systemic absorption does take place. This can be minimised by the use of vaginal tablets and rings. Vaginal absorption of oestrogen decreases as the vaginal mucosa becomes better oestrogenised. The transdermal route does not cause an increase in the risk of thromboembolic events because of bypassing the liver. RCTs have shown that transdermal administration of HRT improved sexual function and activity. With matrix patches, allergic skin reactions decreased, and oestrogen absorption through the skin improved. Oestrogens can also be administrated in the form of implants, but with prolonged use, tachyphylaxis may develop. Oestrogen should be administered daily.

Progestin Use

Progestin must be used with oestrogen if:

- Presence of uterus or cervix
- Endometriosis
- History of endometrial resection or ablation
- History of endometrioid ovarian cancer

The progestin is used to prevent endometrial hyperplasia. The dose will depend upon the dose of oestrogen. A larger oestrogen dose will require a larger progestin dose. A continuous oestrogen regimen will require at least 10 days a month of progestin to prevent endometrial hyperplasia. Progestins may cause mood changes, PMS-type changes, and bleeding. Like oestrogens, progestins can also be administered orally, vaginally, or transdermally. Progestins administered vaginally cause a higher concentration in the uterus without much change in the serum level. Progestin can also be administered through the intrauterine device, such as a levonorgestrel-containing intrauterine device, without many systemic side effects.

Progestins can be administered continuously with oestrogen to prevent any withdrawal bleed or sequentially, up to 10–14 days every month. The latter will cause a withdrawal bleed in 80% of women.

Progestin alone can also be used to ameliorate vasomotor symptoms, if oestrogen is contraindicated or the woman is unwilling to take it. Medroxyprogesterone acetate 20 mg daily or megestrol acetate 40 mg daily are effective to treat vasomotor symptoms.

Combined Oestrogen and Progestin Use

In the presence of the uterus or cervix, oestrogen should always be used with progestin. It is the most common form of HRT administration. HRT should be stopped slowly to prevent rebound of menopausal symptoms.

Testosterone Use

The level of serum testosterone decreases after natural or surgical menopause. The main role of testosterone in menopausal women is in the treatment of hypoactive sexual desire and arousal disorder, especially in younger women. Testosterone also gets converted to oestrogen and hence can be responsible for endometrial hyperplasia if a progestin is not administered simultaneously. Hence testosterone is used with oestrogen and progestin.

Tibolone

Tibolone is a 19-testosterone derivative with oestrogenic, androgenic, and progestogenic characteristics. It causes reduced oestrogenic stimulation of the breast tissue, and hence there is minimal change to breast density and pain. It has been shown to cause recurrence of breast cancer in an oestrogen-receptor-positive group but not in the oestrogen-receptor-negative group (Sismondi P et al., 2011). In a dose of 2.5 mg daily, it helps with vasomotor symptoms, bone density, and libido. Its adverse effects include lower abdominal pain, abdominal hair growth, vaginal discharge, and endometrial hyperplasia.

Selective Oestrogen Receptor Modulators (SERM)

These are a group of drugs (raloxifene, tamoxifen) with oestrogen agonist and antagonist properties in different tissue. Raloxifene (60 mg/day) does not stimulate breast parenchyma and endometrium but has beneficial effects on bones and lipids. It reduces vertebral fractures by about 30–50% but does not prevent hip fractures. It decreases total and low-density lipoprotein cholesterol and hence lowers cardiovascular events. However, tamoxifen may cause endometrial hyperplasia. The incidence of hot flushes, leg cramps, and venous thromboembolism increases 3 times with raloxifene. SERM is now being combined with conjugated estrogen to better treat menopausal symptoms without the risk of endometrial hyperplasia.

Selective Serotonin Reuptake Inhibitors (SSRI) and Serotonin and Noradrenaline Reuptake Inhibitors (SNRI)

These drugs (venlafaxine, citalopram, paroxetine, fluoxetine) exert their beneficial effect on hot flushes by inhibiting the reuptake of serotonin. Both the frequency and the severity of hot flushes are reduced. The dose required for treating hot flushes is much less than that for depression (venlafaxine 75 mg/day, paroxetine 25 mg/day), and the beneficial effect also starts much earlier, within 1–2 weeks. The most common side effects are nausea and insomnia. Paroxetine and fluoxetine induce CYP2D6 and interfere with tamoxifen metabolism, and hence they should not be used in a woman who is already on tamoxifen.

Gabapentin

Gabapentin is a gamma aminobutyric acid analogue that is used for epilepsy and neuropathic pain. In double-blind randomised trials, it has been shown to be of equivalent efficacy to oestrogen in reducing the frequency and severity of hot flushes. It is effective in a dose-dependent manner and has a rapid onset of action. The mechanism of action is not fully understood. The dose is 900 mg/day. An estimated 50% of women have adverse effects.

Clonidine

It is a centrally acting alpha-adrenergic agonist antihypertensive that also alleviates hot flushes after 4–6 weeks of use. The mechanism of its action may involve reduced catecholamine production or reduced peripheral vasodilation. The dose is 0.1 mg/day, which could be increased on a weekly basis up to 0.3 mg/day. The side effects are dizziness, constipation, and insomnia in about 50% of women.

Plant and Nutritional Products

There is no conclusive evidence that these products are of any real benefit.

Summary of Drugs to Treat Menopausal Symptoms

Feature	Drugs
Treat vasomotor symptoms	Oestrogen, progestogen, tibolone, SSRIs, gabapentin, clonidine
Treat decreased libido	Testosterone, tibolone
Treat genitourinary problems	Topical oestrogen
Prevent loss of bone-mineral density	Oestrogen, progestogen, tibolone, SERM, bisphosphonates
May cause endometrial hyperplasia	Unopposed oestrogen, testosterone, tibolone, tamoxifen
Increased risk of VTE	Oestrogen, raloxifene, nonpregnane progestogens, venlafaxine

Table 9.1. Drugs to treat various menopausal symptoms

Chapter 9.2.   Premature Menopause (Premature Ovarian Failure)

Premature menopause (PM) is cessation of menstruation for a continuous period of at least 12 months in a woman aged less than 40 years, due to a complete loss of follicular function. Early menopause is menopause before 45 years of age.

Causes

- Idiopathic: Most common. In the majority, there is sclerosis of the ovary, similar to a normal menopausal change in the ovary. In 30% of women, there is an arrest of development of follicles beyond the antral stage. In the latter, there is some production of oestrogen from the ovaries, which sustains menstrual bleeding for a few years.
- Iatrogenic: Any intervention that results in the depletion of ovarian follicles, such as irradiation, chemotherapy, bilateral oophorectomy, or ovarian surgery.
- Autoimmune disease: Hashimoto's disease, Addison's disease, hypoparathyroidism
- Genetic: Turner's syndrome, Fragile X syndrome
- Enzyme deficiency: galactosaemia

Investigations

- Serum FSH and oestradiol level: If consistent with menopause, repeat after a month
- Serum quantitative hCG
- Serum prolactin and TSH
- Transvaginal ultrasound to exclude haematometra and haematocolpos and to ensure that there is no other pathology

Once the diagnosis of PM is established, the following investigations could be done to find the cause of PM:

- Karyotype
- Tests for autoimmune diseases: autoantibodies for thyroid or adrenal, gastric parietal-cell antibodies, DHEAS
- Other tests:
    - DEXA scan
    - Serum B12, folate, ESR, rheumatoid factor, ANA
    - Fasting glucose, calcium, phosphate, albumin

Management

- Psychological and emotional support:
    - Counselling.
    - Referral to support groups.

- Lifestyle and dietary modifications:
    - Calcium-rich food.
    - Aerobic exercise.

- HRT:
    - There is no consensus on the ideal dose and route of administration of HRT.
    - There is very little data regarding efficacy of HRT for PM in terms of safety and prevention of complication.
    - Therapy should be individualised, started early, and continued at least until 50 years of age.
    - Women desiring menses should be on cyclical HRT.
    - Women not desiring menses should be on continuous HRT.
    - Spontaneous remission or reflex ovulation may occur, with a lifetime chance of conception of 5–10%.
        - Women not desiring pregnancy should be on a low-dose combined contraceptive pill or higher doses of HRT, as usual doses of HRT are not contraceptive.

- Management of complications of PM, such as osteoporosis, cardiovascular disease, cognitive dysfunction, and stroke by HRT:
    - Adverse lipid profile: dietary modifications and lipid lowering drugs.
    - The incidence of recurrent breast cancer is lower in women with PM. There is not much data on the effect of HRT on breast cancer in women with PM.

- Management of complications of diseases causing PM: yearly TSH and fasting glucose.

Chapter 9.3.   Benefits and Risks of HRT

Osteoporosis and HRT

Osteoporosis is diagnosed by dual energy X-ray absorptiometry (DEXA) of the hip bones and spine. The result is expressed as a T-score that represents the number of standard deviations from the mean of healthy young female. A T-score of more than –1 is normal, and a T-score of less than –2.5 indicates osteoporosis.

Oestrogen is effective in preventing and treating osteoporosis. If started soon after menopause and continued long-term, oestrogens reduce osteoporotic fractures by about 50%. The Women's Health Initiative (WHI) study showed a significant reduction (34%) in hip fractures in healthy women on oestrogen therapy. Studies recently have shown that even low-dose oestrogen treatment, such as conjugated equine oestrogen 0.3 mg/day, oestradiol 0.25 mg/day, or transdermal oestradiol 0.025 mg/day, are effective in significantly improving bone-mineral density. The benefits reverse within a few years of the cessation of treatment.

Other treatments, such as bisphosphonates, calcium and vitamin D supplementation, and a healthy lifestyle with cessation of smoking, weight-bearing exercise, and exposure to sunlight, also reduce osteoporosis.

Cardiovascular Disease and HRT

Studies such as the WHI study and the Heart and Oestrogen/Progestin Replacement study (HERS) have not shown any benefit from HRT in terms of cardiovascular health. The WHI study, in fact, showed an increased risk of cardiovascular events with HRT. There is an increase in the risks of coronary heart disease (RR 1.24). The WHI and HERS studies involved conjugated equine oestrogens and medroxyprogesterone acetate, but in the absence of suitable randomised controlled trials, it can be assumed that the other types of oestrogen and progestin regimens will have similar effects.

Venous Thromboembolism (VTE) and HRT

The absolute risk of VTE with HRT is low (Evidence Level IV). The risk is greatest in the first 6 months of use of HRT (Evidence Level IIB). There is very little information on whether the VTE risk differs with the type of oestrogens (Evidence Level IIA). The VTE risk is dose dependent (Evidence Level IIA). Micronised progesterone and pregnane derivatives carry a lower thrombotic risk compared with nonpregnanes. The risk of VTE with SERM is similar to oestrogen (Evidence Level IB). Routine screening for thrombophilias before commencing HRT is unnecessary unless there is a personal or family history (Evidence Level IV). If a woman desires to continue on HRT after a VTE, long-term anticoagulation should be prescribed (Evidence Level IB). The combination of HRT and postoperative changes in coagulation and venous functions significantly increase the risk of VTE (Evidence Level IV); hence thromboprophylaxis must be ensured.

Risk factors for VTE are smoking, increasing age, BMI > 30, past VTE, postthrombotic syndrome, varicose veins with phlebitis, first-degree relative with VTE, immobility for more than 3 days, duration of surgery > 1 hour, malignancy, infections, and sickle cell disease.

Cancers and HRT

The much-publicised risk of oestrogen therapy for menopause is the increased risk of breast cancer to the magnitude of 8/10,000 women per year. There is increased incidence of recurrence of breast cancer following HRT use (HABITS study). The WHI study did not show a significant rise in the incidence of ovarian cancer, but the Million Women Study showed an increased risk of ovarian cancer to the magnitude of 1/2500 women over a 5-year period. The incidence of colorectal cancer decreases (Evidence Level IB).

Alzheimer's disease and HRT

The use of HRT does not affect the existing disease. Observational studies have shown improvement in the disease, but RCTs have shown worse cognitive function in HRT arm.

Other Risks of HRT

The side effects of HRT are breast tenderness, fluid retention (sometimes described as abdominal bloating), and hypertension. Many of these side effects ameliorate after prolonged use or changing the dose or type of oestrogen.

Contraindications of HRT

- Undiagnosed vaginal bleeding
- Presence or suspicion of breast, endometrial, or ovarian carcinoma

- Acute liver disease
- Past venous thromboembolism or family history of VTE in a first-degree relative (Evidence Level IIB)
- Uncontrolled hypertension
- Benign breast disease (relative contraindication)

| Chapter 9.4. | Postmenopausal Bleeding (PMB) |

Definition

Any bleeding from the genital tract after menopause is called postmenopausal bleeding (PMB). Any PMB, irrespective of quantity, colour, and frequency, is abnormal and must be investigated. Use of HRT increases the incidence of PMB fivefold. Women with PMB have a 10–15% chance of having endometrial carcinoma. The likelihood of endometrial carcinoma increases with age at presentation.

Prevalence of PMB is about 3%.

Causes

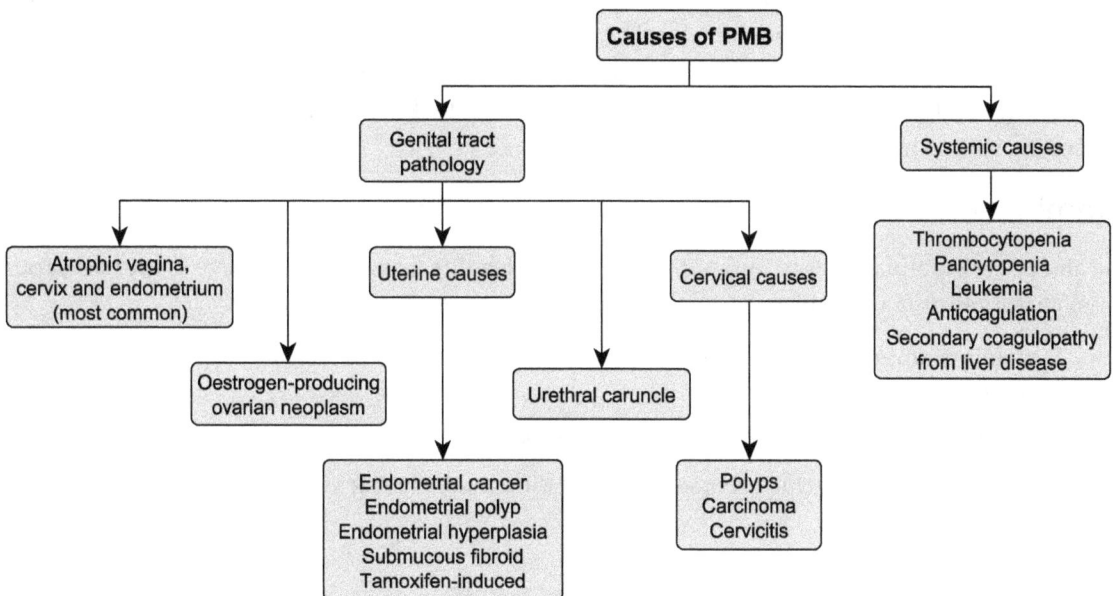

Figure 9.2. Causes of postmenopausal bleeding

Risk Factors

An estimated 20% of women with PMB will have significant genital tract pathology. The aim of investigation is to exclude endometrial carcinoma or atypical endometrial hyperplasia. Hence, the risk factors for PMB are the same as those of endometrial carcinoma. They are:

- Increasing age (1% at 50 years and 25% at 80 years of age)
- Early menarche and late menopause
- Obesity
- Nulliparity
- Unopposed oestrogen
- Systemic disease, e.g., diabetes, hypertension

The type and severity of vaginal bleeding has no diagnostic significance. Pain is uncommon but may signify sarcomatous change in a preexisting uterine myoma.

Tamoxifen

Women on tamoxifen have a three- to sixfold increased incidence of endometrial carcinoma. Hence any PMB in a woman on tamoxifen should be thoroughly investigated.

A thorough history should be taken, keeping in mind the risk factors and causes mentioned above. Vulvovaginal examination will exclude local causes such as atrophic vagina, cervicitis, cervical polyps, and ulcers. Swabs for microbiology and biopsy for histology should be obtained from suspicious lesions. A cervical smear should be done if due or the cervix looks abnormal. Urinary and anal sources of bleeding should be excluded.

Examination

The aim of the examination is to find out any cause of bleeding as mentioned above in the background of risk factors elicited in the history.

- Systemic examination to ascertain general state of health and suitability for anaesthesia or surgery if required
- Abdominal examination for any abnormal mass
- Pelvic examination, including speculum and bimanual, aiming at exploring any pelvic cause of bleeding

Investigations

The aim of the investigations is to find out the cause of the bleeding beyond what was already elicited from the history and examination. The investigations are:

- Cervical cytology, especially if due, bleeding postcoital or the cervix looking abnormal.
- Colposcopy, if bleeding postcoital or cervix looking abnormal.
- A transvaginal ultrasound scan to exclude any uterine or adnexal pathology

Endometrial thickness should be measured in the midsagittal plane, the cut-off for normality is 4 mm without HRT and 8 mm with sequential HRT. Endometrial nodularity or irregularity should also be looked for. Endometrial volume measurement and Doppler study of endometrium do not aid diagnosis. A small amount of fluid in the endometrial cavity is not unusual in this age group. No endometrial thickness threshold completely excludes carcinoma.

With tamoxifen use, the endometrium and adjoining myometrium appear sonolucent, with subendometrial cystic areas. This makes the endometrium look thicker.

MRI has a higher sensitivity in identifying myometrial invasion with endometrial carcinoma but is rarely used because of cost and limited availability.

Blood tests aimed at the systemic causes should be done in a woman with a suggestive history and negative findings on transvaginal or clinical examination.

Endometrial biopsy should be done if endometrial thickness is greater than 4 mm or if there is recurrent bleeding. In outpatient settings, specimens obtained by Pipelle/Vabra are better than a blind curettage. The evaluation of PMB is not complete without a hysteroscopy and curettage (gold standard). Hysteroscopy helps in diagnosing endometrial polyps, hyperplasia, atrophy, and uterine abnormality. However, hysteroscopy and curettage do have surgical and anaesthetic risks. Uterine polyps or submucous myomas can be dealt with at the same time.

Management

It depends upon the cause.

Genital tract atrophy is treated with topical oestrogen for a month or two. Periodic courses may be needed. Vaginal moisturisers help in alleviating vaginal dryness, itching, and irritation.

Causes such as polyps, hyperplasia, carcinoma, and adnexal masses need surgery.

Simple endometrial hyperplasia could be treated by curettage or medically by either sequential or continuous HRT or levonorgestrel-containing IUCD. Endometrial hyperplasia with atypia has a 5–10% risk of malignant transformation, and a complex hyperplasia with atypia has a 25–30% risk of malignant transformation.

Women with recurrent PMB should also undergo TAH BSO, especially if no genital tract pathology is seen.

All women with uterine bleeding on tamoxifen should have a hysteroscopy and endometrial biopsy. There is no supporting evidence to screen the endometrium of asymptomatic women on tamoxifen.

Short-Answer Questions

Question 1

A 64-year-old postmenopausal woman presents with blood-stained, watery vaginal discharge.

Part a

List the differential diagnosis.

Answer:

- Atrophic vaginitis, cervicitis, endometritis
- Endometrial hyperplasia, polyp, or cancer
- Cervical ectropion, polyp, or cancer
- Infective: pessary, foreign body, forgotten IUCD
- HRT: Breakthrough bleeding

Part b

How would you manage this woman?

- History:
  - When did the bleeding occur? Its duration, frequency, volume.
  - Precipitating factors, such as trauma, postcoital.
  - Last Pap smear: When was it done, and was it negative?
  - Any associated symptoms such as pain, fever, or changes in bladder or bowel function.
  - Medical history, such as obesity, bleeding disorders, diabetes, hypertension, hypothyroidism. Previous surgery, such as D&C, endometrial ablation, polypectomy, hysterectomy, or vaginal repair, especially with a synthetic mesh.
  - Drugs, such as unopposed oestrogen, hormone therapy, tamoxifen, anticoagulants.
  - Family history: nonpolyposis colorectal cancer, endometrial or ovarian cancer.
  - Age of menarche and menopause.

- Examination: General including vital signs and BMI, thyroid. Abdominal: any palpable mass, ascites. Speculum: any blood in the vagina, any foreign body, any vaginal or cervical lesions, atrophy, discharge, microbiological vaginal/cervical swabs if sign of infection, Cervical cytology if due or cervix looks abnormal. Any palpable abnormal mass in the vagina or pelvis, uterine contour and size.

- Consider Pipelle endometrial sampling.

- Transvaginal ultrasound scan: Uterine dimensions, fibroids, endometrial thickness and regularity, abnormal adnexal mass.

<u>Treatment</u>:

- If atrophic, normal uterus, endometrial thickness < 4mm: vaginal oestrogen for 1–2 months.
- If abnormal endometrial histology on Pipelle or/and endometrium thickness > 4 mm: hysteroscopy and endometrial biopsy and then treat the cause.
- Optimise medical conditions and drugs.

Question 2

What are the risk factors and types of endometrial hyperplasia (EH)? How will you treat them in a postmenopausal woman?

Answer:

EH can be defined as the irregular proliferation of the endometrial glands with marked increase in the gland-to-stroma ratio. It is the precursor of most types of endometrial cancer.

EH develops when unopposed oestrogen stimulates endometrial cell growth by binding to the receptors in the nuclei of the endometrial cells. The risk factors of endometrial hyperplasia (EH) are as follows:

- Unopposed oestrogen, irrespective of the dose (Evidence Level IIA)
- Obesity
- Anovulation with PCOS or perimenopause
- Oestrogen-secreting ovarian tumours, e.g., granulosa cell tumour (up to 40% prevalence of EH)
- Drug induced, e.g., tamoxifen
- Immunosuppression (twofold increase in women with renal transplant; (Evidence Level III)
- Infection (Bobrowska K et al., 2006)

According to WHO (2014), there are 2 types of EH:

1. Endometrial hyperplasia without atypia
2. Endometrial hyperplasia with atypia

Diagnosis:

1. Transvaginal ultrasound scan shows thickened hyperechoic endometrium, suggestive of endometrial hyperplasia. In a study of premenopausal women, no one had endometrial hyperplasia when the endometrial thickness was less than 7 mm (Cheung A, 2001).
2. Endometrial biopsy as an outpatient; 2% of women will have endometrial hyperplasia despite a negative endometrial biopsy.
3. Hysteroscopy and endometrial curettage: Endometrial biopsy alone may not be able to diagnose hyperplasia of the endometrial polyp. Hysteroscopy is more sensitive in detecting endometrial pathology than excluding.
4. Serum inhibin and oestradiol levels if a granulosa cell tumour is suspected.
5. CT and MRI scans have no role.

Treatment of EH without Atypia:

The risk of malignant transformation without atypia is 5% over a 20-year period (Evidence Level IIA). The majority will regress during follow-up. Reversible risk factors should be addressed and treated. Bariatric surgery for obese women reduces the risk of EH (Evidence Level II). The treatment options are medical and surgical. Among the medical options, levonorgestrel-containing IUCD, continuous progestogens (medroxyprogesterone acetate 10–20 mg/day or norethisterone 10–15 mg/day) are used. Different orally administered progestogens have similar regression rates for endometrial hyperplasia.

Cyclical progestogens fail to cause regression of the hyperplasia and hence are not recommended. Levonorgestrel-containing IUCD is the first line and most effective treatment. Regression of the hyperplasia should be confirmed by at least two endometrial biopsies six months apart before stopping the treatment. Hysterectomy and bilateral salpingo-oophorectomy should be considered if medical treatment has failed, the disease has relapsed or progressed to hyperplasia with atypia, or the surgery is contraindicated or not desired by the woman. Endometrial ablation is not a suitable option because complete and persistent endometrial destruction cannot be ensured.

<u>Treatment of EH with Atypia</u>:

In women undergoing a hysterectomy for atypical EH, 43% were found to have endometrial carcinoma (Evidence Level IIB).

Premenopausal women with EH with atypia who are still desirous of future fertility should be treated as EH without atypia. Once future fertility is no longer desired, such women should be treated with a total hysterectomy and bilateral salpingo-oophorectomy.

Postmenopausal women with atypical EH should be treated with total hysterectomy and bilateral salpingo-oophorectomy, preferably by a laparoscopic approach (Evidence Level IA). A laparoscopic approach shortens hospital stay. Intraoperative frozen section (Evidence Level IIA) and pelvic lymphadenectomy (Evidence Level IIB) are not required. Morcellation of the uterus or a subtotal hysterectomy are not recommended (Evidence Level IV). Such women should not be treated with endometrial ablation (Evidence Level IIA), because the ablation of the entire surface of the endometrium cannot be ensured.

Question 3

A premenopausal woman with atypical endometrial hyperplasia desires to maintain her fertility. List the principles of your management.

Answer:

- Extensive counselling by a multidisciplinary team.
- Exclude endometrial or ovarian cancer (4% risk of simultaneous ovarian cancer) by hysteroscopy, tumour markers, transvaginal ultrasound/MRI. The risk of progression to a higher-stage endometrial cancer is 2%.
- The woman should be treated with levonorgestrel-containing IUCD (Evidence Level IIA). The second medical option would be a continuous progestogen (not sequential).
- Once the disease regression has been established by endometrial biopsy in 3 months, the endometrial biopsy should be repeated every 3 months to ensure that hyperplasia does not recur.
- The woman should be advised to get pregnant as soon as practicable, preferably by IVF because of higher pregnancy rate; 25% of such women achieve a live pregnancy.
- Once the family has been completed, a total hysterectomy and at least bilateral salpingectomy, if not salpingo-oophorectomy, should be offered as soon as practicable.

Question 4

What did the Million Women Study show? How valid were the findings?

Answer:

The Million Women Study, a prospective cohort study, was conducted in the United Kingdom between 1996 and 2001 to study the effects of HRT on women over 50 years of age. It showed that there were different relative risks of breast cancer to the different types of HRT used. The relative risk of breast cancer was significantly higher when combined HRT was used ($p < 0.001$), compared with oestrogen only or tibolone. The study showed that after 10 years of oestrogen-only HRT use, the risk of breast cancer increased to 5 additional cases per 1000 users (95% CI 3–7), whereas with the oestrogen and progesterone HRT use, the risk of breast cancer increased to 19 per 1000 users (95% CI 15–23).

The study has been criticised because the participants were recruited from the National Breast Cancer screening program, which may have led to a detection bias. Additionally, women with breast cancer detected in the beginning were not excluded. Also, the rapid onset of breast cancer, as suggested by the investigators, was not in accordance with the biological course of the disease.

Question 5

A woman with breast cancer that was treated 6 months earlier consults you with severe hot flushes. How will you manage her?

Answer:

This woman should ideally be managed by a multidisciplinary team. The factors that will have a bearing on whether the woman's hot flushes are treated by HRT are as follows:

- The stage of breast cancer at diagnosis
- The oestrogen-receptor status of the original tumour
- Time elapsed since diagnosis
- The size of the original tumour

Prescribing HRT only 6 months after treatment is not advisable. Tibolone has been shown to increase the incidence of the recurrence of breast cancer in oestrogen-receptor-positive cases, but not in oestrogen-receptor-negative cases.

I would prefer to treat her hot flushes with SSRIs, gabapentin, or clonidine.

Question 6

Evaluate the different methods of endometrial assessment.

Answer:

Method	Accuracy	Advantages	Disadvantages
Transvaginal ultrasound scan (TVS)	Sensitivity 80–100%	• Non-invasive • Cheap, easily available • Better patient acceptability • Evaluates myometrium and adnexa	• High false positive • Low sensitivity for endometrial polyps
Pipelle/Vabra endometrial biopsy	Sensitivity > 90% for cancer, 80% for hyperplasia	• Outpatient procedure • Cheap • No anaesthetic need • Can be done with initial consult	• 20% failure due to stenosed cervix and insufficient sample • Does not identify endometrial polyps
Hysteroscopy, D&C	Gold standard	• Increased detection rate of polyps and cancer • Tissue diagnosis possible • Treatment can be done at the same time	• Involves surgery and anaesthesia, each of which can have complications • Expensive
Saline infusion sonohysterography	95% sensitivity and 92% specificity for endometrial polyps	• Outpatient procedure • Cheap • No anaesthetic needed • Identifies endometrial abnormalities better than just TVS	• Involves uterine catheterisation and then injecting water into the endometrial cavity, which is uncomfortable
3D transvaginal ultrasound	Similar to saline sonohysterography	• Can identify endometrial pathology better than 2D • No need for uterine catheterisation	• Requires training to use 3D ultrasound
MRI	As accurate as TVS for endometrial pathology	• For staging endometrial cancer	• Expensive • Not easily available

Table 9.2. Different methods of endometrial assessment

Multiple-Choice Questions

Q1. Which of the following statements regarding PMB is not correct?

   A Unopposed oestrogen for a prolonged period increases the relative risk of endometrial cancer fivefold.

   B. Sequential HRT causes endometrial thickening.

   C. Tibolone does not cause endometrial thickening.

   D. Combined HRT causes endometrial atrophy.

Answer: C

Q2. What percentage of endometrial thickness (between 6–10 mm) in a postmenopausal woman are reported as atrophic on histology?

   A. 11%

   B. 22%

   C. 33%

   D. 44%

Answer: C (Karrlson, 1995)

Q3. Which of the following drugs does not cause endometrial hyperplasia in a postmenopausal woman?

   A. Raloxifene

   B. Testosterone

   C. Tibolone

   D. Tamoxifen

Answer: A

Q4. In reference to menopause, which of the following events occurs first?

   A. Reduced secretion of inhibin

   B. Increase secretion of FSH

   C. Increased secretion of LH

   D. Reduced secretion of progesterone

Answer: A

Q5. In a 60-year-old with postmenopausal bleeding, which of the following is the most probable cause?

   A. Genital tract cancers

   B. Endometrial polyps

   C. Atrophic endometrium

   D. Atrophic vaginitis

Answer: C

Q6. A major histological change in the ovaries after menopause is the proliferation of:

   A. Stromal cells

   B. Granulosa cells

   C. Theca interna cells

   D. Surface epithelial cells

Answer: A

Q7. Which of the following is least likely to help hot flushes?

    A. Clonidine

    B. Phytoestrogens

    C. Fluoxetine

    D. Venlafaxine

Answer: B

Q8. Which is a "placebo effect"?

    A. Improved outcome from an inert therapy

    B. The effect of blinding patients to the nature of therapy

    C. The effect of blinding doctors to the patient's allocation

    D. The effect of blinding those assessing the outcome of allocation

Answer: A

Q9. A 57-year-old has been on oestrogen replacement therapy intermittently for 6 years but none in the past 6 months. She is troubled with severe hot flushes. Everything else is normal except a slightly bulky uterus. The best hormone replacement therapy for her will be:

    A. Conjugated oestrogen 0.625 mg on days 1–25 and medroxyprogesterone acetate (MPA) 10 mg on days 16–25

    B. Conjugated oestrogen 0.625 mg on days 1–25 and (MPA) 10 mg on days 13–25

    C. Conjugated oestrogen 0.625 mg daily and MPA 5 mg daily

    D. Conjugated oestrogen 0.625 mg daily and MPA 2.5 mg on days 21–30

Answer: C

Q10. A woman on tamoxifen complains of hot flushes. Which of the following drugs will you prescribe?

    A. Raloxifene

    B. Fluoxetine

    C. Paroxetine

    D. Gabapentin

Answer: D

Q11. Which of the following does not cause endometrial hyperplasia?

    A. Raloxifene

    B. Tibolone

    C. Tamoxifen

    D. Testosterone

Answer: A

Q12. Which of the following bones is least prone to an osteoporotic fracture?

    A. Vertebrae

    B. Femoral neck

    C. Radius

    D. Tibia

Answer: D

Q13. Which of the following statements is incorrect in relation to menopause?

    A. Synthetic oral oestrogens are more potent than natural oestrogen.

    B. Venlafaxine increases the risk of thrombosis threefold.

    C. Oestrogen alone can be used in a woman who has undergone a laparoscopic subtotal hysterectomy.

    D. Progestin alone will help with vasomotor symptoms.

Answer: C

Q14. In a female, the peak bone density is attained at what age?

    A. 10 years

    B. 20 years

    C. 30 years

    D. 40 years

Answer: C

Q15. The false negative rate in an outpatient endometrial biopsy is:

    A. 2%

    B. 4%

    C. 6%

    D. 8%

Answer: A

Q16. Which of the following will you prescribe to a postmenopausal woman with endometrial hyperplasia without atypia?

    A. Sequential HRT

    B. Continuous HRT

    C. Tibolone

    D. Raloxifene

Answer: B

Q17. Lactobacillus colonisation of the vagina is lowest in:

    A. A neonate of 1 week

    B. A pregnant woman

    C. A nonpregnant woman of 30 years of age

    D. A 60-year-old woman

Answer: D

Q18. Which of the following oestrogens will have the least serum concentration in a 53-year-old menopausal woman of BMI 25?

    A. Oestradiol

    B. Oestrone

    C. Oestriol

    D. Androstenedione

Answer: A

Q19. In obese postmenopausal women, peripheral conversion of oestrogen precursors results mainly in the formation of:

    A. Oestradiol
    B. Oestrone
    C. Oestriol
    D. Androstenedione

Answer: B

Q20. In postmenopausal women, oestrogen treatment is least effective for which of the following conditions?

    A. Osteoporosis
    B. Bowel cancer
    C. Urge incontinence
    D. Skin wrinkling

Answer: D

Q21. Which of the following is correct with reference to HRT in a 50-year-old?

    A. Bone loss is most rapid in the first 3 years after menopause.
    B. HRT is not indicated after the age of 60.
    C. HRT increases the risk of bowel cancer.
    D. HRT increases coronary artery disease incidence.

Answer: A

Q22. Which of the following is the most effective treatment for endometrial hyperplasia without atypia?

    A. Levonorgestrel-containing IUCD
    B. Continuous progestogen
    C. Sequential progestogen
    D. Observation

Answer: A

Q23. The probability of endometrial cancer is reduced to < 1% when the endometrial thickness is less than:

    A. 10 mm
    B. 8 mm
    C. 6 mm
    D. 4 mm

Answer: D

Chapter **10**
Urogynaecology

Chapter 10.1. | Pelvic Organ Prolapse

Definition

Pelvic organ prolapse (POP), also referred to as uterovaginal prolapse, is the descent of the uterus, cervix, or any part of the vagina from its anatomical position in a caudal direction through the vaginal orifice, due to weakening of the normal supportive mechanisms. It is seen in 30–50% of parous women.

Clinical Anatomy

The vagina has ligamentous, fascial, and muscular supports that have been studied and are described in detail by DeLancey as level 1, 2, and 3 supports, respectively.

The pelvic floor consists of the parietal pelvic peritoneum, endopelvic fascia, levator ani muscles (iliococcygeus, pubococcygeus, and puborectalis muscles), perineal membrane (previously called the pelvic diaphragm), and superficial perineal muscles.

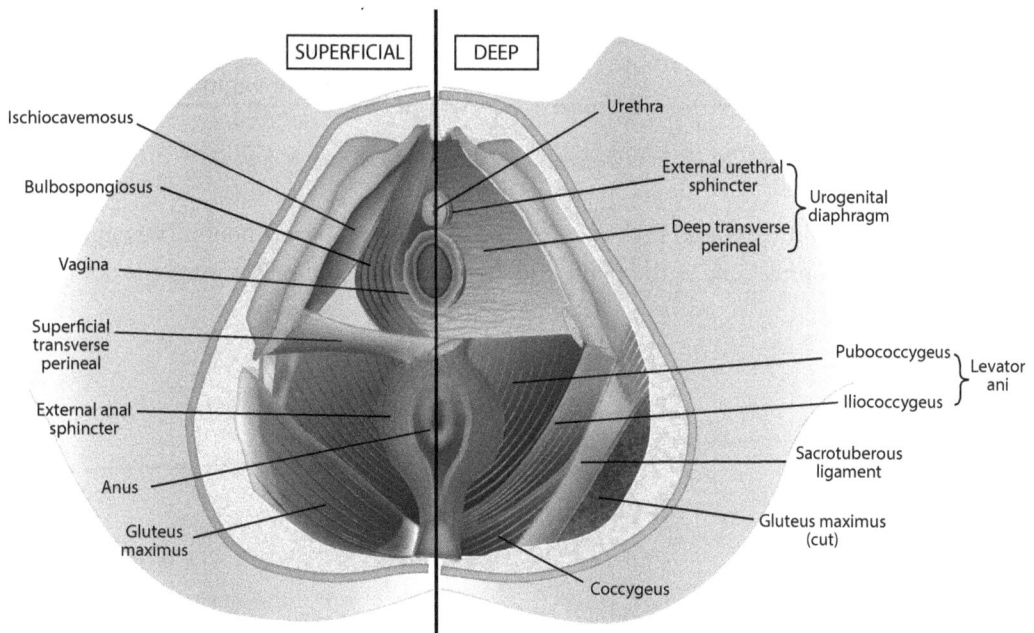

Figure 10.1. Anatomy of the female perineum

The levator muscles are the most caudal part of the pelvic floor. The cervix, vagina, and urethra are connected and supported by the levator ani muscles as they pass through the perineal membrane. This constitutes the DeLancey level III support (muscular) of the vagina. The levator ani muscles have short-twitch and long-twitch fibres. The short-twitch fibres provide the resting tone of the pelvic floor, whereas the long-twitch fibres provide support when the intraabdominal pressure increases suddenly.

Arcus tendineus is a band of condensed connective tissue on either side of the pelvic wall and runs from the lower and lateral part of the pubic bone to the ischium, just above the ischial spine. The midvagina is directly attached to the lateral pelvic walls (arcus tendineus) and constitutes the DeLancey level II support (fascial).

The uterosacral and cardinal ligaments are made up of smooth muscle, loose and dense connective tissue, blood and lymphatic vessels, and nerves. In the standing position, the uterosacral ligament is more dorsal, whereas the cardinal ligament is vertical in orientation. The DeLancey level I support (ligamentous) consists of the uterosacral and cardinal ligaments, which support the uterus, cervix (vaginal vault in its absence), and upper one-third of the vagina.

The following table shows the clinical effects of the defects of each level of support:

DeLancey Level	Anatomical structure involved	Resulting defects
I (ligamentous)	Upper vagina, cervix, uterus	Uterine prolapse Enterocoele Apical/vault prolapse
II (fascial)	Mid vagina	Cystocoele Rectocoele
III (muscular)	Lower third of the vagina	Urethrocele Deficient perineum Gaping vagina

Table 10.1. Clinical effects of the defects of each level of support

The female pelvis is mainly divided into anterior and posterior compartments. The vagina and uterus, through their lateral connections to the pelvic side walls, divide the pelvis into anterior and posterior compartments.

Anterior Compartment

Support of the anterior compartment depends upon the midvaginal attachment to the arcus tendineus (AT). Lateral detachment from the arcus tendineus results in stress incontinence and anterior prolapse. Anterior vaginal prolapse is further divided into "distension" or "displacement" groups. The clinical implications of such a division are shown in the following table:

Group	Reason	Attachment to AT	Examination findings
Distension	Passage of fetal head Menopause	Attachment to arcus tendineus preserved	Central defect Rugae absent Lateral vaginal sulcus present
Displacement	Iatrogenic	Attachment to arcus tendineus not preserved	Paravaginal defect Rugae present Lateral vaginal sulcus absent

Table 10.2. Clinical implications of distension or displacement

Posterior Compartment

The upper third of the posterior vagina is supported by DeLancey level I support (ligamentous), similar to the anterior vaginal support.

The midposterior third of the vagina receives its support from the DeLancey level II support system (fascial), which prevents vaginal prolapse during increased abdominal pressure.

The lower third of the vagina receives its support from the DeLancey level III support system (muscular), perineal membrane, and perineal body. The perineal membrane fibres fuse in the midline with each other and also with the perineal body. This attachment presents the prolapse of the lower third of the posterior vaginal wall. Hence, surgical repair of a prolapse of the lower third of the posterior vagina must include reattachment of the separated fibres of the perineal membrane and perineal body.

Defects of level I or III support systems cause a central defect, whereas a defect of the level II support system leads to a paravaginal defect.

Types of Uterovaginal Prolapse

	Type	Description
1	Uterine prolapse	Prolapse of the uterus and cervix
2	Apical/vault prolapse	Prolapse of the vaginal apex after hysterectomy
3	**Anterior vaginal wall prolapse**	
	Cystocoele	Prolapse of the anterior vaginal wall with urinary bladder attached to it; affects the upper two-thirds of the anterior vaginal wall
	Urethrocoele	Prolapse of the urethra; affects the lower one-third of the anterior vaginal wall
4	**Posterior vaginal wall prolapse**	
	Enterocoele	Herniation of the parietal peritoneum of the pouch of Douglas with or without small bowel loops; affects the upper third of the posterior vaginal wall
	Rectocoele	Prolapse of the posterior vaginal wall with rectum closely attached to it; affects the lower two-thirds of the posterior vaginal wall
5	Procidentia	Prolapse of the uterus and cervix or vault to a level outside the vaginal orifice
6	Cervical elongation	Marked cervical elongation in the presence of a normally positioned uterus and good pelvic support

Table 10.3. Types of prolapse

Grading

There are many grading systems. Two of these systems will be described.

Traditional System

This is the most widely used method in which the cervix is the reference point.

- Normal (0°)   Cervix at or above the level of the ischial spine
- First degree (1°)   Cervix below the ischial spine but above the vaginal introitus
- Second degree (2°)   Cervix at the level of vaginal introitus
- Third degree (3°)   Cervix below (outside)the vaginal introitus
- Procidentia   Uterus and cervix outside the vaginal introitus

In the absence of an immobile reference point, there is built-in subjectivity and hence a lack of reproducibility and standardisation in this system of POP grading.

POP-Q System

This system has been developed by the International Continence Society, and it brings in reproducibility and objectivity due to fixed reference points. Hence, it is suitable for comparison of pre and postsurgical outcomes.

In this system, the hymenal ring is the fixed point. Distance above the hymenal ring is shown as negative and the distance below as positive. The distance from the hymenal ring to six predetermined reference points is measured in centimetres by a scale in supine or left lateral positions, while the patient is performing a Valsalva manoeuvre. The results are then shown in a 3x3 table. The range of measurement is –3 to +3 cm, except for a total vaginal length.

Total vaginal length is measured at rest after reducing the vaginal prolapse.

Aa Anterior wall	Ba Anterior wall	C Cervix or vaginal vault
gh Genital hiatus	pb Perineal body	tvl Total vaginal length
Ap Posterior wall	Bp Posterior wall	D Posterior fornix

Table 10.4. POP-Q system abbreviations

Once the measurements are done, stages are assigned according to the most dependent part of the prolapse.

Stage 0	No demonstrable prolapse. All measurements on the anterior and posterior vaginal walls are at –3 cm.
Stage I	All points are more than 1 cm above the hymenal ring.
Stage II	Lowest point of the anterior/posterior vaginal-wall prolapse is within 1 cm of the hymenal ring.
Stage III	Lowest point of the prolapse > 1 cm is below the hymenal ring.
Stage IV	Complete prolapse is evident, with lowest point equalling tvl−2 cm.

Table 10.5. POP staging according to POP-Q

Risk Factors

POP has multifactorial aetiology.

Damage to the support system of the pelvic floor leads to prolapse at the damaged site. Most often, more than one site is involved, and hence women present with different types of prolapse simultaneously.

There is no racial predisposition. The following are risk factors:

- Pregnancy and delivery
  - Pregnancy and vaginal delivery cause direct trauma to fascial, muscular, and nervous supply to the muscles (S2, S3, and S4).
  - Levator ani muscles get detached from their bony attachment on one or both sides.
  - The incidence of prolapse increases with forceps delivery, macrosomia, and a prolonged second stage of labour.
  - Multiparity is the strongest risk factor.
  - Protection to the pelvic floor by a caesarean delivery only lasts a few years.
- Aging
  - With aging, there is increased denervation of the pelvic support and conversion of muscle tissue to fascial tissue. Hence, prolapse is occasionally seen in nulliparous women too.
- Connective tissue disorders
  - For example, myopathies, neuropathies, Marfan's syndrome.
  - Collagen disorders predispose to POP.
  - Changes in collagen metabolism may be associated with prolapse.
  - An increased level of collagen leads to weakened pelvic support and stress incontinence.
  - Hydroxyproline content is lower by 40% in women with stress incontinence.
- Menopause
  - With menopause and lack of oestrogen, connective tissue atrophies.
- Raised intra-abdominal pressure
  - Obesity, chronic cough, smoking, constipation, and weight-lifting exercises lead to increased intra-abdominal pressure, which damages the pelvic floor and hence predisposes to prolapse.
- Iatrogenic
  - Pelvic surgery may damage, distort, or denervate the pelvic floor.
  - For example, an enterocoele may develop after colposuspension, a vault prolapse after a hysterectomy, and cystocoele after a sacrospinous colpopexy.

Factors Predisposing to Recurrent Prolapse

- Poor surgical technique
  - As described above, poor surgical technique can lead to recurrence or a different type of prolapse. Surgical complications such as a haematoma and infection can also lead to suboptimal outcomes.

- Poor surgical preparation
  - In menopausal women, the vagina should be oestrogenised by topical oestrogen at least 6 weeks before surgery and 3 months after surgery.
- Patient factors
  - As described above, an increase in intra-abdominal pressure will lead to prolapse.
  - Women who are young when they first develop POP have a greater risk of recurrence due to their greater longevity.
  - Aging also causes loss of muscle, collagen, and denervation.

Examination

The following describes a general approach to examining a patient with suspected POP.

- Instruments
  - Sims speculum.
  - Bivalve speculum if cervix not visualised.
  - Goniometer to measure urethral angle with the help of a Q-tip (rarely used now).
- Accessories
  - Gloves.
  - Jelly.
  - Good light.
  - A chaperone when required.
- Consent
  - A verbal consent after proper explanation of the proposed examination.
  - Ensure privacy.
- Position of the patient
  - In most cases, the patient will be supine.
  - It is easier to introduce a Sims speculum in the left lateral position or when the buttocks are at the end of the couch.
  - Very rarely, a patient may need to be examined in a standing position with one foot on a stool and an empty bladder.

With the help of a Sims speculum, anterior and posterior walls are examined sequentially when the patient is performing a Valsalva manoeuvre. Measurements are taken if the POP-Q method of quantification is being used. Presence of rugae, asymmetry, and the state of the paravaginal sulci on both sides is noted. Cervical and uterine descent is also assessed at the same time. Rectal examination may be needed to differentiate a rectocoele from an enterocoele. Presence of atrophy, decubitus ulcers (due to pressure or friction of two tissue surfaces), or vaginal discharge is noted. Uterine size should be assessed. A Pap smear or HPV test and a high vaginal swab may be done, if needed.

Kegel's manoeuvre: With two examining fingers in the vagina, the patient is asked to squeeze the fingers with her vaginal muscles. This test provides an assessment of the levator tone.

Role of Imaging

The role of imaging is very limited. The diagnosis and quantification of POP is clinical. However, 2D/3-D perineal/translabial ultrasound scans are being increasingly used in research centres. Injury to the levator muscles and the position of mesh or sling used in surgery can be seen with 2D/3-D ultrasound scans, and the outcomes can be objectively compared.

Chapter 10.1.1.	Anterior Vaginal Wall Prolapse (Urethrocoele and Cystocoele)

History

Symptoms can be disproportionate to the size and site of prolapse. It's a disease of parous women, but, rarely, nulliparous women can also present with prolapse symptoms. The common symptoms are a sensation of something falling out through the vaginal orifice and feeling a bulge or fullness in the vagina. In severe cases, difficulty sitting or walking is experienced, and it can cause dyspareunia or obstruction to the penile penetration of the vagina.

Occasionally, urinary urgency or voiding difficulty is felt on prolonged standing. Some women complain of stress urinary leakage due to urethral hypermobility. Some other women have no stress incontinence due to the kinking of the urethra following severe prolapse.

In the evening hours, many women feel a dragging pain in the pelvis radiating to the vagina that is relieved by lying down. Valsalva manoeuvre accentuates the prolapse.

Examination

Examination of a woman with prolapse has already been described. If the bladder neck is well supported, the urethra is also well supported. However, if the bladder neck is not well supported, a cystocoele and urethrocoele will be present. They feel soft, pliable, and nontender. If a cystocoele or urethrocoele is present, its severity should be quantified.

Differential Diagnosis of Urethrocoele

- Inflamed/enlarged Skene's glands
  - These are tender, and there will be pus coming from the urethra.
- Urethral diverticula
  - Pus may be expressed from the urethra secondary to chlamydial or gonococcal infection.

Differential Diagnosis of Cystocoele

- Bladder tumour
- Bladder diverticula
  - Both of these conditions are rare. Radiological imaging or cystoscopy will be needed to exclude these pathologies.

Management

The treatment of any type of POP should start with lifestyle changes, such as weight reduction if obese, giving up smoking, and treating chronic cough or constipation.

Physiotherapy

The role of physiotherapy is limited to reducing the rate of worsening of prolapse. Kegel's exercises and pelvic-floor-muscle training have been used as the starting point in the management of urethrocoele and cystocoele, although there is no direct evidence to support them. However, they may help in other symptoms, such as urinary or faecal incontinence, since often there are multiple types of prolapse causing multiple symptoms.

The frequency and technique of pelvic-floor-muscle training are very important, and hence there needs to be emphasis on involving a physiotherapist.

Vaginal Pessary

The indications for use of a vaginal pessary are:

- Frail and elderly women unfit for surgery and/or anaesthetic
- Younger women whose families are not complete
- Recurrent prolapse
- Woman's choice

<u>Types of pessary</u>

There are several types. The commonly used ones are as follows:

- Ring
- Shelf
- Smith-Hodge
- Inflatable

The pessary must be large enough to be retained in the vagina but not so large as to cause discomfort, pain, and necrosis of the vaginal walls. The pessary, if retained, should be changed at least every six months to prevent vaginal erosion and fistula formation. Women with a large prolapse or wide subpubic arch will not be able to retain the pessary. Pain on bleeding necessitates removal of the pessary, and any local cause of bleeding should be excluded.

Surgery

Indications

- Family is complete
- Failed conservative therapy
- Recurrent prolapse
- Woman's choice
- Woman medically fit to undergo surgery

Types of Surgery

<u>Vaginal Approach</u>

Anterior colporrhaphy is still the most commonly performed surgery for this prolapse. It is done by opening the anterior vaginal wall and then reinforcing the underlying fascia, pubocervical fascia (anatomists call it the muscularis and adventitial layers of the vaginal wall) by one or more layers of suturing using dissolvable suture material (mostly polyglycol). If the urethrocoele is present, similar suturing is done over the urethra. The vaginal mucosa is trimmed, and the vaginal wall is then closed.

The use of mesh to provide level I and II support, which started around 1996, has considerably decreased in recent years due to legal action against the manufacturers.

A simultaneous posterior colpoperineorrhaphy may be needed because often the defect in the pelvic support affects more than one area.

Childbirth after prior surgery for POP should be preferably by a caesarean.

The recurrence rate of prolapse after surgery is 20–30%.

<u>Abdominal Approach</u>

Sacrocolpopexy is used to treat anterior vaginal-wall prolapse, but because the surgery involves a laparotomy, it is not the first choice. In this surgery, the vaginal vault is attached to the sacral promontory through a graft, which is then retroperitonealised. The important complications to this surgery are damage to the median sacral artery causing profuse haemorrhage and ureteric trauma. The graft may get infected or detach from its vaginal attachment. This surgery is only for apical prolapse and lateral cystocoeles.

<u>Laparoscopic Approach</u>

This is used for a level I pelvic-floor-support defect. A paravaginal repair is performed with laparoscopic suturing. This is only done by certain advanced laparoscopic gynaecologists in selected centres, and the evidence behind its effectiveness in comparison to a vaginal approach is not strong. Laparoscopic sacrocolpopexy has a lower failure rate and less dyspareunia.

| Chapter 10.1.2. | Posterior Vaginal Wall Prolapse (Rectocoele and Enterocoele) |

History

Posterior vaginal-wall prolapse can cause bowel, bladder, and sexual dysfunction. Women often complain of a bulge in the vagina that can affect sitting down or walking. They may also feel incomplete emptying of the rectum and may learn to splint the posterior vaginal wall with their fingers (vaginal digitation) to empty the rectum completely. Constipation is not a symptom of rectocoele. A large rectocoele can press upon the bladder and urethra and cause urinary voiding difficulty.

Like a large cystocoele, a large rectocoele or enterocoele may also cause dyspareunia or difficulty in vaginal penetration during coitus.

Examination

As mentioned earlier, a rectocoele can be seen after retracting the anterior vaginal wall with one half of the Sims speculum. The prolapse accentuates on Valsalva manoeuvre or straining.

Management

Nonoperative treatments are similar to that in anterior vaginal-wall prolapse.

Vaginal Surgical Approach

Posterior colpoperineorrhaphy is the mainstay of surgical treatment for this condition. The principles of this surgery are similar to that of an anterior colporrhaphy. In this surgery, instead of pubocervical fascia, the rectovaginal septum (Denonvilliers fascia) is reinforced with dissolvable suturing. A perineorrhaphy (approximation of the levator muscles with reconstruction of the perineal body) is mostly needed due to a low rectocoele, an absent perineal body, or a gaping vagina.

If an enterocoele is present, its sac is identified and opened, and the contents are replaced into the peritoneal cavity. The neck of the sac is sutured in a purse-string fashion. A properly repaired enterocoele does not usually recur.

Chapter 10.1.3.   Uterine Prolapse

History

The symptoms of a uterine prolapse are heaviness, fullness in the vagina, and the sensation of something coming out of the vagina. Often in a supine position, the prolapse retracts and symptoms transiently disappear. It is common for the patient to have concurrent symptoms of a cystocoele and/or rectocoele.

A decubitus ulcer may cause bloody vaginal discharge.

Examination

A diagnosis is made by inspection, as mentioned in earlier sections.

Management

Physiotherapy and vaginal pessaries may be helpful if the prolapse is up to a grade II. A vaginal hysterectomy should be offered if there are no contraindications and conservative treatment has failed. Some women directly request a vaginal hysterectomy. If a vaginal hysterectomy is not possible or is contraindicated, a laparoscopic-assisted vaginal hysterectomy or an abdominal hysterectomy could be done.

An anterior and posterior colporrhaphy with perineorrhaphy is also often needed.

In elderly women with associated comorbidities who are not sexually active, a Le Fort's colpocleisis (suturing opposing areas of anterior and posterior vaginal walls together with delayed absorbable sutures, causing closure of the vagina with small openings on either side) is a suitable option, requiring a much shorter operative time. The prognosis in terms of surgical outcome is excellent.

Women wanting to conserve their uteri will benefit from either uterosacropexy or another surgery in which the uterosacral ligaments on both sides are sutured to the ipsilateral sacrospinous ligaments. Such women should always deliver by a caesarean section in future pregnancies.

Chapter 10.1.4.   Vaginal Apical Prolapse

This occurs as a result of an unsatisfactory level I support, usually as the result of a hysterectomy. It can be total (complete vault prolapse, complete vaginal eversion) or partial. It is usually accompanied by different grades of cystocoele, enterocoele, and rectocoele. The incidence is 0.1–0.8%.

History

- Vaginal fullness
- Heaviness
- Backache
- Sensation of a bulge coming out of the vagina
- Urinary voiding problems, urgency, and incontinence
- Sexual discomfort

Examination

Diagnosis is made by visual inspection and examination as noted in earlier sections. Any associated cystocoele, enterocoele, or rectocoele should also be noted.

Management

Vaginal pessaries could be used, but in a large prolapse, they are mostly expelled. Shelf pessaries are better retained when the prolapse is large or the perineum is deficient. Pessaries are more likely to fail with previous hysterectomy (Evidence Level II).

Vaginal oestrogen in a postmenopausal woman, 6 weeks before surgery, will make the vaginal wall healthier (atrophic changes will vanish), and the decubitus ulcers will also heal.

Surgery

Types of Surgery

Abdominal Approach

Sacrocolpopexy is the gold standard surgery (Evidence Level IA). This involves fixation of the vaginal vault to either the anterior abdominal wall or the sacral promontory or the sacrospinous ligament and various tendons in the true pelvis. Fixation to the anterior abdominal wall and sacral promontory needs a graft. Unfortunately, this procedure opens up the pouch of Douglas posteriorly and facilitates an enterocoele. Fixation to the sacrospinous ligament is a very effective method among these surgeries; however, sacrocolpopexy has lower rates of dyspareunia and stress incontinence (Evidence Level IA). There are risks of intraoperative bleeding and infection of the graft.

<u>Vaginal Approach</u>

The different techniques used in the vaginal approach attach the vaginal vault to the sacrospinous ligament with a nondissolvable suture. This surgery is called sacrospinous colpopexy. The success rate is 65–97%. The surgical outcome is better when the vagina is nearly horizontal. This surgery can be performed directly under vision using a Miya hook or with the aid of a needle-fixing device. Doing colpopexy bilaterally makes the vagina nonanatomical, stretches the vault corners, and sometimes the stitches cut through the vaginal walls.

A concomitant anterior vaginal repair should be done to reduce the incidence of a cystocoele. Other types of prolapse which are often present must be addressed at the same time, including a perineorrhaphy.

A unilateral sacrospinous colpopexy maintains the vaginal length and makes the vagina retroverted and deviated to one side, but coitus is still possible. Complications of this surgery include damage to pudendal nerves and vessels, causing heavy bleeding. Fortunately, these are not common. Buttock pain usually lasts a few weeks and can be treated by simple analgesic.

When a shorter operative time is required in a frail, elderly woman, a Le Fort's or modified Le Fort's colpocleisis affords good symptomatic improvement.

Chapter 10.1.5. Summary of History and Examination

	Anterior vaginal wall prolapse (urethrocoele and cystocoele)	Posterior vaginal wall prolapse (rectocoele and enterocoele)	Uterine prolapse	Vaginal apical prolapse
History	• Sensation of something falling out through the vaginal orifice • Bulge in vagina, difficulty sitting or walking • Dyspareunia • Obstruction to penile penetration of vagina • Urinary urgency or voiding difficulty, after prolonged standing • Stress urinary leakage due to urethral hypermobility • Otherwise, no stress incontinence due to urethral kinking • Dragging pain in pelvis in evening; radiates to vagina; relieved by lying down	• Bulge in vagina, affecting sitting down and walking • Incomplete rectal emptying, vaginal digitation • Urinary voiding difficulty • Dyspareunia • Difficulty in vaginal penetration during coitus	• Heaviness • Fullness in vagina • Sensation of something coming out of vagina • Decubitus ulcer may cause bloody discharge	• Vaginal fullness • Heaviness • Backache • Sensation of a bulge coming out of the vagina • Urinary voiding problems, urgency and incontinence • Sexual discomfort
Examination	• Urethrocoele and cystocoele feel soft, pliable and nontender • Valsalva manoeuvre accentuates the prolapse • If prolapse present, severity should be quantified	• Rectocoele can be visualised when anterior vaginal wall retracted with Sims' speculum • Prolapse accentuates with Valsalva manoeuvre	• Prolapse retracts, may disappear in supine position	• Prolapse is observed using techniques described above

Table 10.6. Summary of history and examination for different types of POP

Chapter 10.1.6.   Summary of Management

	Anterior vaginal wall prolapse (urethrocoele and cystocoele)	Posterior vaginal wall prolapse (rectocoele and enterocoele)	Uterine prolapse	Vaginal apical prolapse
Lifestyle	• Weight reduction if obese • Give up smoking • Treating chronic cough or constipation			
Physiotherapy	• Kegel's exercises • Pelvic floor muscle training • Pelvic floor strengthening exercises help symptoms such as urinary or faecal incontinence and slow progression of prolapse, but do not cause regression of disease			
Pessary	• Must be large enough to be retained in vagina but not so large as to cause discomfort, pain, and discomfort			• In large prolapse, pessaries are mostly expelled • Shelf pessary may be most suitable

Surgery	• Anterior colporrhaphy (vaginal approach) to reinforce pubocervical fascia with sutures
	• Sacrocolpopexy by laparotomy
	  o Complications: haemorrhage, ureteric trauma, infection of graft or detachment of graft
	• Laparoscopic approach for level I support defect, only performed by gynaecologists with advanced skills in laparoscopic surgery
		• Posterior colpoperineorrhaphy by vaginal approach to reinforce rectovaginal septum with sutures
		• A perineorrhaphy (approximation of the levator muscles with reconstruction of the perineal body) is mostly needed due to a low rectocoele, an absent perineal body, or a gaping vagina
		• Sac of an enterocoele is sutured in a purse-string fashion after bowel contents are replaced into peritoneal cavity
			• Vaginal hysterectomy is first option
			• Alternatively, vaginal hysterectomy or abdominal hysterectomy
			• Anterior and posterior colporrhaphy with perineorrhaphy is also often needed
			• Le Fort's colpocleisis suitable in elderly women who are not sexually active
			• Uterus-sparing operations include utero-sacropexy or one where uterosacral ligaments are sutured to ipsilateral sacrospinous ligaments on both sides
				• Vaginal oestrogen 6 weeks before surgery make vaginal wall healthier and decubitus ulcers heal
				• Sacrocolpopexy by abdominal approach is gold standard
				  o Risk of intraoperative bleeding, infection of graft
				• The alternative is sacrospinous colpopexy by a vaginal approach, with concomitant anterior vaginal repair
				  o Unilateral sacrospinous colpopexy makes coitus still possible
				• Le Fort's colpocleisis suitable in elderly women

Table 10.7. Summary of management options for different types of POP

Short-Answer Questions

Question 1

Discuss the advantages and disadvantages of a vaginal pessary for the treatment of POP.

Answer:

Advantages:

- Easily available
- Can be inserted in the outpatient setting without any fasting or anaesthesia
- Well-tolerated procedure
- No pain/discomfort, if correctly positioned
- Works immediately
- Suitable for elderly, frail women who are not fit for surgery/anaesthesia
- Not expensive

Disadvantages:

- No guarantee that it will work, and may fall out (usually posthysterectomy)
- Visit to the gynaecologist every 6 months to get it washed and changed
- Causes pain and discomfort if not correctly positioned or size too big
- Can cause vaginal ulceration and bleeding
- In some women, interferes with coitus, depending upon type of pessary
- May unmask urinary incontinence
- Foul vaginal discharge in prolonged neglected cases

Question 2

List the treatments for vault prolapse and an important advantage and disadvantage for each method of treatment.

Answer:

The following is the list of treatments available together with their one advantage and disadvantage.

	Advantage	**Disadvantage**
Pelvic floor exercises	No need for surgery and anaesthesia	No guarantee that symptoms will improve
Vaginal pessary	Can be fitted in outpatient clinics without pain or need for anaesthesia	Visit to the gynaecologist every 6 months
Vaginal sacrospinous colpopexy	Vaginal approach without any graft	May damage pudendal nerve and vessels
Iliococcygeal fixation	Vaginal approach with lower risk of prolapse recurrence	
Colpocleisis	Simple vaginal surgery requiring shorter operative time	Coitus impossible
Abdominal treatments		
Abdominal sacrocolpopexy	Gold standard surgery for vault prolapse	Abdominal approach makes it more invasive and risk of severe intraoperative haemorrhage and damage to ureters
Laparoscopic sacrocolpopexy	Better and shorter abdominal scar	As above
Robotic sacrocolpopexy	As above	As above
Abdominal sacrospinous colpopexy	As per sacrocolpopexy	As per sacrocolpopexy

Table 10.8. Advantages and disadvantages of different treatment options of vault prolapse

Question 3

All POP surgery must include a hysterectomy. Briefly discuss this statement.

Answer:

This discussion encompasses two facets of POP treatment.

First, does routine hysterectomy improve the surgical outcome of prolapse surgery? Historically, a rationale to perform a hysterectomy in a perimenopausal or menopausal woman was to remove an organ that was not of use and that had the potential to become diseased. At present, there is a lack of evidence to support the notion that not doing a hysterectomy at the time of prolapse surgery negatively impacts on the surgical outcome. A normal uterus does not damage the pelvic floor. Alternatively, a hysterectomy may interfere with the level I support mechanism. So, on this score, there is no merit in a routine hysterectomy, so long as uterine pathology has been excluded.

Second, does a hysterectomy affect sexual enjoyment? Masters and Johnson stated that a total hysterectomy could cause sexual and orgasmic dysfunction. However, randomised trials have shown that there is no difference in sexual enjoyment. Some other studies have shown improved sexual function after a total hysterectomy, possibly due to resolution of prolapse and restoration of vaginal anatomy (Roovers JP et al., 2003).

On balance, it appears that there is no merit in doing a routine hysterectomy at the time of prolapse surgery. A patient's expectation from surgery should be balanced with the medical indications.

Question 4

How do pregnancy and vaginal childbirth affect the pelvic floor?

Answer:

The pelvic floor is affected by stretch, avulsion, tearing, and pressure necrosis during childbirth.

Effect of pregnancy on the pelvic floor:

- Pregnancy, especially in the third trimester, causes hypermobility of the urethra and bladder neck, resulting in stress incontinence. The endopelvic fascia becomes more elastic and hence more likely to cause stress incontinence. According to Thorpe et al. (1999), the frequency of incontinence episodes peaks in the third trimester.

- The lordosis of pregnancy exposes the anterior perineum to the abnormally high pressures of the gravid uterus and intra-abdominal contents.

Effect of childbirth on the pelvic floor:

- The hypermobility of the urethra and bladder neck is accentuated.

- The maximum trauma to the pelvic floor happens in the first vaginal childbirth. The puborectalis muscle of the levator ani group bears the brunt and avulses from its bony attachment, which increases the genital hiatus dimensions by 20–30%. This causes the ballooning of the genital hiatus. The genital hiatus ballooning is clinically diagnosed when the total of genital hiatus (gh) and perineal body (pb) measurements exceeds 7 cm. Ballooning and avulsion of the puborectalis, while often associated, are independent predictors of prolapse and its recurrence.

- About 10–30% of women suffer from macroscopic trauma to the levator ani muscles. A far greater proportion of women suffer "microtrauma," the significance of which is unclear at present.

- The length of second stage of labour, birth weight, head dimensions, and forceps delivery are risk factors for levator trauma.

Clinical effect of puborectalis avulsion:

- It is associated with signs and symptoms of vaginal prolapse, increased vaginal laxity, and reduced tone on coitus. In the medium to long term, it is associated with anterior and central compartment prolapse. The larger the avulsion, the more pronounced are the symptoms and signs of prolapse.

Effect of vaginal childbirth on the anal sphincter:

- The trauma to the anal sphincter is much more common than clinically diagnosed or reported. Endoanal ultrasound has shown that up to 35% of primiparous women have anal sphincter trauma due to a vaginal delivery.

Effect in pudendal neuropathy:

- According to Professor HP Dietz (*O&G Magazine*, Autumn 2014), evidence for pudendal neuropathy secondary to vaginal childbirth is inconsistent. Nerve regeneration does occur. Nerve damage is also seen in nulliparous women and with aging.

Question 5

How will you reduce the damage to the pelvic floor as a result of a vaginal delivery?

Answer:

The following will reduce the damage to the pelvic floor from a vaginal delivery:

- Screening for gestational diabetes and managing diabetes optimally to reduce the risk of macrosomia.
- Active management of the first and second stages of labour.
- Using Ventouse in preference to a forceps delivery.
- Using mediolateral episiotomy when needed.
- Use of the Epi-No device, perineal massage, and a birthing stool have been shown to reduce pelvic-floor damage during vaginal childbirth.
- Early recognition and optimum repair of 2nd- and 3rd-degree perineal tears and follow-up by a colorectal surgeon for 3rd- and 4th-degree tears.

Question 6

A 25-year-old woman presents with vaginal prolapse two years after having a vaginal childbirth. Briefly describe your management.

Answer:

My management will start with a focused history, which will cover the following areas:

- Details of labour
  - Duration of the second stage of labour.
  - Any forceps used.
  - Baby's birth weight and head circumference.
  - Any associated perineal tear and whether it was repaired in the birth suite or operating theatre.
  - I will also seek the woman's opinion about whether it was a traumatic birth or a normal birth.
- Whether she would like to have more children
- Any history of uterovaginal prolapse in the family, suggesting connective tissue disorders or a gynecoid pelvis

- Any precipitating factors, such as smoking, chronic cough, obesity, or constipation
- Any associated urinary symptoms—stress or urge incontinence, frequency, dysuria
- Other symptoms, such as perineal pain or pressure, bulge, backache, or a dragging pelvic pain

My examination will include a general examination of the cardiorespiratory system and abdomen and then a vaginal examination. The aim of a vaginal examination will be to detect:

- The type of prolapse(s)
- Degree of prolapse, using the POP-Q system
- Tone of the levator muscles
- Any urethral hypermobility

My investigations will be:

- MSU
- Transvaginal pelvic ultrasound scan, if there is any suspicion of a big uterus, abnormal bleeding, or abnormal adnexal mass
- Urodynamics if urinary incontinence is present

Management: The fact that she is very young indicates that she will most likely have more children in the future, and the benefit of any surgery will be either fully or incompletely lost after future pregnancies and childbirth. Hence, the most suitable option will be the use of a vaginal pessary with pelvic-floor exercises under the guidance of a physiotherapist. Definitive surgery should take place once the family has been completed. Given her young age, a synthetic graft should not be used in her prolapse surgery.

According to the US National Institutes of Health (NIH), there is only weak evidence to support a preventative role for elective caesarean delivery, and the existing data do not adequately answer the question of whether elective caesarean delivery can reduce the incidence of PFDs. Even if a reduction in PFDs could be demonstrated, other harms and benefits of elective caesarean delivery need to be weighed against this benefit.

Question 7

A 62-year-old woman, having had a hysterectomy 5 years ago, presents with vaginal-vault prolapse. Discuss your assessment and available treatment options. If this woman also has genuine stress incontinence, what will you do differently?

Answer:

My assessment of this woman will start with a focused history, including the following points:

- Type of hysterectomy—abdominal or vaginal
- Any associated prolapse repair, with or without a graft
- Any predisposing factors, such as smoking, constipation, obesity, or chronic cough increasing intra-abdominal pressure
- Any associated urinary symptoms, such as urge, stress, frequency, and dysuria
- Any back pain, dragging pelvic pain, or a lump between the thighs

- State of general health—other surgeries, medical problems, drug use, allergies, etc.

After obtaining the history, I will obtain verbal consent to examine the woman, ensuring privacy in the presence of a chaperone. The aim of my examination will be to detect:

- The type of prolapse(s)
- Degree of prolapse, using the POP-Q system
- Tone of the levator muscles
- Any urethral hypermobility

I will then request the following investigations:

- MSU
- Transvaginal pelvic ultrasound scan if there is any suspicion of a big uterus, abnormal bleeding, or abnormal adnexal mass
- Urodynamics if urinary incontinence is present

<u>Management options</u>:

I will start her on vaginal oestrogen.

If there is only vault prolapse (with or without cystocoele or rectocoele) and no urinary incontinence, I will recommend a sacrospinous colpopexy with anterior colporrhaphy and posterior colpoperineorrhaphy. This is a very commonly performed surgery by most gynaecologists with a success rate approaching 100%.

Since the woman is only 62 years old, colpocleisis will not be an option.

Vaginal pessaries are also options if they do not fall out. But the woman will have to see a gynaecologist every 6 months for the replacement of the pessary. If the woman does not want surgery, then a pessary is the only option.

While there are many abdominal surgical options, they are performed by only a small number of gynaecologists. The options are:

- Sacrocolpopexy (gold standard)
    - Open
    - Laparoscopic
- Sacrospinous colpopexy

<u>If this woman has genuine stress incontinence</u>:

Assuming that her MSU is normal, I will first refer her to a physiotherapist for pelvic-floor exercises, for nearly 3 months. I will also prescribe vaginal oestrogen therapy. I will defer any prolapse surgery until a review in 3 months. If, at the review, the woman requests surgery or does not have any benefit from the pelvic-floor exercises, then I will combine the prolapse surgery, as described above, with either a vaginal midurethral sling surgery or a Birch colposuspension.

Question 8

Briefly discuss the controversy around the use of synthetic mesh in gynaecological prolapse surgery.

Answer:

Synthetic mesh has been used in gynaecological prolapse surgery since 1955, but there was a sudden increase in the number of such surgeries since the early 2000s. Simultaneously, there was a mushroom growth of mesh kit manufacturers who indulged in indiscriminate marketing and suboptimal mesh kit designs. This increase was not accompanied by adequate evaluation of mesh kit safety and efficacy. The initial confidence in the use of synthetic mesh was derived from the use of mesh in surgical herniorrhaphy. However, within the last decade, there has been a plethora of lawsuits by women who had mesh surgery, on account of pain, dyspareunia, recurrence of prolapse, and bowel and renal tract injuries. Consequently, major manufacturers withdrew from the market due to legal and commercial implications.

The 2016 Cochrane review showed that the synthetic mesh did reduce the rates of awareness of recurrent prolapse, when compared with native tissue repairs, but it caused a 2.5-fold increase in reoperation rates for prolapse and mesh exposure in both apical and posterior compartments. The risk-benefit profile was similar for recurrent anterior vaginal-wall prolapse, with a higher rate of mesh erosion (Ow L et al., 2016). Studies have also shown that the use of synthetic mesh in the posterior compartment did not improve either the anatomy or function (Maher C et al., 2013). It has also been shown that hysterectomy with simultaneous vaginal mesh repair has a high rate of mesh erosion (Collinet P et al., 2006). All these unintended consequences of vaginal mesh surgery have been attributed to the properties and function of the vagina, inadequate surgical techniques, and poor patient selection. Mesh characteristics, such as weight, pore size, porosity, pore geometry, and stiffness also have roles in the genesis of unintended consequences. There is no study yet that shows better outcomes with newer meshes.

In the last decade, apart from the body habitus, levator avulsion, and consequent hiatal ballooning have been identified as the major risk factors for prolapse recurrence (Dietz H et al., 2010). Studies on prolapse recurrence have shown an odds ratio of 2–3 in women with levator avulsion (Model A et al., 2010). Rodrigo N et al. (2014) have shown that anteriorly anchored mesh could partially compensate for the effect of levator avulsion and significantly reduce the risk of vaginal prolapse recurrence in women with avulsion. They have shown that women with levator avulsion and hiatal area of 40 cm^2 on Valsalva will have a prolapse recurrence risk of 80% with conventional surgery and 45% with anterior mesh repair. So, with proper patient selection and mesh kit design, vaginal mesh surgery has a definite place in treating prolapse recurrence. It should not be used as the primary repair procedure. Women with risk factors for prolapse recurrence, such as obesity, young age, chronically raised intra-abdominal pressure, and with stage 3–4 prolapse may find the risk-benefit profile of vaginal mesh surgery acceptable. Women should also be counselled regarding other evidence-based treatment options, such as sacral colpopexy. Ensuring adequate apical support at the time of colporrhaphy reduces risk of recurrence.

Multiple-Choice Questions

Q1. In the POP-Q system, what does Bp –3 mean?

    A. The most dependent part of the posterior vaginal wall is 3 cm above the hymenal ring.
    B. The reference point of the posterior vaginal wall is 3 cm above the hymenal ring.
    C. The reference point of the anterior vaginal wall is 3 cm above the hymenal ring.
    D. The most dependent part of the anterior vaginal wall is 3 cm above the hymenal ring.

Answer: A

Q2. Stage II of the POP-Q system corresponds with which degree of the conventional grading system of prolapse?

    A. 0th degree
    B. 1st degree
    C. 2nd degree
    D. 3rd degree

Answer: C

Q3. Which of the following diseases predisposes to POP?

    A. Holt-Oram syndrome
    B. Sjogren syndrome.
    C. Ehlers-Danlos syndrome
    D. Down syndrome

Answer: C (connective tissue disorder)

Q4. Which muscles are cut during a mediolateral episiotomy?

    A. Bulbospongiosus and Kallman syndrome
    B. Bulbospongiosus and transverse perineal muscles
    C. Ischiocavernosus and transverse perineal muscles
    D. Ischiococcygeus and bulbospongiosus

Answer: B

Q5. Which of the following statements is correct for a normal woman in the standing position?

    A. The levator plate forms a gutter in the midline.
    B. The levator plate is inclined anteriorly, and the urethra rests on it.
    C. The levator plate is inclined posteriorly, and the rectum rests on it.
    D. The levator plate is horizontal, and the cervix, urethra, and rectum rest on it.

Answer: D

Q6. Which of the following operations leads to an enterocoele?

    A. Sacrospinous colpopexy
    B. Rectocoele repair
    C. Manchester repair
    D. Trans-obturator sling surgery

Answer: C (posterior apical vagina not supported)

Q7. Which of the following operations leads to a cystocoele?

    A. Sacrospinous colpopexy
    B. Rectocoele repair
    C. Manchester repair
    D. Trans-obturator sling surgery

Answer: A (anterior vaginal wall not supported)

Q8. Which of the following predisposes to a urethrocoele?

    A. Android pelvis
    B. Anthropoid pelvis
    C. Platypelloid pelvis
    D. Gynaecoid pelvis

Answer: C (wide subpubic arch)

Q9. The lifetime risk of surgery for urogenital prolapse is:

    A. 11%
    B. 22%
    C. 33%
    D. 44%

Answer: A

Q10. The risk of ureteric trauma in a McCall culdoplasty is:

    A. 5%
    B. 10%
    C. 15%
    D. 20%

Answer: A

Q11. The recurrence rate of vault prolapse after a vaginal sacrospinous colpopexy is:

    A. 11%
    B. 22%
    C. 33%
    D. 44%

Answer: C

Q12. Which of the following is **not** part of vaginal histology?

    A. Adventitia

    B. Muscle layer

    C. Basement membrane

    D. Epithelium

Answer: C

Q13. Which of the following is a true hernia of the peritoneal cavity?

    A. Rectocoele

    B. Enterocoele

    C. Urethrocoele

    D. Cystocoele

Answer: B

Q14. Injury to which of the following structures does **not** cause uterine prolapse?

    A. Round ligament

    B. Uterosacral ligament

    C. Cardinal ligament

    D. Endopelvic fascia

Answer: A

Q15. Injury to which of the following structures is most likely to cause uterine prolapse?

    A. Ischiocavernosus

    B. Ischiococcygeus

    C. Puborectalis

    D. Transverse perineal muscles

Answer: C

Q16. A 55-year-old presents with an everted vagina 10 years after a vaginal hysterectomy. She is sexually active. How would you treat her?

    A. Portex pessary

    B. Posterior colpoperineorrhaphy

    C. Sacrospinous colpopexy

    D. Colpocleisis

Answer: C

Q17. In Australasia, what is the most common cause of a vesicovaginal fistula?

    A. Radiation

    B. Anterior colporrhaphy

    C. Abdominal hysterectomy

    D. Vaginal hysterectomy

Answer: C

Q18. In a nulliparous woman with no prolapse, the normal vaginal axis in standing position is:

A. Upward and backward at 135 degrees

B. Upward and backward at 230 degrees

C. Upward and backward at 310 degrees

D. Upward and backward at 90 degrees

Answer: A

Q19. In a randomised controlled trial of a new surgical technique for rectocoele, the most appropriate method for determining the outcome of the procedure is:

A. Sims speculum examination by the surgeon at 3 months

B. Bimanual examination by a blinded external assessor at 3 months

C. Validated POP-Q questionnaire assessed by the surgeon at 3 months

D. POP-Q score by blinded external assessor at 3 months

Answer: D

Chapter 10.2.   Urinary Incontinence

Definitions

Detrusor overactivity	Premature contraction of detrusor muscle during filling or on provocation when the woman is trying to stop urinating
Enuresis	Repeated inability to control urination
Frequency	> 8 voids in the day
Mixed incontinence	A combination of symptoms, such as frequency, urgency, urge, and stress incontinence
Nocturia	Getting up more than once at night to urinate
Overactive bladder	Urgency with or without urge incontinence, usually with frequency and nocturia; often used synonymously with urge incontinence
Painful bladder syndrome (interstitial cystitis)	Suprapubic pain due to bladder filling with daytime frequency and nocturia with the absence of infection or pathology
Rhabdosphincter	The outer, circular, striated muscle layer of the urethra, which works as sphincter urethrae
Stress incontinence	Involuntary leakage of urine on sudden increase in intra-abdominal pressure such as coughing or sneezing
Urethral syndrome	Recurrent urethral pain, usually on voiding, with daytime frequency and nocturia in the absence of infection or any other pathology.
Urge incontinence	Involuntary leakage of urine, which is immediately preceded by urgency
Urgency	Sudden, uncontrollable desire to urinate

Table 10.9. Chapter 10.2. Definitions

Chapter 10.2.1.   Incontinence

This is the involuntary loss of urine. It can occur at any age, but the incidence increases with age.

Types

- Stress incontinence
- Urge incontinence
- Overflow incontinence
- Continuous incontinence
- Mixed incontinence

Clinical Physiology of Continence

The urinary bladder, which has a capacity to hold 400–500 mL of urine, has three histological layers: outer serosa, middle detrusor muscles (smooth muscle), and inner transitional epithelium. When the bladder starts to fill up, the first sensation to void is experienced when it has around 150–200 mL of urine.

A female urethra is 4 cm long. Apart from the inner mucosal layer, which consists of transitional epithelium in the upper half and stratified squamous epithelium in the lower half, it has a complex muscular layer that contributes to the continence mechanisms. The inner smooth muscle, which is continuous with the detrusor muscle of the bladder, acts as the intrinsic sphincter. The outer, circular, striated muscle layer, which acts as the extrinsic sphincter, has two components—the sphincter urethrae and the levator ani. The sphincter urethrae, also known as rhabdosphincter, surrounds the upper two-thirds of the urethra and is responsible for urethral closure. The fibres of the distal one-third of the urethra come from levator ani.

Nerve	Muscle	Function
Sympathetic (T11-L2)	Detrusor	Relaxation
	Intrinsic sphincter	Contraction
Parasympathetic (S2-S4)	Detrusor	Contraction
	Intrinsic sphincter	Relaxation
Pudendal nerve (S2-S4)	Sphincter urethra	Contraction
	Levator ani	Contraction

Table 10.10. Innervation of urinary bladder and urethra

The micturition reflex occurs with the following process. Detrusor contractility is mediated by the parasympathetic system through acetylcholine, and detrusor relaxation is mediated by the sympathetic system through the β-receptors in the bladder wall. The sympathetic nervous system also affects urethral muscle sphincter contraction through the α-receptors in its wall. When the bladder volume exceeds the threshold volume, the stretch receptors in the bladder wall send sensory signals to the micturition centre in the pons. The pons has neuronal connections with the cerebellum, which controls

302

the rate, force, and range of detrusor contractions. The pons communicates with the upper cerebral cortex, which has inhibitory influence on the micturition centre. The upper cerebral cortex permits the pontine micturition centre to send efferent signals through the spinal cord to the sacral micturition centre. The sacral micturition centre sends signals through the parasympathetic nerves (S2–4) to the detrusor muscles, which contract, and the sphincter vesicae, which relaxes, allowing the urine to come out. This is the micturition reflex.

There are many other receptors in the bladder and urethra, including oestrogen and progesterone, but their role in continence is unclear. The urinary bladder and urethra act as one unit, and continence depends on the equilibrium between urethral closure and detrusor contraction.

For urine to come out through the urethra, the maximum urethral pressure must be lower than the intravesical pressure. The resting pressure in the bladder is 20–30 cm of water. Intravesical pressure depends upon:

- Urine volume in the bladder
- Intra-abdominal pressure affecting the bladder
- Bladder-wall tension

The intraurethral pressure depends upon:

- Muscular layers in the urethral wall
- The pressure in the urethral submucosal cavernous plexus containing oestrogen receptors
- The fraction of the intra-abdominal pressure that is exerted on the proximal urethra
- The passive elasticity of the urethra

From the continence point of view, the functional part of the urethra is the part in which the urethral pressure is greater than the intravesical pressure. Urethral pressure increases up to 20 years of age (25 cm of water), declines until menopause (5 cm of water), and then declines rapidly after menopause. The highest pressure zone in the urethra is around the centre of the functional length, which is about 5 mm above the urogenital diaphragm.

Investigations

Microbiological Examination of Midstream Urine

The presence of bacteria in uncontaminated midstream urine suggests urethritis, an infected urethral diverticulum, cystitis, or even pyelonephritis. To diagnose clinical infection, there should be at least 10^5 mL bacteria in the urine. White blood cells are always seen in the urine (pyuria) in cases of UTI, and red blood cells may be present (haematuria). It can result in urinary urgency, frequency, dysuria, and incontinence.

Residual Urine Volume

A normal residual urine volume is 100–150 mL. A large volume indicates voiding difficulty.

Bladder Diary (Frequency-Volume Chart)

The woman records volume and time of fluid intake, and volume and time of urination, including incontinence accidents. It is a cheap and effective way of diagnosing detrusor overactivity.

Urodynamics

It is an objective tool to measure the function of the lower urinary tract. Intravesical and urethral pressures are measured by a multichannel recorder at different anatomical points in standing and supine positions, at rest, and with Valsalva manoeuvre. The intravesical pressure is reflected by intra-abdominal pressure, which is measured by a vaginal or rectal pressure sensor. The addition of a video recorder to the multichannel device facilitates the live recording of urination and any anatomical changes under stress or at rest.

Chapter 10.2.2. Urinary Tract Infection

Female Risk Factors

A urinary tract infection (UTI) is predominantly a bacterial infection of any part of the urinary tract. Almost half of all women will have a UTI at some time in their lives. UTIs are more common in women because of the following reasons:

- Anatomical position of urethra close to vagina and anus, organs that harbour bacteria
- Shorter length of urethra compared with men
- Coitus facilitating entry into the urethra
- Pregnancy
  - o Progestogenic effect on smooth muscles of the bladder and ureters causing stasis
  - o Venous engorgement in the pelvis applying pressure on the ureters
  - o Pregnancy is a hyperglycaemic and immunocompromised state
- Puerperium
- Urogenital prolapse—incomplete voiding
- Menopause due to oestrogen deficiency—higher incidence of asymptomatic bacteriuria
- Postoperative period
- Bladder stones, diabetes mellitus, meatal stenosis, etc.

Causative Bacteria

- *Escherichia coli*: most common, usually community acquired
- *Proteus mirabilis*
- *Pseudomonas aeruginosa*
  - o Both of these are often hospital acquired or due to prolonged catheterisation
- *Klebsiella*
- *Streptococcus faecalis*

- *Enterococcus*
- *Staphylococcus saprophyticus*

Asymptomatic Bacteriuria

This is the presence of bacteria in the urine without symptoms. It is more common in postmenopausal women. It should only be treated if surgery is planned.

Pyelonephritis

This is an infection of the kidneys due to ascent of bacteria from the lower urinary tract.

History

- Frequency, urgency, and dysuria are characteristic.
  - The dysuria is at the end of urination as opposed to dysuria of vulvitis, which happens at the start of urination.
- Pain.
  - Usually suprapubic; backache, loin pain if pyelonephritis.
- Haematuria.
- Fever.

Investigations

- Urine dipstick.
  - Shows white blood cells and nitrites, which are metabolic products of pathogenic bacteria.
  - A presumptive diagnosis of UTI can be made on the basis of a positive urine dipstick.
- MSU.
  - Any presumptive diagnosis of UTI should be confirmed by a microbiological examination of a clean-catch midstream urine sample. A bacterial count of 100,000/mL or greater of urine usually indicates a UTI.
- Urethroscopy and cystoscopy.
  - Needed only in cases of recurrent or chronic infection.

Management

- Cystitis and urethritis.
  - Oral norfloxacin, 400mg twice daily for 5 days.
  - Oral ciprofloxacin, 250 mg twice daily for 5 days.
- Persistent or recurrent cystitis.
  - Oral cefuroxime, 250 mg two daily for 5 days.
- Fever or pyelonephritis.
  - Intravenous antibacterial agent.

The antibacterial agents must be altered according the microbiological sensitivities.

Prevention

This includes behaviour modification, such as increased oral fluid intake, frequent voiding, voiding after coitus, and topical oestrogen if postmenopausal.

Chapter 10.2.3. Urethral Syndrome (Urethral Pain Syndrome)

This condition is defined as recurrent urethral pain, usually on voiding, with daytime frequency and nocturia in the absence of infection or any other pathology.

The prevalence is 20–30% of all women.

The cause is unknown. It is thought that possibly an infection of paraurethral glands by organisms such as *Mycoplasma*, *Ureaplasma*, or *Chlamydia* may cause pain.

Urethroscopy may show an inflamed urethra with spasm at the bladder neck.

Since the cause is unknown, many therapies have been tried with varying success. These include progressive urethral dilatation, antispasmodics, topical oestrogen in postmenopausal women, and cryotherapy.

Chapter 10.2.4. Painful Bladder Syndrome (Interstitial Cystitis)

This is defined as suprapubic pain related to bladder filling, with daytime frequency and nocturia, in the absence of infection or any other pathology.

The prevalence is around 16% of all women.

The cause is unknown. There are many theories, however, such as increased epithelial permeability, mast cell activation, and upregulation of sensory afferent nerves.

Cystoscopy may reveal petechial haemorrhages that resemble glomeruli and that appear with bladder distension. Oozing of blood may be seen.

As the cause is not known, the treatments are nonspecific:

- Behavioural:
  - o Stress management.
  - o Avoid acidic or spicy foods, alcohol, tea, coffee, tobacco, tomatoes, etc.
  - o Bladder retraining to increase the duration between voids.

- Pharmacological:
  - o Anticholinergics suppress detrusor contraction.
    - ▪ Effectiveness is 70%.
  - o Tricyclic antidepressants (amitriptyline) inhibit neural activation leading to pain.
  - o Topical oestrogen.

- Surgical:
  - Bladder hydrodistension, with or without instillation of heparin, dimethyl sulfoxide (DMSO), local anaesthetic agents, and steroids.
    - This is therapeutic with water alone in 20–30% of cases.
    - DMSO is an antiinflammatory drug that causes bladder sedation, mast cell inhibition, and may dissolve collagen.

The approach to treatment will be multidisciplinary, involving all of the above options over a prolonged period.

Chapter 10.2.5. Stress Incontinence

This is defined as involuntary leakage of urine when the intra-abdominal pressure (IAP) suddenly increases and when there is no detrusor contraction. With a sudden increase in the IAP, if the intravesical pressure becomes greater than the maximum urethral closure pressure, stress incontinence (SI) will occur. It happens after coughing, sneezing, and sudden activity, and usually the leaked urine volume is small.

It is the most common type of urinary incontinence in women, accounting for 50% of cases.

Types

I. Urine loss without urethral hypermobility.

II. Urine loss with urethral hypermobility.

- This is the most common type, and it responds well to surgery. It results from the following:
  - Lack of urethral supports
  - Intra-abdominal urethra becoming extra-abdominal
- Hence the increased IAP due to descent of the bladder neck is not transmitted to the proximal urethra equally.
  - Posterior urethrovesical angle > 120°
  - Leak-point pressure > 60 cm H_2O

III. Urine loss with urethral intrinsic sphincter weakness.

- The urethral sphincter remains open at rest.
- Patients with this type of SI do not respond well to surgery.
- It results from childbirth, nerve damage, and radiotherapy.
- Leak-point pressure < 60 cm H_2O.

Risk Factors

- Age.
- Multiparity in younger women.
  - Levator ani strength decreases.
- Vaginal delivery, especially with forceps, large baby.

- Obesity.
  - A dose-response relationship has been seen.
- Menopause.
- Increased intra-abdominal pressure due to chronic cough, smoking, constipation, ascites, obesity, etc.
- Previous surgery causes scarring and rigid urethra, resulting in intrinsic urethral sphincter weakness.
- Drugs: diuretics.

History

A thorough history should be obtained, covering the following aspects:

- Most troubling symptoms
  - Frequency, duration, timing of urinary leakage
- Precipitating factors
  - Leakage with coughing, sneezing, or physical activity
- What improves or worsens the leakage
- Any treatment in the past
- Any associated symptoms, such as frequency, urgency, nocturia, hesitancy, dysuria, haematuria, and suprapubic pain
- Review general medical and surgical history (e.g., diabetes mellitus, COPD, stroke)
- Drug history
- Quality of life

Examination

- Neurological
  - Perineal and patellar reflexes
  - Perineal sensation
  - Gait
- Cardiorespiratory
  - Heart failure
  - COPD
- Abdominal
  - Any palpable mass, especially arising from the pelvis
  - Ascites
- Pelvic
  - Pelvic organ prolapse
  - Vulval or vaginal atrophy
  - Levator function

- o   Anal sphincter function
- o   Urethral hypermobility (Kegel's test, Q-tip test)

Investigations

- MSU for microbiological examination
- Residual urine volume
  - o   Higher volume can cause SI
- Urodynamics
  - o   Especially if other urinary symptoms are present

Management

1. Behavioural modification
   - Weight loss.
   - Eliminate causes of increased intra-abdominal pressure.
   - Avoid caffeine, alcohol, and smoking.
   - Restrict fluid intake to 2 L per 24 hours.
2. Review medications
   - Avoid diuretics.
3. Supervised pelvic-floor exercises
   - The Cochrane Incontinence Group has shown that pelvic-floor muscle training is consistently better than placebo or no treatment.
   - Intensive, persistent, and repetitive therapy with correct technique yields better results than standard pelvic-floor training (40–60% improvement).
   - The benefit of conservative therapy following previous continence surgery is not proven.
   - Electrical stimulation of the pelvic-floor muscles by putting a probe into the vagina and rectum has yielded mixed results.
4. Behavioural therapy
   - Its aim is to suppress the urge to void rather than changing bladder function.
   - It comprises voiding schedules (void every 30–60 minutes), fluid management, and urge-suppression strategies (e.g., solving mathematical problems, singing, deep breathing, etc.)
5. Pessaries and urethral plugs
   - This is suitable for those women who are unfit for surgery due to age or comorbidities or those who want to delay surgery because of child-bearing desire in future. It offers an acceptable solution with mixed results.
6. Drugs
   - Sympathomimetics and α-agonists can theoretically improve SI by enhancing the intrinsic sphincter mechanism of the urethra, but they are rarely used because of side effects.
   - Oestrogen has shown to not improve SI in randomised trials (Evidence Level IA).

7. Surgery

- Surgery elevates and supports the bladder neck and urethra, thereby restoring the urethrovesical angle. It sometimes improves urethral closure as well. It is the treatment for moderate to severe SI.
- Surgery could be performed laparoscopically, abdominally, vaginally, or by a combination of approaches.
- Anterior colporrhaphy: It has been largely superseded by sling procedures. It is less effective than retropubic procedures (Evidence Level IA). It is combined with Kelly suturing.
- Burch colposuspension: It is the most effective surgery for SI, with a continence rate of 85–90% at one year. In this surgery, through the abdominal retropubic space, the paravaginal tissue at the level of the bladder neck is sutured to the iliopectineal ligament (Cooper's ligament) bilaterally.

  Voiding difficulty is reported to occur in 10.3% of women postsurgery and detrusor overactivity in 17% of women. The incidence of rectocoele and enterocoele at 5 years is about 13.6%. Open or laparoscopic approaches have similar results.
- Suprapubic surgery: The role of procedures such as Marshall-Marchetti-Krautz and paravaginal repair is unclear (Evidence Level IA).
- Sling procedures: These, with either autologous or synthetic materials, produce a continence rate of approximately 80% with little reduction in continence over time (Evidence Level IA). For autologous grafts, rectus fascia or fascia lata are the most commonly used. Allogenic grafts from cadavers or porcine dermal implants are not widely used these days. Synthetic grafts are associated with sling erosion (0–16%) and sinus formation. Urethral erosion can be 0–5%. De novo detrusor overactivity ranges from 3.7–6.6%.

  It has a similar success rate as colposuspension.

  Sling procedures could be retropubic or trans-obturator. In the former, a polypropylene sling is placed under the midurethra, which passes through the retropubic space and is fixed to the rectus fascia just superior to the pubic symphysis. In the trans-obturator method, the polypropylene sling is passed under the midurethra to the obturator membrane, avoiding the bladder and vessels in the retropubic space. Retropubic slings are most efficacious but have a slightly higher rate of voiding difficulty.
- Injectable agents: Many bulking agents (bovine collagen, Teflon, fat, silicon) have been injected in a retrograde or antegrade fashion into the periurethral tissue and bladder neck to increase urethral coaptation. They have a lower success rate, a short-term continence rate of 48%, and an improvement rate of 76%. There is a continuous decline in continence over a longer period. This has a role when other methods have failed, when diagnosis of intrinsic sphincter deficiency has been made (Evidence Level III), or when drainpipe urethra is present.
- Artificial sphincters: These are used when other treatments have failed. They have higher morbidity.

Chapter 10.2.6. | Urge Incontinence

It is defined as involuntary and painless leakage of urine, which is immediately preceded by urinary urgency. In contrast to SI, urine loss can occur at any time during sleep. The incidence increases with age.

Risk Factors

- Increasing age
- Obesity, constipation
- Functional and cognitive impairment
- Medical conditions (e.g. DM, CVA, spinal cord injuries)
- Hysterectomy

Causes

1. Detrusor overactivity: Approximately 20% of adult women suffer from it. It results from involuntary and premature detrusor contraction during the filling phase of the micturition cycle.
2. Involuntary bladder contraction may be due to certain neurological diseases, such as CVA, Parkinson's disease, multiple sclerosis, spinal cord trauma, and prolapsed intervertebral disc.
3. Urge incontinence can also accompany outflow obstruction.
4. Bladder irritation/infection.
   - Chronic UTI
   - Bladder calculus
   - Bladder neoplasm
5. Psychosomatic.

History

Symptoms include:

- Urinary urgency
- Frequency
- Nocturia
- Lack of sleep
- Cognition impairment
- Social isolation
- Depression

A focused history should include questions about:

- Duration and severity of symptoms
- Any previous therapy

- Any precipitants
- Associated urinary symptoms: SI, frequency, nocturia, voiding difficulty, weak urinary stream, dysuria, haematuria
- Fluid intake: type of fluid such as tea, coffee, beer; quantity and frequency
- Other systems: neurological, bowel, sexual
- General health: diabetes mellitus, chronic cough, obesity
- Drugs: diuretics, anticholinergics, psychotropics

Examination

- General
  - BMI
  - Chronic cough
  - Cardiorespiratory exam
- Vaginal
  - May be completely normal
  - A degree of any associated vaginal prolapse, atrophy, pelvic mass, levator and anal sphincter tone and integrity
- Neurological
  - Perineal sensation and pelvic-floor muscle-contraction strength

Investigations

- MSU
- Urinary diary
- Urodynamics if mixed symptoms
- Transvaginal ultrasound scan if abnormal pelvic mass suspected on clinical examination or history of pain or recurrent UTIs
- Cystoscopy if bladder inflammation or haematuria present

Management

It requires a multidisciplinary approach.

1. Behavioural modification.
   - To limit fluid intake to 1.5–2 L per 24 hours.
   - Avoid caffeine and alcohol.
   - Weight reduction (when BMI > 30) and constipation reduction, if present

2. Supervised pelvic-floor exercises.

- Behavioural changes and bladder retraining are the first-line therapy. Up to 90% of women become continent.
- Exercises with a physiotherapist for at least 6 weeks.
  - Can help reduce detrusor overactivity.
  - Bladder retraining.
  - Improve ability to suppress urgency.
  - Improve bladder capacity and continence.
  - Biofeedback.

- Cochrane review has shown that bladder training is more effective than placebo.

3. Medical therapy

- It should be started in conjunction with the above treatments. It is the mainstay for urge incontinence therapy. The following group of drugs are in use:
- Anticholinergics/antimuscarinic agents: They cause symptomatic improvement by 70% by blocking the parasympathetic nerves, and hence suppressing detrusor contractions and reducing intravesical pressure.
  Detrusor contraction is due to the action of acetylcholine on mainly M3 muscarinic receptors. Anticholinergic drugs block the action of acetylcholine on all muscarinic receptors (M1-M4), including M3. M3 receptors are also found in salivary glands and intestine—hence side effects such as dry mouth and constipation. Side effects are covered in the "Short-Answer Questions" section.
  The following drugs are equally effective, but solifenacin has the fewest side effects:
  - Propantheline   15–30 mg   oral   QID
  - Oxybutynin   2.5–5 mg   oral/transdermal patch   up to TDS
  - Tolterodine   2 mg   oral   BD
  - Solifenacin   5 mg   oral   daily
  Contraindication for these group of drugs is closed-angle glaucoma.
- Mirabegron: 50 mg   oral   daily
  It is a potent and selective β_3-adrenoceptor agonist. It causes detrusor relaxation and improves urinary storage. Tachycardia, UTI, and nausea are side effects.
- Tricyclic antidepressants: These are used because of their anticholinergic and sedative effects. They are useful in nocturia and nocturnal enuresis.
  - Imipramine   10–50 mg   oral   nocte
  It increases the concentration of serotonin or norepinephrine in CNS and down-regulates β-adrenergic receptors.

- Synthetic vasopressin: Desmopressin is used for primary nocturnal enuresis and nocturia due to its antidiuretic effect.
  - Desmopressin   10 µg nasal spray (10 µg/spray) nocte
- Topical oestrogen: This improves collagen synthesis and blood flow to the urethra. It is used to treat urge incontinence, frequency, and nocturia (Evidence Level IA).

4. Surgery.

- · It is used when other treatments have not worked.
- <u>Hydrodistension of the bladder</u>: This is done for two hours under regional analgesia. It acts by causing ischemic nerve damage. Bladder pressure is maintained between systolic and diastolic arterial pressure. There is an improvement rate of 50%. It can be repeated at 3 to 6 months. The main complication is bladder rupture.
- <u>Botox (botulinum toxin A)</u>: It paralyses muscles and interacts with the bladder epithelium. It is injected cystoscopically. It is mainly used for interstitial cystitis and OAB. The effect lasts for 3 to 6 months. It should be used only in those women who have not responded to other treatments and who are able to self-catheterise.
- <u>Augmentation cystoplasty</u>: Bladder capacity is augmented by anastomosing a segment of small bowel. The continence rate is up to 90%. Side effects include diarrhoea, metabolic acidosis, and adenocarcinoma in the enteric segment.
- <u>Sacral-nerve modulation</u>: It is offered on the basis of response to prior percutaneous nerve evaluation. It is extremely expensive.
- <u>Urinary diversion</u>: This is a treatment of last resort when nothing else has worked.

Chapter 10.2.7. Mixed Incontinence

A large percentage of women present with mixed symptoms of stress and urge incontinence, frequency, and nocturia. It results from detrusor overactivity in combination with an incompetent rhabdosphincter.

Investigations are similar to urge and stress incontinence.

In urodynamically proven cases, urgency is treated first by behavioural change, bladder retraining, and medical treatment, before embarking on surgery for the stress incontinence component. Imipramine is especially suited because of its anticholinergic, noradrenergic, and serotonin reuptake inhibitor properties.

Chapter 10.2.8. Overflow Incontinence

Chronic urinary retention eventually leads to involuntary leakage (overflow) of urine.

History

Trouble in starting to urinate, weak stream, incontinence when changing position, and dribbling after stopping urinating.

Causes

Neurogenic deficit causing detrusor atony due to diabetes mellitus, lumbosacral nerve disease, and high spinal cord injury.

Outflow obstruction due to urethral scarring, urethral angulation from a large cystocoele, or meatal stenosis is seen in very young and elderly women.

Differential Diagnosis

- Stress incontinence
- Urge incontinence

Diagnosis

A history suggestive of the causes mentioned above will help. Any association of incontinence with change of position or straining should be explored.

Examination

A detailed examination as described in the previous section should be carried out. Any mass arising from the pelvis and felt abdominally that is dull on percussion should indicate the possibility of a bladder distension. Catheterisation of the bladder with disappearance of the mass will confirm a diagnosis of urinary retention.

Investigations

- Postvoid residual urine ≥ 500 mL indicates chronic urinary retention and overflow as opposed to stress incontinence.
- Pelvic ultrasound scan may show a hugely dilated bladder or a large pelvic neoplasm such as a leiomyoma pressing upon the bladder.
- Cystoscopy may show urethral scarring, stricture, or meatal stenosis.
- Urodynamics may show absent or weakened bladder contraction, urethral abnormalities, the site of obstruction, or abnormal urethral angulation.

Management

Any associated UTI should be treated. Medical treatment has no role otherwise.

Surgery

- <u>Urethral dilatation</u>: For urethral stricture and correction of urethral angulation.
- <u>Sphincterotomy</u>: For women with spinal cord injury who are not able to relax the sphincter.
- <u>Clean intermittent self-catheterisation</u>: When other treatments have failed, this is the last resort. It should be done four times a day.

Short-Answer Questions

Question 1

A 70-year-old woman is complaining of constant leakage of urine, all the time. She finds the problem unmanageable now. List the differential diagnoses.

Answer:

- Detrusor overactivity
- Urge incontinence

- Stress incontinence
- Retention with overflow
- Mixed stress and urge incontinence
- Functional
  - ○ Delirium, infection, pharmacological agents (diuretics), psychological, excessive fluid intake, restricted mobility, stool impaction
- Fistula
  - ○ Ectopic ureter, bladder exstrophy, pelvic cancers
- Incontinence secondary to prolapse
- Fistula following
  - ○ Gynaecological surgery (hysterectomy, anterior colporrhaphy, laparoscopic pelvic surgery)
  - ○ Obstetric trauma in developing world
- Diabetes mellitus
- Neurological disorders (multiple sclerosis, cerebrovascular accident, spinal cord tumour)

Question 2

List the causes of acute urinary retention in a 32-year-old female.

Answer:

Most common causes:

- Genital herpes infection
- UTI
- Severe constipation

Less common causes:

- Post bladder-neck surgery
- Postoperative spinal/epidural anaesthesia
- Obstetric postpartum, impacted retroverted uterus
- Pelvic mass (fibroid, neoplasm)
- Anticholinergic therapy
- Neurological disease (stroke, multiple sclerosis, spinal cord tumour)
- Psychological
- Pregnancy

Question 3

What is a bladder diary? Discuss its use.

Answer:

A bladder diary, also known as a frequency-volume chart, records:

- Time and volume of all fluid intake
- Time and volume of all fluid output, including accidents
- Urgency with agency score 0–4

It is usually used for 2 to 3 days prior to a urodynamic study, as part of it or alone.

Use:

- It is a noninvasive, simple, and cheap tool to diagnose detrusor overactivity.
- It reflects bladder function in a natural environment and quantifies the information.
- It reveals urinary frequency and nocturia.
- It helps in counselling the patient; 35% of patients improve with this alone.

Question 4

What is cystometry? What are its indications?

Answer:

Cystometry measures the pressure-volume relationship of the bladder and differentiates between cough-induced detrusor overactivity and stress incontinence.

Indications of cystometry:

- Mixed symptoms
- Voiding problems (hesitancy, poor stream, straining)
- Recurrence of symptoms after incontinence surgery
- Neuropathic bladder

Question 5

List the anatomical features that help in maintaining urinary incontinence.

Answer:

1. Support of proximal urethra and bladder neck
   - Levator ani muscles
   - Arcus tendineus fascia
   - Anterior vaginal wall
   - Pubourethral ligaments

2. External urethral sphincter

3. Internal urethral factors

- Mucosal folds
- Smooth muscle of the urethral wall
- Urethral submucous cavernous plexus
- Passive elasticity of the urethra
- Length of the intra-abdominal urethra

4. Reflux pelvic-floor contraction

- Occurs in response to sudden increase in intra-abdominal pressure
- Causes increased urethral closure

Question 6

List the causes of urinary fistulae.

Answer:

- Surgical
  - From tissue necrosis due to excessive diathermy, clamping, or suturing during surgery
- Neoplastic
  - Due to malignant invasion of bladder and urethral tissue
  - Biopsy the fistula site
- Radiotherapy
  - From ischemic changes due to vascular injury
- Inflammatory
  - Crohn's disease
- Obstetric
  - Poorly managed labour, and developing world

Question 7

A 48-year-old woman has been referred to you with symptoms of stress incontinence.

Part a

Critically evaluate the bladder investigations available for these symptoms (i.e., when are they indicated, advantages and disadvantages).

Answer:

Test	Advantages	Disadvantages
MSU (Level D, GPP)	Detect occult UTI, glucose may indicate diabetes Up to 50% of incontinent women may have UTI Negative result excludes UTI with high NPV	Treatment of UTI makes little difference to incontinence
Frequency-volume chart/bladder diary (over 3 days, Level D, GPP)	Reasonable reproducibility Gives reference point for outcome May initiate behavioural modification (in case of OAB)	Inconvenience May make no difference, and may add additional visit to the process
Q-Tip (if moves > 30°), Bonney or Marshall test	Indicates urethral hypermobility If negative Q-tip, then higher failure rate of procedure	Little evidence to support benefit routine practice
Residual Urine (indicated if symptoms of difficulty with flow, incomplete emptying or palpable bladder)	Identifies chronic retention, a risk factor for failure	No agreed definition of what constitutes a substantial residual
Pad Testing (little evidence to support, Evidence Level IV)	May demonstrate volume & frequency of urine lost	Little diagnostic or therapeutic value
Urodynamics (cystometry, urethral pressure profile, flowmetry). No value prior to conservative management Not required in women with symptoms of pure stress incontinence and no voiding difficulties Indicated if mixed symptoms, previous surgery to bladder neck or anterior compartment or voiding dysfunction	Low urethral closure pressure or Valsalva leak point pressure may predict failure of procedures Poor initial flow (< 20 mL/s) associated with delayed voiding in some (but not all) studies High closure pressures associated with de novo OAB on one study (but not another)	One RCT and 2 observational studies have shown no difference in symptoms or severity in women having urodynamics or not Cost of procedure, invasive, delay in surgery Inconsistent data showing identification of likely complications or failure
Cystoscopy (only indicated if pain or recurrent UTI)	May identify chronic cystitis or bladder pathology	No evidence of benefit in routine assessment

Table 10.11. Advantages and disadvantages of different bladder investigations

Part b

After your assessment, she is interested in having a suburethral sling procedure. What factors are associated with a likelihood of having complications from this surgery?

Answer:

Patient factors	Chronic strain or intra-abdominal pressure
	Age (older women may have more retention)
	Obesity, chronic cough, smoking
	Clotting disorders (retropubic haematoma)
Bladder factors	Preexisting OAB symptoms or proven detrusor overactivity
	Low urethral closure pressures— (failure if pressure < 20 cm H_2O)
	High preoperative residual or voiding difficulty (if flow < 15 mL/sec)
Operative factors	Type of mesh—polyfilament or tight mesh weave
	Previous surgery, especially retropubic surgery, hysterectomy, continence surgery in some studies
	Concomitant surgery (e.g., repair)—more likely to have retention and perforation, vault suspension associated with voiding dysfunction
	Surgical experience—bladder injury
	Surgical technique—inappropriate bladder-neck deviation

Table 10.12. Factors associated with complications from suburethral sling procedure

Part c

She undergoes an uncomplicated suburethral sling procedure. A catheter is inserted at the time of the surgery and removed the following day. She is unable to pass urine. Outline the options available for the short- and long-term management of this problem.

Answer:

Full history	Pain, haematuria
	Passage of any urine at all?
	Previous history of voiding dysfunction
Examination	Surgical complications—vital signs (temperature, pulse, and blood pressure), bruising, infection
	Vaginal examination (bruising, haematoma)
Assessment	MSU, if possible
	Bladder residual after any voids
	If anuric focus on causes of renal failure, bladder perforation, ureteric injury
Initial nonsurgical management	Treat UTI, analgesia, constipation
	If unable to void then catheterise immediately with either: recatheterisation for 48 hrs, commence ISC or suprapubic catheter
	Aim for residual less than 150 mL
Follow-up in 48 hrs—trial of void	Either recatheterise for 7–10 days or pursue ISC
	Diazepam may help relax pelvic floor if passing some urine
If unsuccessful after 2 weeks conservative management, consider surgical management	Simple sling incision (others stretch or loosen, but incision preferred), 84% success rate in one study
	Formal urethrolysis (mobilise urethra off pubic bone)
Extreme situations	Long-term intermittent self-catheterisation
	Ileal conduit

Table 10.13. Management of a patient with urinary retention postsuburethral sling surgery

Question 8

A 49-year-old presents with urinary leakage 5 weeks after a Burch colposuspension (or any stress-incontinence surgery). She was discharged on day 4. Discuss steps of your management.

Answer:

- Possible causes
  - De novo detrusor overactivity
  - UTI
  - Overflow incontinence
  - Vesicovaginal fistula (VVF)
  - Failed surgery (incidence 10%)

- Focused history
    - Symptoms of urinary leakage, and in particular if they are new or the same as before surgery
    - Leakage all the time or with stress
    - Associated dysuria, haematuria, frequency, and urgency
    - Onset of symptoms with reference to the date of surgery

- Examination
    - Demonstrable leakage from the urethra or vagina
    - Pool of urine seen in the vagina/VVF
    - Distended bladder

- Investigation
    - Catheter-specimen urine (CSU)
    - Residual urine volume
    - Cystoscopy
    - Urodynamics, if no cause identified

- Treatment
    - Treat UTI, urinary retention, and vesicovaginal fistula if seen
    - Intermittent self-catheterisation, if in retention
    - Surgery for vesicovaginal fistula (VVF)
    - If urodynamics shows genuine stress incontinence (GSI), treat with a different surgery
    - If detrusor overactivity, treat with bladder retraining and anticholinergics

Question 9

A 60-year-old woman presents 5 years after a colposuspension for genuine stress incontinence with urinary leakage. Discuss the steps of your management.

Answer:

I will proceed on the following lines:

- Focused history
    - Details of the previous surgery and urodynamics. I will get the relevant medical notes of the previous surgery.
    - Ask about current symptoms such as dysuria, haematuria, frequency, urgency, nocturia, and stress and urge incontinence.
    - Duration of the symptoms and whether they are worsening.
    - Symptoms of prolapse such as feeling of a vaginal lump, any bowel or bladder dysfunction, or a dragging pain in the perineum.

- Examination
    - General examination: chronic cough, diabetes mellitus, obesity.
    - Abdominal examination: any pelvic mass, urinary retention.
    - Vaginal examination: prolapse, atrophy, presence of any fistula, any incontinence on coughing or sneezing, any palpable pelvic mass.
    - Neurological examination: plantar reflex, perineal sensation, and anal reflex.

- Investigation
  - MSU.
  - Blood glucose.
  - Bladder diary.
  - Urodynamic study.
  - Pelvic ultrasound scan from postvoid residual, any abnormal pelvic mass, type, and positioning of a sling/mesh if used in the previous surgery.

- Treatment
  - It will depend upon the above findings.
  - Treat UTI if present.
  - Add topical oestrogen.
  - For OAB, I will suggest behavioural changes, bladder retraining, and one of the anticholinergic drugs.
  - For genuine stress incontinence, a different type of surgery, preferably by a urogynaecologist, will be considered. The complications of surgery should be discussed, emphasising that the recurrence rate of incontinence following repeat surgery is about 60% after 5 years.
  - Any uterovaginal prolapse requiring surgery will be combined with the stress incontinence surgery.

Question 10

A 65-year-old woman complains of wetting herself while shopping.

Part a

List the possible causes.

Answer:

Possible causes:

- UTI
- Mixed incontinence
- Urge incontinence
- OAB
- Stress incontinence, less common in older woman than urge incontinence
- Urinary fistula

Part b

What questions should be asked to make a differential diagnosis?

Answer:

Relevant questions:

- UTI
  - Any pain, burning or stinging at the end of micturition?
  - Any blood in the urine?

- Mixed incontinence
    - Leakage of urine on coughing or sneezing?
    - How often do you pass urine during the day and night?
    - Do you have to run to the toilet when you get the urge?
    - Do you wet yourself on the way to the toilet or if the toilet is busy?

- Urge continence
    - Do you run to the toilet to urinate?
    - Do you wet yourself on the way to the toilet or if the toilet is busy?
    - Do you suddenly get an irresistible desire to pass urine?

- OAB
    - Is there trouble in getting started when there is an urge to urinate?
    - Is the urinary stream weak?
    - Is there dribbling after the cessation of urination?

- Stress incontinence
    - Leakage of urine on coughing or sneezing?
    - Is the volume of such leakage small?
    - Does it happen during sleep? (SI does not usually happen during sleep)

- Urinary fistula
    - Do you get the urge to urinate?
    - Do you feel wet all the time?
    - Do you have any marks of excoriation/itching as a result?

Part c

List the tests to confirm the diagnosis.

Answer:

Tests:

- MSU for UTI
- Bladder diary for frequency, urgency, and accidents suggesting detrusor overactivity (DO)
- Urodynamics to differentiate between GSI and DO
- Cystourethroscopy and CT urogram will show the site and nature of any fistula

Question 11

List the clinical features of urethral diverticulum. List the appropriate investigations. Discuss the management options and their advantages and disadvantages.

Answer:

- Aetiology of a urethral diverticulum
  - From the distal two-thirds of the urethral wall.
  - From the periurethral glands.
  - From childbirth trauma, surgical trauma, or infection of the urethral gland.
  - They can be associated with vaginal cysts.
  - The incidence is about 1%.

- History
  - Postmicturition dribbling.
  - Dysuria.
  - Dyspareunia.
  - Frequency, urgency, and incontinence.
  - Haematuria.

- Examination
  - Palpable anterior vaginal wall mass, when compressed, exudes pus or urine from the urethral meatus.
  - Periurethral tenderness.
  - Recurrent UTI.

- Investigation
  - Ultrasound—transvaginal or translabial.
  - Urethroscopy—direct visualisation.
  - MRI—very sensitive.

- Management
  - Expectant.
    - Only for small asymptomatic diverticulum, with prophylactic antibiotics.
  - Ultrasonic lithotripsy.
    - If stones are present in the diverticulum.
  - Surgery.
    - Transvaginal excision is the main treatment.
    - The complication rate is 5–46%.
    - Common side effects are recurrence, fistula, and strictures.

Question 12

List the drugs used for OAB and their main benefits, weaknesses, and side effects.

Answer:

Drug	Benefits	Weaknesses	Side effects
Oxybutynin oral	Cheap	Marked dryness of mouth	Constipation, diarrhoea, dry mouth (88%), blurred vision, voiding difficulty, drowsiness, photosensitivity
Oxybutynin patch	Reduced side effects		
Tolterodine	Newer anticholinergic	Not as effective as solifenacin Expensive	Act on muscarinic receptors and hence generalised side effects very uncommon
Solifenacin	Reduced side effects	Expensive	
Darifenacin	M$_3$ selective	Expensive	Dry mouth and eyes, drowsiness, mild constipation, fever
Trospium	Does not cross the blood-brain barrier	Broad-spectrum anticholinergic	
Propiverine	Calcium antagonist action	Only for treating the frequency component of OAB	Dry mouth, constipation, blurry vision, tiredness, dizziness
Imipramine	Helps sleep Useful for nocturia and enuresis	Should not be used if working due to the risk of drowsiness	Drowsiness, postural hypotension, urinary retention, sedation
Desmopressin	Useful for primary nocturnal enuresis, and nocturia	Antidiuretic	Hyponatraemia in elderly, water retention, nausea

Table 10.14. Comparison of drugs for OAB

Multiple-Choice Questions

Q1. In a standing, normal, continent woman, the bladder base is:

   A. Horizontal

   B. Vertical

   C. Inclined anteriorly

   D. Inclined posteriorly

Answer: A

Q2. In genuine stress incontinence, which has the least pressure?

    A. Intra-abdominal pressure

    B. Intravesical pressure

    C. Urethral closure pressure

    D. Rectal pressure

Answer: C

Q3. Which of the following structures does not support the urethra?

    A. Arcus tendineus fascia pelvis

    B. Anterior vaginal wall

    C. Levator ani

    D. Cardinal ligament

Answer: D

Q4. Which of the following is not associated with UTI?

    A. Urinary frequency

    B. Urinary urgency

    C. Urinary incontinence

    D. Urethral syndrome

Answer: D

Q5. Which of the following can cause urge incontinence in a 65-year-old?

    A. Loss of posterior urethrovesical angle

    B. Increase in posterior urethrovesical angle

    C. Chronic UTI

    D. Myasthenia gravis

Answer: C

Q6. With regard to tension-free vaginal tape, which of the following statements is correct?

    A. The risk of overactive bladder postoperatively is 12–15%.

    B. The risk of needing to perform self-catheterisation is 0.5–1%.

    C. The cure rate on 24-hour pad test at 3 years is 94–96%.

    D. The vaginal erosion rate within 3 years is 10–11%.

Answer: B

Q7. Which of the following statements is incorrect?

    A. Nearly 60% of all women may suffer some degree of urinary incontinence during their lives.

    B. Continence is the balance between forces maintaining urethral closure and factors affecting detrusor function.

    C. Acetylcholine is responsible for detrusor contraction.

    D. Anticholinergic agents decrease detrusor activity.

Answer: A

Q8. Resting pressure in a normal urinary bladder is between

    A. 10 and 20 cm H_2O

    B. 20 and 30 cm H_2O

    C. 30 and 40 cm H_2O

    D. 40 and 50 cm H_2O

Answer: B

Q9. Use of an indwelling catheter for more than 24 hours causes bacteriuria in what percentage of women?

    A. 30

    B. 40

    C. 50

    D. 60

Answer: C

Q10. Which of the following treatments of GSI does not have a long-term cure rate of approximately 80%?

    A. Marshall-Marchetti-Krantz operation

    B. Burch colposuspension

    C. Midurethral slings

    D. Anterior urethro-colporraphy

Answer: D

Chapter 11

Benign Diseases of the Uterus

Chapter 11.1.　Fibroids

The term *fibroid* is a misnomer and histologically represents a leiomyoma. In this book, *fibroid*, *leiomyoma*, and *myoma* have been used interchangeably.

Definition

It is a benign neoplasm of the smooth muscle of the uterine wall.

The term *fibroid* comes from the small amount of fibrous tissue in the leiomyoma and results from the atrophy and degeneration of the smooth muscles due to vascular insufficiency.

Incidence

Uterine leiomyoma occurs in 30–50% of women in the reproductive age group. It is the most common neoplasm in women.

Clinical Physiology

The leiomyoma arises from a single myocyte. Depending on its direction of growth, it can be either:

- subserous—growing toward the serosal layer of the uterus,
- submucous—growing toward the endometrium, or
- intramural—confined mainly in the wall of the uterus.

It can also extend into the broad ligament or cervix. There are often multiple leiomyomas of different sizes. The neoplastic transformation of the myocyte results from a somatic mutation in a single progenitor cell. This mutation affects cytokines that stimulate neoplastic transformation. The neoplastic transformation is also affected by oestrogen and progesterone levels. There is a higher concentration of oestrogen and progesterone receptors in the leiomyoma. The interaction of leiomyoma growth and oestrogen and progesterone levels is complex. Leiomyomas develop during the reproductive years and stop growing or diminish in size postmenopausally, when there is relative hypoestrogenism.

A growing leiomyoma compresses the surrounding myometrium, which forms a pseudocapsule that helps shelling off during a myomectomy.

The vascular supply to the leiomyoma is significantly less than the adjoining similar-sized myometrium. Sometimes, a subserosal or pedunculated leiomyoma attaches to the adjoining organs, such as the omentum or bowel, and receives an additional blood supply. With continued proliferation, the leiomyoma outgrows its blood supply and starts to degenerate.

Microarray analysis has shown that leiomyomas have multiple chromosomal abnormalities. The most common ones are translocation between chromosome 12 and 14 and deletion of chromosome 7.

Risk Factors

- Aging
- Early menarche
- Low parity
- Dark-skinned woman
- Tamoxifen use
- Obesity
- High-fat diet

Protective Factors

- Childbearing
- Smoking, thus creating a hypoestrogenic state
- Long-term use of oral contraceptive pills
- Depot medroxyprogesterone use long-term
- Levonorgestrel-containing IUCD

Recent Changes to Understanding

Contrary to popular notions, recent evidence has shown that:

- Most leiomyomas do not increase in size during pregnancy.
- Oral contraceptive pills do not cause an increase in leiomyoma size.
- Progestogens do not cause a reduction in leiomyoma size.
- HRT and tibolone do not cause an increase in leiomyoma size.
- Sarcomas have a distinct origin (Parker W, 2007) because of different cytogenic profile.
- Increased endometrial surface area due to fibroid does not cause increased bleeding.

History

Nearly two-thirds of women with fibroids are asymptomatic. The history should be taken in the same way as described in the History section for DUB.

Abnormal Bleeding

This occurs in 30% of cases. It may either cause heavy menstrual bleeding or intermenstrual bleeding. It is mainly caused by submucous leiomyomas but also sometimes by intramural leiomyomas. The following explanations have been put forward to explain abnormal uterine bleeding from a leiomyoma:

- Abnormal microvascular growth and function
- Decreased myometrial contractility
- Surface ulceration, rare
- Endometrial hyperplasia

Pressure

A large anterior leiomyoma may press on the bladder, causing urinary frequency, urgency, and rarely retention. A large broad-ligament leiomyoma may cause hydroureter. Rectal pressure symptoms are uncommon. It may also increase abdominal girth.

Pain

It is an uncommon symptom of leiomyoma. The onset of pain in a woman with preexisting leiomyoma, alongside increasing uterine bleeding and increased leiomyoma size, is an indication of sarcomatous change. Leiomyomas may cause pain from secondary dysmenorrhoea or red degeneration during pregnancy or COC use. Pedunculated leiomyomas may undergo torsion and cause severe, acute pain.

Infertility and Recurrent Miscarriage

Submucous leiomyomas distorting the endometrial cavity may cause lower ongoing pregnancy rates by either interfering with sperm transport or implantation. Women with intramural fibroids experience a higher miscarriage rate. Large leiomyomas may occlude the proximal fallopian tube. There is no conclusive evidence that fibroids decrease fecundity.

Symptoms in Pregnancy

Adverse obstetric outcomes are rare; however, fibroids can lead to preterm labour, abruption, malpresentation, or red degeneration. Intrapartum, they can cause an obstructed or dysfunctional labour, caesarean delivery, and postpartum haemorrhage.

The important determinants of the effects of leiomyomas on pregnancy are the size and site (distance from the placenta) of the leiomyoma. A large leiomyoma in the lower uterine segment or in the cervix can obstruct labour.

Abruption, preterm labour, and postpartum haemorrhage have a higher incidence if the placenta is on or very close to the leiomyoma.

Types

Leiomyomas are classified on the basis of their location with reference to the endometrial cavity. The size and location of the leiomyoma largely determines the symptomatology.

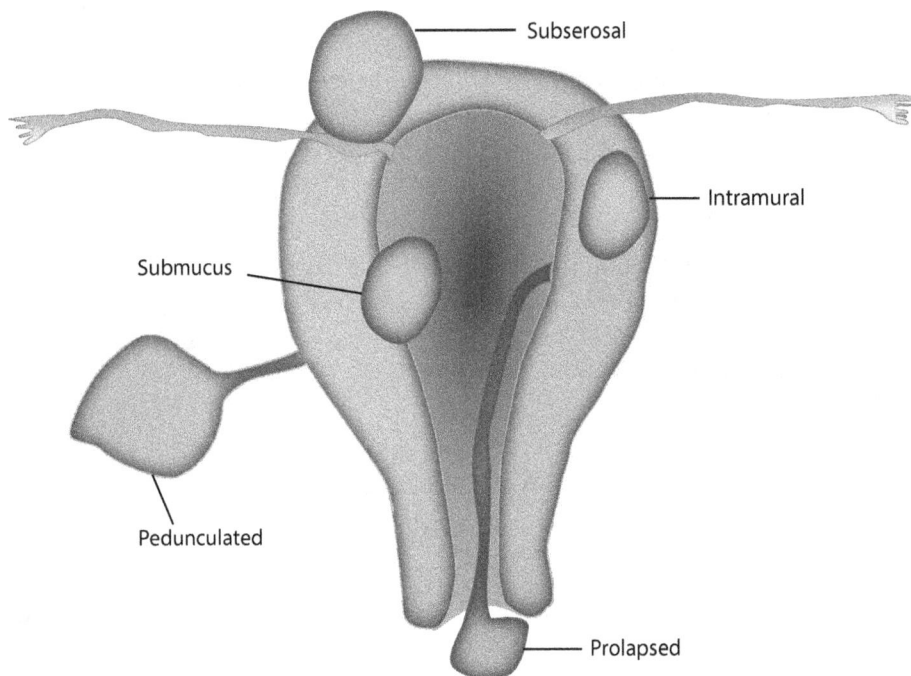

Figure 11.1. Different types of leiomyomas

Intramural leiomyomas (most common): These are centred within the myometrium and are surrounded by normal myometrium for more than 180° of their margins. They may sometimes cause bleeding, infertility and postpartum haemorrhage. When larger than 5 cm, they may cause pressure symptoms.

Submucosal leiomyomas (5%): These protrude into the endometrial cavity to varying degrees, from a minor indent to almost entirely within the endometrial cavity. These leiomyomas cause dysmenorrhoea, bleeding, infertility, and complications in pregnancy. When on a large peduncle, they may prolapse outside the cervix.

Subserosal leiomyoma: The main bulk of these leiomyomas are outside the uterine wall, and when pedunculated, they can undergo torsion. If large, they can cause pressure symptoms.

Cervical leiomyomas (5%)

Broad-ligament leiomyomas (5%)

Fallopian tube and round-ligament leiomyomas (< 1%)

Examination

The process for examination should also follow that described in the DUB and HMB sections.

A medium-sized leiomyoma will make the uterus bulkier, irregular, and can often be palpated in a thin woman by bimanual vaginal examination.

A large leiomyoma can be palpated abdominally if it has come above the pelvic brim. It feels firm, has some mobility, and is continuous with the uterus. Submucous leiomyomas, which are responsible for most symptoms, cannot be diagnosed by clinical examination.

Differential Diagnosis

- Pregnancy
- Adenomyosis
- Ovarian neoplasm
- Endometrial polyp (for submucous leiomyoma)

A clinical examination will only have a limited role in differentiating between the above conditions. However, a transvaginal ultrasound scan can easily distinguish between these conditions.

Complications

- Torsion:
  - A pedunculated leiomyoma may undergo torsion and cause severe, acute abdominal pain. An ultrasound scan will aid in making a diagnosis by either showing the torted pedicle of the myoma or a relative ground-glass, atypical, oedematous appearance of the myoma.

- Infection:
  - Submucous leiomyomas, and intramural leiomyomas during the puerperial period, may get infected and cause severe pain and an offensive vaginal discharge.
  - An ultrasound scan will aid in making a diagnosis. The appearance of leiomyoma undergoing any of the complications is different from the typical leiomyoma appearance.

- Malignant transformation:
  - The onset of pain, vaginal bleeding, and a finding of an enlarging leiomyoma strongly suggests a malignant transformation.
  - The incidence of malignant transformation (sarcomatous change) is 0.5%.

Degeneration: The following types of leiomyoma degeneration have been recognised:

- Hyaline (65%) — most common, mildest form, whorled pattern on histology, cellular details are lost.
- Myxomatous (15%) — consists of fluid-filled spaces.
- Calcific (10%) — in elderly women, calcified to different degrees but remains asymptomatic.
- Cystic.
- Fatty.

- Red (corneous)—occurs in up to 10% of pregnant women and with COC use; this is the most acute form, causing severe pain, peritoneal irritation, and haemorrhagic discoloration. It is also seen in nonpregnant uteri sometimes.
  - ○ Large leiomyomas, due to vascular insufficiency, show liquified areas of degeneration, making the sonological appearance complex.

Investigations

- FBE and iron studies for anaemia and iron deficiency. Rarely, polycythaemia may be seen due to the increased level of erythropoietin.
- Ultrasound scan with/without saline sonohysterography:
  - ○ It is the primary investigation, as it shows the number, site (type), and size of the leiomyoma(s).
  - ○ It also can suggest any complication, such as torsion or degeneration.
  - ○ It will also show any adnexal pathology.

    Saline sonohysterography will differentiate between a submucous and intramural leiomyoma, and it will help in excluding an endometrial polyp. It also helps in planning for a hysteroscopic resection of the leiomyoma by determining the portion of the submucous myoma protruding into the endometrial cavity.

  - ○ Ultrasound appearance of a leiomyoma:
    - Uterine leiomyomas are well-circumscribed, hypoechoic, solid, spherical lesions with very little peripheral vascularity.
    - They may be multiple and of different sizes.
    - With an increasing content of fibrous or fatty tissue, leiomyomas become hyperechoic.
    - In some elderly women, they are also calcified.
    - Leiomyomas undergoing degeneration will show cystic areas interspersed among the solid tissue.
    - Since leiomyomas affect blood-flow velocity in the uterine arteries, blood-flow velocity measurement is of little use in differentiating a benign from a sarcomatous leiomyoma.

- Hysteroscopy:
  - ○ An outpatient or inpatient hysteroscopy will differentiate between a submucous leiomyoma and an endometrial polyp.
  - ○ A therapeutic procedure can be combined with it.

- Laparoscopy:
  - ○ This can confirm the presence of a subserosal or pedunculated leiomyoma and any torsion, and it will also be of value in investigating pelvic pain and infertility.

- MRI:
  - ○ Its routine use is not recommended.
  - ○ It has no advantage over an ultrasound scan.
  - ○ It has greater precision and less interobserver variation when dealing with larger leiomyomas.
  - ○ Gadolinium-enhanced MRI is used when there is a suspicion of a leiomyosarcoma.

Management

Asymptomatic leiomyomas do not need to be treated. Anaemia, if present, should be treated. The treatment should be individualised, depending on the symptoms and requirement for fertility.

Medical

Leiomyomas with a uterine size up to 10 weeks of pregnancy could be treated medically. The aim of treatment is to either reduce bleeding or to create a lower level of circulating oestrogen.

Nonhormonal Treatment

- NSAIDs do not reduce HMB secondary to a uterine leiomyoma but do help with pain from degeneration, including red degeneration.
- Tranexamic acid has been shown to reduce bleeding by 50%.

Hormonal Treatment

- COC pills, in high doses and in the absence of anaemia, can reduce HMB associated with a leiomyoma by 50%. Long-term use has a preventative effect on leiomyoma growth.
- Levonorgestrel-containing IUCD reduces blood loss when the leiomyomas are small and the endometrial cavity is not distorted.
  - With endometrial cavity distortion, the risk of expulsion of the device is higher.
- Progestogens reduce blood loss if used cyclically but do not affect leiomyoma size.
  - Long-term use of depot medroxyprogesterone acetate prevents leiomyoma development but does not treat the symptoms.
- Danazol and gestrinone reduce leiomyoma size as well as resultant blood loss.
- Antiprogesterone agents, such as mifepristone at a dose of 5–10 mg daily for 3–6 months, significantly decrease blood loss but do not decrease leiomyoma size.
- Selective progesterone receptor modulator (SPRMs), such as ulipristal acetate in a dose of 5–10 mg daily, significantly decrease blood loss and decrease leiomyoma size by 25%.
- GnRH agonists decrease leiomyoma size by 40–50%, most of which happens in the first 3 months of the commencement of treatment.
  - After cessation of treatment, leiomyomas attain their previous size by 6 months.
  - Their principal use is prior to surgery in the reduction of intraoperative blood loss at the time of a myomectomy or hysterectomy. However, they may obliterate the tissue plane and make shelling off the myoma difficult.
  - Vasomotor symptoms are treated by either lose-dose COC pill or tibolone.
  - Because it reduces leiomyoma size, surgery after GnRH agonist use is possible by a conservative Pfannenstiel incision rather than a big, midline vertical incision (midline laparotomy).

Radiological Treatment

- Uterine artery embolisation (UAE)
  - This technique, performed by an interventional radiologist, reduces uterine arteriolar blood flow, causing ischaemic necrosis and shrinkage of the uterine fibroids, while allowing the surrounding myometrium to recover.
  - HMB resolves in 85–95% of women.
  - It should only be done once any sarcomatous change in the fibroid has been excluded.
  - UAE is controversial in women desirous of maintaining fertility but may have a limited role because of surgical risk, failed previous surgery, or the woman's choice.
  - Because of a lack of good-quality evidence, its routine use in the younger age group is not advocated.
  - The effects of UAE on fertility and pregnancy are uncertain.
  - Advantages of UAE compared with other surgical methods are as follows:
    - No significant difference in patient satisfaction and quality of life
    - No difference in short- or long-term complications
    - Significantly reduced length of stay and recovery time
    - No difference in the rate of premature menopause
  - Complications of UAE:
    - Vaginal discharge and fever (4%)
    - Failed procedure (4%)
    - VTE (0.3%)
    - Groin haematoma
    - Allergy to contrast
    - Artery dissection
  - Two randomised control trials (REST and EMMY) have shown reintervention rates between 28.4–32% at 5 years for UAE, compared with 2–10.7% for the surgical methods.
- Magnetic-resonance-guided focused-ultrasound surgery (MRgFUS)
  - This is a noninvasive technique for large fibroids and is not commonly available.
  - It employs a MRI thermal-imaging system to continuously measure temperature changes inside the uterus.
  - A high-intensity ultrasound beam is focused in the different areas of the fibroid, where it raises the temperature, causing necrosis.
  - Its effect on future pregnancies is not yet established. However, it does result in symptomatic improvement in HMB that is caused by large fibroids.

Surgical Treatment

- Hysteroscopic resection
  - This is suitable only for symptomatic submucous leiomyoma.
  - More than one attempt at resection may be needed.
  - It reduces HMB in 69–85% of women.
  - Its effectiveness can be further improved by simultaneous endometrial resection, if future fertility is not desired.

- o   Prior treatment with a GnRH agonist reduces the volume of distending medium and treatment failure.
- o   This surgery will also improve the conception rate in an infertile woman.

- Myomectomy
  - o   This surgery results in nearly 80% reduction of symptoms.
  - o   A laparoscopic approach is suitable if the leiomyoma is pedunculated, subserous, or intramural, and not more than 8 cm in diameter.
  - o   Use of an electrical morcellator is best avoided because of unintended intraperitoneal seeding of an undiagnosed sarcoma.
  - o   The recurrence rate of leiomyoma is 62% in a 5-year period.
  - o   Emergency hysterectomy is needed in 1% of cases to stop haemorrhage.
  - o   The following table compares laparoscopic and open myomectomy:

	Laparoscopy	Laparotomy
Operation time	Longer	Shorter
Blood loss	Less	More
Recovery	Shorter	Longer
Complication rate	Lower	Higher
Menstrual blood loss	Nil	Nil
Pregnancy rate	Similar	Similar
Recurrence	Similar	Similar
Scar rupture during pregnancy	Similar	Similar
Cost	Similar	Similar

Table 11.1. Comparison between laparotomy and laparoscopy for myomectomy (Jin C et al. 2009)

- Hysterectomy
  - o   It is an option only when future fertility is not desired.
  - o   It is associated with a 90% patient satisfaction rating and is cost-effective in the long term.
  - o   It is preferable to use GnRH agonists preoperatively if the leiomyoma is large. It has been shown to reduce operative time and intraoperative blood loss.

Short-Answer Questions

Question 1

How will you reduce blood loss during a myomectomy?

Answer:

The following measures can reduce the blood loss at myomectomy:

- Preoperative
  - Treat anaemia prior to surgery
  - Bilateral uterine artery embolisation
  - GnRH agonists for at least 3 months preoperatively
  - Misoprostol, tranexamic acid, and gelatin-thrombin matrix
- Intraoperative
  - Pericervical tourniquet
  - Large volume of diluted vasopressin injected into the myometrium
  - Use of myomectomy clamps
  - Uterine arteries ligated
  - Laparoscopic approach

Question 2

Justify the treatment of uterine leiomyoma.

Answer:

Asymptomatic leiomyomas less than 16 weeks in size do not need to be treated.

Treatment should be individualised with a clear goal. There is a definite resolution of symptoms following treatment, although the 5-year cumulative recurrence rate of the leiomyoma is around 62%. Side effects or complications following treatment are not high. Medical treatment ameliorates symptoms when the uterine size is less than 10–12 weeks. Drugs like tranexamic acid, COC pill, levonorgestrel-containing IUCD, progestogens, and antiprogestogens all reduce blood loss significantly. Danazol, gestrinone, SPRMs, and GnRH agonists also reduce leiomyoma size, in addition to reducing blood loss.

Radiological intervention, such as UAE and MRgFUS, reduce leiomyoma as well as reducing blood loss, are well tolerated, and avoid surgery.

Surgery does improve blood loss, pressure symptoms, and conception rates, but the live pregnancy rate is not increased. It also reduces the incidence of some pregnancy-related complications of leiomyomas, such as malpresentation, preterm labour, abruption, obstructed labour, and PPH. So there is a clear justification for treatment of leiomyomas in a symptomatic woman, as long as the treatment is directed at the symptoms.

Question 3

What factors will influence your choice of treatment of leiomyomas?

Answer:

Asymptomatic leiomyomas are not treated. The following factors will influence my choice of treatment:

Symptoms: The symptoms would dictate the treatment. For example, HMB due to a small leiomyoma could be treated medically, whereas HMB due to a large leiomyoma will need surgery. Ulipristal reduces HMB and also reduces myoma size by 25%. Pressure symptoms are best treated with surgery or with EUA/MRgFUS, which could progressively achieve a reduction of up to 60% in size in a period of 6 months.

Fertility needs: When future fertility is desired, a hysterectomy is not an option. Medical treatment does not improve conception rates, but resection of a submucous leiomyoma does.

Age: In perimenopausal women, when medical treatment has not been successful, a hysterectomy will be a reasonable option.

Type, number, and size of leiomyoma: These factors play an important role in selecting the most appropriate treatment option. Small leiomyomas could be treated medically. A submucous leiomyoma could be treated by hysteroscopic resection. A large leiomyoma will either need a myomectomy or a hysterectomy.

Prevention: Long-term use of COC pills or depot medroxyprogesterone acetate protect against leiomyoma development. (Smoking also protects against leiomyoma development, but this should not be encouraged.)

Comorbidities: In the presence of comorbidities making surgery or anaesthesia risky, radiological interventions should be considered.

Question 4

A 40-year-old Jehovah's Witness is due to have a hysterectomy for an 18-week-size uterine leiomyoma. How will you counsel her? How would you reduce haemorrhage intraoperatively?

Answer:

I would provide the following counselling for this patient:

- Treat anaemia preoperatively. Arrange anaesthetic consult.
- Explore which drugs she will accept:
  - Some will accept recombinant clotting factors.
  - Some will accept the use of cell-saver.
  - Some will accept blood products in the event of impending death.
- Discuss alternative options with her, for example:
  - UAE.
  - MRgFUS.
  - Further trial of a different medical treatment such as GnRH agonists or SPRMs.

- Explain the potential source of haemorrhage during surgery and the steps that will be taken to prevent such an occurrence.
- Clear and detailed documentation of the discussion.
- Informed written consent, clearly documenting possible complications, such as heavy bleeding, CVA (5–10%), and death, and the patient's refusal to receive blood products.
- Possible ICU admission if heavy bleeding occurs.

In order to reduce haemorrhage intraoperatively, I would undertake the following measures:

- Preoperative measures:
  o Treat anaemia prior to surgery.
  o Bilateral uterine artery embolisation.
  o GnRH agonists for at least 3 months preoperatively.
  o Misoprostol, tranexamic acid, and gelatin-thrombin matrix.
- Intraoperative measures:
  o Have experienced anaesthetic and surgical teams available, with an experienced colleague assisting the surgery.
  o Keep cell-saver ready if acceptable to the patient.
  o Use oxygen 100%.
  o Meticulous haemostasis:
    ▪ Don't rush.
    ▪ Double clamping of pedicles.
    ▪ Double ligation of pedicles.
    ▪ All cutting under direct vision.
  o Use appropriate IV fluids for volume replacement.

Question 5

You are consulting a 32-year-old female with secondary infertility. She had a vaginal delivery 4 years ago, following spontaneous conception. She is now known to have a uterine leiomyoma, according to her family doctor.

Part a

Evaluate the options available to assess the leiomyoma.

Answer:

See investigations of leiomyomas mentioned in the text.

Part b

When would you treat these leiomyomas, given the above information?

Answer:

Leiomyomas that distort or occlude the fallopian tube will need to be treated by a myomectomy to increase the conception rate.

Intramural leiomyomas reduce fertility and increase miscarriage rate, but there is no evidence that treatment improves fertility.

Resection of submucous leiomyomas, especially if they are distorting the endometrial cavity, improves the conception rate but not the live birth rate.

In terms of outcomes for fertility, a laparoscopic myomectomy has no advantage over an open myomectomy.

Subserosal leiomyomas and submucous/intramural leiomyomas that are 1–2 cm in diameter do not need to be treated.

There is no evidence that medical therapy of leiomyomas improves fertility.

Question 6

Critically appraise the available treatments for leiomyomas in the context of a planned pregnancy.

Answer:

Evidence shows that medical treatment does not improve fertility.

There is no evidence behind MRgFUS for its use as treatment for a uterine leiomyoma to improve fertility.

UAE is ideally avoided as a treatment for uterine leiomyoma, when a pregnancy is planned in the future, because of the increased risks of pregnancy complications, such as IUGR, preterm birth, and miscarriage. UAE has a 3% risk of premature ovarian failure due to unintended embolisation of the ovarian vessels. In a systematic review by Sud et al. in 2009, in the UAE cohort, the rates of ongoing pregnancy and live birth rates were 63.7% and 57.8%, respectively. The same rates in the myomectomy cohort were 77.9% and 77.4, respectively.

Myomectomy has been shown to improve conception rate if the leiomyoma is occluding the fallopian tube, if it is a submucous leiomyoma, and if this is also distorting the endometrial cavity. Resection of such a leiomyoma improves the conception rate and reduces the chance of a miscarriage.

Compared to an open myomectomy, a laparoscopic myomectomy has less intraoperative haemorrhage and a shorter recovery. But in terms of recurrence rate, pregnancy rate, or scar dehiscence rate, it is similar to the open myomectomy.

There is no evidence of benefit in treating an asymptomatic leiomyoma, unless it is 16 weeks or more in size.

Multiple-Choice Questions

Q1. Which is the primary investigation for a uterine leiomyoma?

    A. MRI

    B. Hysteroscopy

    C. Transvaginal ultrasound

    D. Saline sonohysterography

Answer: C

Q2. A saline sonohysterography should be done when:

    A. A well-demarcated normal endometrial stripe is clearly seen

    B. An endometrial stripe is indistinctly seen

    C. Investigating any type of uterine leiomyoma

    D. A submucous leiomyoma is suspected

Answer: D

Q3. In which of the following cases is MRI not indicated?

    A. When there is doubt about the nature of the uterine mass

    B. When a leiomyosarcoma is suspected

    C. When UAE is being planned

    D. When a hysteroscopic resection of leiomyoma is planned

Answer: D

Q4. COC pills, when used in the presence of a uterine leiomyoma:

    A. Reduce blood loss by 25%

    B. Reduce leiomyoma growth, if used for a long period and in high dosage

    C. Mostly cause an increase in the size of the leiomyoma

    D. Reduce blood loss irrespective of anaemia

Answer: B

Q5. Which of the following does not stop a leiomyoma from growing?

    A. Long-term COC

    B. Long-term depot medroxyprogesterone acetate

    C. Progesterone-only pill

    D. Gestrinone

Answer: C

Q6. After UAE, the prevalence of new leiomyoma growth is:

    A. 7%

    B. 14%

    C. 21%

    D. 28%

Answer: A

Q7. After myomectomy, the prevalence of new leiomyoma growth is:

    A. 20%

    B. 40%

    C. 60%

    D. 80%

Answer: C

Q8. On ultrasound scan, a uterine leiomyoma appears:

    A. Hypoechoic

    B. Isoechoic

    C. Hyperechoic

    D. Heterogenous

Answer: A

Q9. In terms of distinction between a leiomyoma and adenomyosis, which of the following is not correct?

    A. A leiomyoma has central vascularity.

    B. A leiomyoma is discrete.

    C. Adenomyosis is more vascular than a leiomyoma.

    D. Adenomyosis is heterogenous.

Answer: A

Q10. A woman, at 28 weeks of pregnancy and with a 4-cm left-sided leiomyoma, develops acute pain with low-grade pyrexia and mild leucocytosis. What is the most likely explanation for her symptoms?

    A. Infection in the leiomyoma

    B. Torsion of the leiomyoma

    C. Red degeneration of the leiomyoma

    D. Preterm labour

Answer: C

Q11. How does an anterior cervical leiomyoma initially present?

    A. Vaginal bleeding

    B. Constipation

    C. Frequency of micturition

    D. Faecal incontinence

Answer: C

Q12. Which of the following complications can result from uterine leiomyomas in a woman who is 20 weeks pregnant?

    A. Fetal malpresentation

    B. Preterm labour

    C. Uterine rupture

    D. Corneous degeneration

Answer: C

Q13. Which of the following is not caused by a uterine myoma?

    A. Infertility

    B. Recurrent miscarriage

    C. Pain

    D. Amenorrhoea

Answer: D

Q14. The prevalence of uterine leiomyoma is highest in which decade of life?

    A. 2nd
    B. 3rd
    C. 4th
    D. 5th

Answer: D

Q15. What is the most frequent complaint in women with a uterine leiomyoma?

    A. Dysmenorrhoea
    B. HMB
    C. DUB
    D. Midcycle bleeding

Answer: A

Q16. A 58-year-old woman with a BMI of 52, hypertension, and diabetes presents to you with vaginal bleeding. An ultrasound scan shows multiple large fibroids and an endometrial thickness of 15 mm. What will you do?

    A. Total abdominal hysterectomy
    B. Uterine artery embolisation
    C. Myomectomy
    D. Start her on continuous combined HRT

Answer: A

Q17. Red degeneration of a uterine fibroid:

    A. Only occurs in pregnancy
    B. Causes leucopenia and lymphocytosis
    C. Causes a rise in ESR
    D. Is due to emboli occluding blood vessels supplying the fibroid

Answer: C

Q18. Which of the following is true regarding uterine leiomyoma?

    A. Rate of sarcomatous change is 1%.
    B. Associated with nulliparity.
    C. Characteristically causes pain.
    D. Should be removed by caesarean section if > 2 cm.

Answer: B

Chapter 11.2.   Adenomyosis

Definition

Adenomyosis is defined as the presence of endometrial glands and stroma in the myometrium with surrounding myometrial hyperplasia and hypertrophy.

Epidemiology

The prevalence is 21–30%.

Clinical Physiology

Adenomyosis forms as a result of the abnormal ingrowth and invagination of the basal layer of the endometrium due to a weakness at the endometrial-myometrial interface. The reason for the weakness of the endometrial-myometrial interface is not clear, but various factors are thought to be contributing, such as increased pressure inside a gravid uterus, surgical trauma, greater invasive potential of the endometrial cells, and, lastly, altered myometrial contractility.

The endometrial glands and stroma are at least 2.5 mm deeper than the basal layer's position. These endometrial glands do not undergo the cyclical physiological proliferative and secretory changes, despite having oestrogen and progesterone receptors. Bleeding does occur among the invading, ectopic endometrium. The surrounding myometrium reacts to the ectopic endometrial glands by hyperplasia and hypertrophy, which causes uterine enlargement. The uterus enlarges in a way that its contour is not lost. It is the posterior myometrium that is often affected. In contrast to a leiomyoma, adenomyoma does not have a capsule, is diffuse, and is more vascular, and hence surgical enucleation becomes more difficult.

Nearly two-thirds of women with adenomyosis will have other pathologies, such as leiomyoma, endometriosis, endometrial hyperplasia, and salpingitis isthmica nodosa. It has also been associated with preterm delivery.

Risk Factors

- Increasing age and parity
- Surgical insult: caesarean section, endometrial curettage
- Obesity

History

An estimated 50% are asymptomatic.

- Dysmenorrhoea
- Heavy menstrual bleeding
- Pelvic pain
- Deep dyspareunia in midline

The severity of symptoms is proportional to the bulk of the disease and depth of invasion of the endometrial cells.

The history is to be taken as in DUB and HMB.

Examination

As in DUB and HMB.

The uterus is enlarged, nodular, and tender. History and examination findings are nonspecific.

Investigations

- Transvaginal ultrasound scan
  - The following features can be seen:
    - Heterogenous myometrium
    - Thickened posterior myometrium or rarely anterior myometrium
    - Displaced endometrial stripe
    - Myometrial glands (5–7 mm)
    - Myometrial linear striations ("venetian blind" appearance)
    - Diffuse in two-thirds of women
    - Scattered vessels

- MRI
  - Widening of junctional zone (subendometrial myometrium) > 12 mm.
  - A junctional zone < 8 mm excludes adenomyosis.
  - The role of MRI:
    - Prior to surgery, to differentiate between a leiomyoma and adenomyosis in a woman wishing to maintain her fertility
    - Prior to UAE

There is no difference in the sensitivity and specificity between transvaginal ultrasound scan and MRI (Maheshwari, 2012); however, MRI is less observer-dependent.

Management

Medical

The evidence of effectiveness of medical treatment of adenomyosis is lacking. There is no proven drug treatment. Hence, all the drugs listed under HMB are used with different degrees of improvement of symptoms.

The expulsion rate of a levonorgestrel-containing IUCD was higher (16%) in adenomyosis.

The evidence is lacking for any role of UAE or MRgFUS in the treatment of adenomyosis.

It is an incurable disease.

Surgical

Endometrial ablation has a higher failure rate due to regeneration of the endometrium from deeper lesions. The levonorgestrel-containing IUCD is preferred in this situation.

Surgical excision of an adenomyoma is also practiced, but because of its diffuse nature, it is impossible to enucleate it completely.

Hysterectomy is the only definitive treatment, but it can only be done when future fertility is not desired.

Multiple-Choice Questions

Q1. The severity of symptoms of adenomyosis is proportional to:

A. Increasing age
B. Increasing weight
C. Increasing parity
D. Increasing depth of invasion

Answer: D

Q2. Which of the following is not caused by adenomyosis?

A. Secondary dysmenorrhoea
B. Infertility
C. Deep dyspareunia
D. Heavy menstrual bleeding

Answer: B

Q3. Which of the following statements regarding adenomyosis is incorrect?

A. It is usually not well defined.
B. It is usually less vascular than a leiomyoma.
C. It may coexist with a leiomyoma.
D. The rate of malignant transformation is higher than a leiomyoma.

Answer: B

Chapter 11.3. Endometrial Polyp

Definition

It is the focal hyperplastic outgrowth of endometrial glands and stroma with a vascular core, projecting into the endometrial cavity to different degrees.

Incidence

Endometrial polyps occur in:

- 10% of asymptomatic women
- 24–41% of symptomatic women

Clinical Physiology

The aetiology of endometrial polyps is poorly understood. However, it is believed that the polyps do not have apoptotic regulation and overexpress oestrogen and progesterone receptors, avoiding the normal control mechanisms (McGurgan P et al., 2005). Endometrial polyps are mostly asymptomatic. With aging, the incidence increases, peaking in the fifth decade of life.

Risk Factors

- Increasing age
- HRT use
- Tamoxifen use
- Diabetes mellitus
- Hypertension
- Obesity

Predictors of Malignancy

The risk of malignant transformation is 0.5% of malignancy. The predictors include the following:

- Postmenopausal age
- Abnormal uterine bleeding
- Size > 1 cm with bleeding, or > 1.8 cm without bleeding
- Concurrent use of HRT
- Coexistent endometrial hyperplasia

Hysteroscopic Markers of Malignancy

- Surface necrosis
- Whitish thickened area on the surface
- Vascular irregularity

History

Most endometrial polyps are asymptomatic and are discovered incidentally. When symptomatic, they cause the following:

- Heavy menstrual bleeding
- Premenstrual and postmenstrual staining
- Scanty postmenopausal spotting
- Infertility when large
- Miscarriage

Examination

This will be a routine gynaecological examination. However, a clinical examination will not be able to help in making a diagnosis of an endometrial polyp. An endometrial polyp is only diagnosed by either imaging or a hysteroscopy.

Investigations

	Sensitivity	Specificity
Hysteroscopy	90%	93%
Transvaginal ultrasound	91%	90%
Saline sonohysterography	95%	92%
MRI of pelvis	95%	92%

Table 11.2. Features of investigations for endometrial polyp

Management

Medical

Very small endometrial polyps can slough out with medical curettage (pharmacologically induced withdrawal bleeding). Otherwise, medical therapy has no role.

Surgical

Endometrial polyps that meet any of the following criteria should be removed:

- Polyps in the postmenopausal age group
- Symptomatic polyps
- Polyps > 1 cm in size

Asymptomatic endometrial polyps < 1 cm in size in the premenopausal age group can be observed.

Hysteroscopic resection is much preferable to blind avulsion of the polyp. The recurrence rate of endometrial polyps with the blind avulsion technique is 15%.

Criteria for removal of asymptomatic polyp in the premenopausal age group:

- Size > 1 cm
- Multiple polyps
- Polyp prolapsed through the cervix
- Infertility

Chapter 11.4.   Uterine Perforation during Hysteroscopy/Curettage

Incidence

Hysteroscopy	1%
Suction curettage	0.5%
Endometrial ablation	1%
Endometrial resection	2%
D&C in the postmenopausal age group	2.6%
D&C in the immediate postpartum period	5%

Table 11.3. Incidence of uterine perforation from various gynaecological procedures

Risk Factors

- Cervical stenosis
- Scarring of endocervical canal due to prior surgery
- Extremely retroverted or anteverted uterus
- Postmenopausal age
- Prolonged use of depot medroxyprogesterone acetate injection
- Postradiation

Prevention

- Vaginal oestrogen prior to the procedure to postmenopausal women where atrophy is suspected, women on prolonged depot medroxyprogesterone acetate or postradiation if not contraindicated
- Misoprostol PV/PR 4 hours prior to surgery
- Intraoperative measures
  - Straightening of uterine axis by pulling on the cervix with a vulsellum
  - Smaller instruments
  - Gentler and careful approach
  - Intracervical injection of vasopressin
  - Simultaneous use of ultrasound or laparoscopic guidance

Diagnosis

Intraoperatively:

- Uterine sound or dilator does not meet resistance and keeps going into the peritoneal cavity
- Direct visualisation of perforation/omentum/bowel
- Fatty tissue obtained on curettage
- Heavy vaginal bleeding that does not stop

Postoperatively:

- Combination of abdominal pain, distension, vaginal bleeding, haematuria, fever within 1–3 days of surgery

Risk of Bleeding

- Fundal perforations usually do not bleed.
- Lateral perforations bleed due to trauma to uterine artery or its branches.
- Cervical perforations can traumatise the lower descending branch of uterine artery. It can cause delayed bleeding, if the artery undergoes spasm.
- Perforation due to the use of blunt instruments does not bleed much, and risk of visceral trauma is also low.

Management

- Administer IV antibiotic intraoperatively.
- Stop doing any further hysteroscopic surgery.
- If bleeding, laparoscopic or open suturing.
- If not bleeding and no suspicion of other visceral trauma—observe overnight.
- If trauma to other viscera suspected/cause to be excluded, a laparoscopy should be done.
- Open disclosure to the patient once she is awake.
- Reevaluate indication for surgery. If surgery is still needed, plan after 3 months.

Short-Answer Questions

Question 1

Discuss the evidence for doing a bilateral oophorectomy in a premenopausal woman who is going to have a hysterectomy for a benign condition.

Answer:

Bilateral oophorectomy (BO) at the time of hysterectomy neither increases the operative time nor the recovery time. There used to be a popular notion that by combining the hysterectomy with BO, the future risk of the development of ovarian diseases and consequent morbidity and mortality were reduced. A modelling study in 2005 showed that at no age was there a clear benefit of prophylactic BO (Parker W et al., 2005). A subsequent observational study, popularly known as the Nurses' Health

Study, which had 30,000 women enrolled over a 28-year median follow-up period, showed that BO, when combined with a hysterectomy for benign condition in a premenopausal woman, was associated with a decreased risk of breast and ovarian cancers but an increased risk of all-cause mortality and fatal and nonfatal coronary disease (hazard ratio 0.06, 95% confidence interval 0.02 to 0.21) (Parker W et al., 2009). This study also showed that at no age was BO associated with increased survival.

Another prospective cohort study of over 24,000 women with a median follow-up period of 7.6 years showed that although BO with hysterectomy decreased the risk of ovarian cancer compared with hysterectomy alone, it did not increase the risk of coronary heart disease, hip fracture, or death (Jacoby V et al., 2011).

A recently published retrospective data analysis of English hospitals involving 113,679 women with a 10-year follow-up period concluded that women who did not have BO had a significantly lower hazard of all-cause mortality and lower death rates from ischaemic heart disease and cancer, when compared with those who had BO with a hysterectomy (Mytton J et al., 2017). According to the Royal Australian and New Zealand College of Obstetricians and Gynaecologists (RANZCOG, 2014), there are increased risks of cognitive dysfunction, dementia, depression, and anxiety symptoms following prophylactic BO.

Premenopausal women having a hysterectomy for a benign condition should be advised that although prophylactic BO protects against future development of ovarian cancer, this advantage comes at the cost of an increased risk of cardiovascular disease and higher overall mortality.

Question 2

List the advantages and disadvantages of doing a bilateral salpingo-oophorectomy concurrently with a hysterectomy for heavy menstrual bleeding in a 45-year-old woman.

Answer:

Advantages:

- Improvement in premenstrual symptoms
- Risk of ovarian cancer is reduced 100-fold
- No possibility of residual ovary syndrome
- Will treat endometriosis, if present
- Will eliminate ovulation pain

Disadvantages:

- Surgical menopause induced, with menopausal symptoms starting very quickly after the operation
- Psychological morbidity, such as cognitive dysfunction, dementia, depression, and anxiety symptoms

Question 3

Discuss the evidence behind opportunistic bilateral salpingectomy (OS) at the time of a hysterectomy for a benign condition.

Answer:

Recently accumulated evidence (Hanley E et al., 2015; Society of Gynaecological Oncology 2013) has overwhelmingly indicated that the fimbrial ends of the fallopian tubes are the site of origin for the majority of high-grade serous ovarian or peritoneal carcinomas. Hence, it is quite justified to perform an OS without oophorectomy at the time of a hysterectomy for a benign condition. Performing a bilateral salpingectomy in preference to tubal occlusion is also justified on the same ground. There is insufficient evidence to support interim salpingectomy in women with BRCA 1 and 2 mutations who want to delay BO for other reasons.

There is no known benefit of retaining fallopian tubes in women who do not desire future fertility. Salpingectomy also does not worsen operative morbidity.

RANZCOG (2014) states that in the absence of population-based data to quantify the risk-benefit profile, it is not clear whether an OS will reduce the incidence of ovarian carcinoma in the general population. The American College of Obstetricians and Gynaecologists (2015) recommends that in the absence of randomised controlled trials, gynaecologists should discuss the potential benefits of OS with their patients.

Chapter 12
Benign Diseases of the Cervix

Chapter 12.1. Clinical Physiology of the Cervix

The cervix is formed by the fusion of the Müllerian ducts. Endocervical glans develop between the 13th and 15th week of pregnancy. It measures about 5 cm in length and 2–3 cm in width in the reproductive age group. In a nulliparous woman, the external cervical os faces toward the posterior vaginal wall.

Blood supply of the cervix: descending branch of the uterine artery.

Lymphatic drainage: to paracervical and parametrial lymph nodes and then to obturator, internal iliac, and external iliac lymph nodes.

Definitions

Dysplasia	Disordered maturation and differentiation of epithelial cells with nuclear changes; a histological term
Dyskaryosis	Disordered maturation and differentiation of the nucleus, with unchanged cytoplasm
Metaplasia	Transformation of one mature differentiated cell type into another in response to altered cellular milieu
Radical trachelectomy	Removal of cervix up to the internal os and paracervical tissue

Table 12.1. Chapter 12, Definitions

Histology

The cervix is principally made up of collagen tissue, elastic tissue, and smooth muscle to some extent.

The ectocervix (vaginal part of the cervix) is covered by stratified, nonkeratinised, squamous epithelium, similar to the vaginal epithelium.

The cervical canal is lined by columnar epithelium. The squamous-columnar junction is the junction of the squamous epithelium covering the ectocervix and the columnar epithelium that lines the cervical canal. This junction can often be identified by the change in colour from a pale pink colour (squamous epithelium) to a bright red colour (columnar epithelium). It can be on the ectocervix in the prepubertal and adolescent girls, or in the cervical canal in postmenopausal women.

Chapter 12.2. Cervical Intraepithelial Neoplasia

This is also referred to as cervical dysplasia.

Precancerous changes of the cervix are known as cervical intraepithelial neoplasia (CIN). These changes are confined to the squamous epithelium layer of the cervix and do not extent beyond the basement membrane. The changes at the cellular level are:

i. Altered nuclear/cytoplasmic ratio

ii. Nuclear atypia

iii. Excessive mitotic activity and the presence of immature cells

The following grading system is used in clinical practice:

- Low-grade change—CIN I, low-grade squamous intraepithelial lesion (LSIL).
- High-grade change—CIN II and CIN III, high-grade squamous intraepithelial lesion. CIN III used to be known as carcinoma-in-situ.

This grading of CIN was thought to be a continuum from low-grade to high-grade changes, but this concept is now being challenged.

Histologically, when the precancerous changes only involve the deeper one-third of the epithelium, it is known as CIN I. When the precancerous changes involve the deeper two-thirds of the epithelium, it is known as CIN II. When the entire thickness of the epithelium is involved, it is known as CIN III. These changes occur in the area of the cervix known as the transformation zone.

Transformation zone (TZ): The squamocolumnar junction at birth is in the endocervical canal and is known as the original squamocolumnar junction. This squamocolumnar junction shifts outward under the influence of oestrogen (puberty, pregnancy, contraceptive pill) or change in the vaginal pH. The shifted squamocolumnar junction is known as the new squamocolumnar junction. The area in between the old and new squamocolumnar junctions is called the transformation zone. It is the area of actively dividing cells. Cervical neoplasia originates from this area.

There are three types of TZ:

- Type 1—TZ is confined to the ectocervix and hence completely visible.
- Type 2—TZ has endocervical component and can be still completely visualised.
- Type 3—The endocervical component of the TZ extends deeper into the endocervical canal and hence is not completely visible.

Clinical Physiology

Human papilloma virus (HPV) is a circular, double-stranded DNA virus that has an affinity for epithelial cells. More than 100 strains are known to exist, 30–40% of which infect the lower genital tract. This virus is sexually transmitted. These strains can cause benign lesions of the cervix, such as condylomata and CIN, or cervical cancer. The strains that cause benign lesions are low-risk HPV strains (6 and 11), and those that cause cervical carcinoma are high-risk HPV strains (16, 18, 45, 56, and 58).

Up to 80% of sexually active women will have HPV infection at some time in their lives. This incidence is rising. Most of the HPV infections are transient and are cleared off by the cell-mediated immunity of the host within 2 years. Most of the HPV infections cause CIN I, and 60% of these clear without treatment. Approximately 10% of these HPV infections will lead to CIN II–III, and 36% of CIN III will progress to invasive cancer in 10–20 years if left untreated. The rate of progression is uncertain, but nearly 11% of CIN I will progress to CIN III.

Progression or regression of the CIN is not well understood, but it is believed to be affected by the following factors:

i.   Integration of HPV genome:
   o   If the virus is in the cytoplasm of the host cell (episomal), it gets cleared by the host's immune system.
   o   Once the viral DNA enters the nucleus of the host cell, it "integrates" with the host-cell DNA, and the process of oncogenesis starts.
   o   This process of oncogenesis is aided by the degradation of the suppressor proteins by oncoproteins E_6 and E_7. This results in uncontrolled proliferation of the cell, due to complete disruption of regulation of the cell cycle.

ii. Smoking suppresses local immunity in the cervix and acts as a cofactor in the development of cervical cancer.

iii. Women with some HLA types are more susceptible to cervical cancer.

iv. Impaired cell-mediated immunity, e.g., women with HIV or immunosuppression following organ transplant, is associated with higher rates of cervical cancer.

	Regression (%)	Progression to cervical cancer (%)
CIN I	60	1
CIN II	40	5
CIN III	30	36

Table 12.2. Rates of regression to normal and progression to cervical cancer from different stages of CIN

The cells that are infected with HPV show the following characteristics:

• Koilocytosis (large cytoplasmic vacuole)
• Hyperkeratosis
• Parakeratosis
• Papillomatosis
• Multinucleation
• Dyskeratosis (keratinisation of individual cells)

Risk Factors

The risk factors for CIN are the same as those for cervical cancer:

- Squamous carcinoma of the cervix
  - HPV infection
  - Early and frequent coitus
  - Multiple sexual partners
  - Immunosuppression
  - Smoking
  - High parity
  - Low socioeconomic status
- Adenocarcinoma of the cervix
  - Oral contraceptive use
  - Lack of cervical cytological screening
  - HPV infection

Screening

Pap Smears

Cervical neoplasia screening was started by Papanicolaou in the 1950s and hence the name Pap smear. In developed countries, where there are well-structured screening programmes, cervical screening has succeeded in reducing the incidence of cervical cancer by half. It involves collecting the exfoliated cells from the transformation zone by "cervical broom" and then quickly making a smear of the collected cells on a glass slide. The smear is then fixed by a fixative (alcohol) before transporting it to the laboratory. Each slide usually has around 20% of the collected cells. Cervical smears have a false positive rate of 7–27% (high specificity) and false negative rate of 20–50% (low sensitivity).

The cytological examination of a Pap smear is based largely on the abnormal features of the nuclei (dyskaryotic). These features are as follows:

- Disproportionate nuclear enlargement
- Irregular shape
- Hyperchromasia
- Abnormalities of number and size of nucleoli
- Multinucleation

Modified Bethesda System of Reporting

This system of reporting of Pap smears ensures uniformity of evaluation and management. The reporting under this system is done under the following headings:

- Adequacy of sample

- Squamous cell abnormalities
  - ○ Atypical cells
  - ○ Low-grade changes
  - ○ High-grade changes
  - ○ Squamous cell carcinoma
- Glandular cell abnormalities
- Other cancers

Occasionally, Pap smears show normal or abnormal endometrial cells. The most common squamous cell abnormality is atypical squamous cell of undetermined significance (ASC-US). These cells show some features of squamous cell lesions, but either they are very few in number or the changes are not consistent with any precise category of reporting.

Follow-up of Abnormal Pap Smears

- LSIL (once)—repeat after 12 months
- Persistent LSIL—colposcopy
- ASC-US—colposcopy
- HSIL—colposcopy
- Glandular abnormalities—colposcopy

Liquid-Based Cytology (LBC)

The conventional Pap smear collection on a glass slide has many limitations, such as the following:

- Low sensitivity
- Only 20% of cells transferring from the cervical broom to the glass slide
- Problems with delayed fixation (drying distortions)
- Blood obscuring the smear

LBC is now increasingly being used as a routine in many developed countries. The cells collected are placed directly, with the end of a cervical broom, into a small bottle with a liquid medium and then transported to the laboratory for cytological examination. LBS has the following advantages:

- Drying distortions are eliminated.
- The chance of blood cells obscuring the cervical cells is reduced from 87% to 1%.
- Improved reporting times.
- HPV DNA testing is possible on the same sample.
- Detection of certain STIs is possible on the same sample.
- There is a higher sensitivity than glass-slide method (Evidence Level IA).

The frequency of cervical screening in normal women has remained controversial. In most developed countries, women who are or have been sexually active are advised to have their cervical cytology screened every 2–5 years. Cervical cytology screening is stopped in most countries when the woman is aged between 65–70 years.

Changes to the National Cervical Screening Program in Australia from December 2017

In Australia, it is planned that beginning in December 2017, conventional Pap smears will be replaced with HPV testing, with partial genotyping combined with LBC triage for HPV-positive women. This system will have the following advantages over the conventional screening program:

- Higher sensitivity, specificity, and positive-predictive value.
- Allows for identification of high-risk HPV strains.
- Incidence of false negatives will be reduced.
- A negative HPV test has a very high negative-predictive value, which allows for a 5-year screening interval.

The salient features of this program are as follows:

- The entry age for the program will be 25 years.
- Women will be invited to screen until 69 years of age.
- Women will be invited to exit the program if they have a further negative HPV test between 70–74 years of age.

- To improve participation, self-collection of a cervical sample for HPV testing will be available for underscreened or never-screened women.

- A national registry will be established. Invitation and recall letters will be sent out.

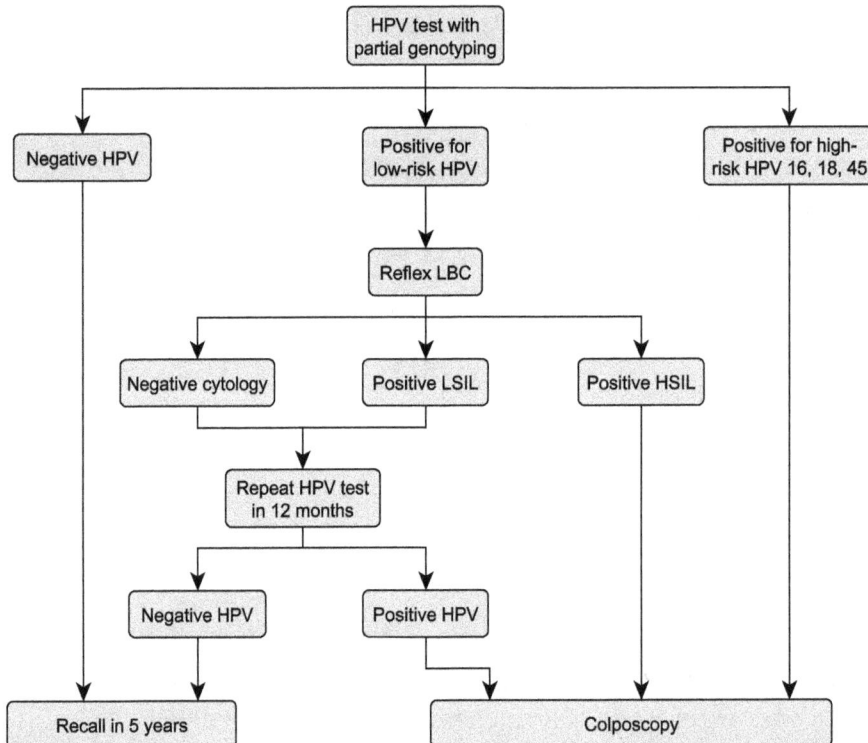

Figure 12.1. Summary of changes to HPV testing in Australia from December 2017

Colposcopy

Colposcopy is a diagnostic procedure in which the cervix is examined by a colposcope for predefined indications. A colposcope is a low-powered (3–25 times) binocular microscope on a mobile stand with a powerful light source. The light source has a green filter that helps the visualisation of the capillaries.

With the help of a bivalve speculum, the cervix, with its transformation zone, is visualised with the colposcope using the correct focal length. The transformation zone should be completely visualised. The application of specific dyes enables identification of the area with CIN in the transformation zone.

Acetic acid (3–5%) is one of the commonly used dyes that makes the nuclei of the dysplastic cells very prominent by desiccating the cytoplasm of the cells. The reflected light of the colposcope makes the area with the CIN look white (acetowhite).

Depending on the characteristics of the acetowhite area, gradation of CIN is done. The acetowhite area takes about 30 seconds to appear, and it disappears after 60–90 seconds.

Another dye that could be used after acetic acid is Lugol's (aqueous) iodine. Lugol's iodine stains the normal epithelium dark brown to black because of the high glycogen content in these cells. The cells with CIN, due to their poorer glycogen content, do not take the Lugol's iodine stain and appear unstained. The areas that do not take Lugol's iodine are called iodine negative or Schiller positive. Conversely, the areas that take up iodine are called iodine positive or Schiller negative.

Targeted biopsies are taken from the acetowhite or iodine-negative areas.

Acetowhite appearance on colposcopy is also seen in certain non-CIN conditions, such as regenerating epithelium, subclinical HPV infection and metaplasia. The colposcopic gradation of CIN is done by the presence of the following features in the acetowhite area:

- Raised and prominent margin—HSIL
- Dense acetowhite area—HSIL
- Presence of vascular pattern such as mosaic, punctation, atypical capillaries—HSIL
- Iodine negative

Current indications for colposcopy:

- HSIL on Pap smear
- Persistent LSIL on Pap smear
- Follow-up of LLETZ/cone biopsy
- Abnormal-looking cervix
- Postcoital bleeding

Other technologies that are being trialled for cervical assessment are the dynamic spectral imaging system (DySIS) and Niris. They are not in common use yet. NICE does not recommend Niris because of higher cost implications.

Management

The management of biopsy-proven CIN is as follows:

- LSIL (CIN I): Repeat Pap smear in 12 months; 60% resolve spontaneously.
- HSIL (CIN II and CIN III): The aim of treatment for HSIL is either to ablate or excise the entire transformation zone. Colposcopy should be done just prior to surgery. Large-loop excision of the transformation zone (LLETZ) or cone biopsy are in common practice.
  - There should be yearly follow-up for 2 years with HPV DNA testing.
  - When the upper limit of the transformation zone is not visible at colposcopy, a cone biopsy should be done (conisation).
  - If there is a normal cervical biopsy but Pap smears persistently show CIN II or CIN III, a cone biopsy or a deep LLETZ should be done with follow-up as above.
- Adenocarcinoma in situ: cone biopsy.

Studies on different methods of treating CIN do not show that one technique is overwhelmingly superior to another (Evidence Level IA). LLETZ is performed in some centres in an outpatient setting. The value of prophylactic antibiotic is uncertain. CIN is not treated during pregnancy, and pregnancy does not affect its course. The lesions often disappear after pregnancy. However, a conisation could be considered in pregnancy if there is an indication of invasive disease.

The following is a comparison between different treatment modalities:

	Cryotherapy	LLETZ	LASER	Cone biopsy
Cost	Cheap	Cheap	Expensive instrument and costly to maintain	Cheap
Location of procedure	Outpatient	Inpatient or outpatient	Inpatient or outpatient	Inpatient
Ease of learning	Easy to learn	Easy to learn	Requires special training	Easy to learn
Indications	HSIL	HSIL	HSIL or large, irregular lesions	HSIL, discrepancy in findings of biopsy/Pap smear, upper limit of TZ/ lesion not seen, AIS
Mode of action	Frozen N2O (-89°C) in 2 sequential freeze-thaw cycles; ablation up to 5 mm, destroys cells by crystallising intracellular fluid	Excision by loop diathermy, up to a depth of 5–6 mm	Ablation by CO_2 laser up to 5–7 mm	Excision by cold knife up to 10–20 mm depth

	Cryotherapy	LLETZ	LASER	Cone biopsy
Criteria	Entire lesion visible	Entire lesion visible	Entire lesion visible	As described in indications
Contraindications	Large cervix, large lesion, pregnancy, glandular involvement	AIS, pregnancy	AIS, pregnancy	Pregnancy
Advantages	• Cheap • Outpatient procedure • Easy to learn	• Cheap • Outpatient procedure • Easy to learn • Histological diagnosis possible	• Outpatient procedure • Area of destruction can be minimised • No troublesome vaginal discharge	• Cheap • Histological diagnosis possible • Cut margins not destroyed by diathermy
Specific risks	• Ongoing vaginal discharge	• Surgical procedure • Secondary haemorrhage • Cervical stenosis/ incompetence (8%) • Lesion may extend up to the diathermy margin • Accidental damage to adjoining structures	• Accidental damage to adjoining structures	• Surgical procedure • Secondary haemorrhage • Cervical stenosis/ incompetence (8%)
Thermal artefact	Very little	Less than laser	Greatest	None
Rate of haemorrhage	Very little	Similar	Similar	Similar
Success rate	95%	95%	95%	95%
Rate of CIN recurrence	17%	Less than cryotherapy		
Rate of secondary haemorrhage	–	0–8%	2–10%	5–15%
Rate of infection	9%	0–2%	0–2%	0.2–6.8%

Table 12.3. Comparison of the different techniques to treat HSIL

Postoperative Follow-up

- Women are discharged home with the advice to not have sexual intercourse, use tampons, bathe, or bathe in a spa for 3–4 weeks.
- Some vaginal discharge is expected for 3–4 weeks.
- Review at 6 weeks to ensure that the cervix has healed well and to review the histology.
- Follow-up with colposcopy, cervical smear, and biopsy (if necessary) at 4–6 months.
- Annual follow-up for 2 years with cervical smear and HPV DNA (test of cure).
- For cervical glandular intraepithelial neoplasia, 6-monthly smears for 5 years and then annual smears for another 5 years should be taken.

Chapter 12.3. Cervical Polyps

A cervical polyp can arise from the ectocervix or cervical canal. It can be single or multiple and look like fleshy, dark-red, soft (and sometimes mobile) masses from a few millimetres to 1–2 cm in size. They may be sessile or pedunculated.

The aetiology is not well understood. Chronic cervicitis or hormonal factors may play a role.

It is often seen at the time of cervical smear. It is often not detected by a pelvic ultrasound scan. It may be asymptomatic, or it can cause postcoital bleeding or excessive discharge.

A cervical polyp is removed by polyp forceps, using a continuous twisting motion with gentle traction. If bleeding, the base may need cautery. Even though the rate of malignant transformation is extremely low, the removed polyp must be sent for histological assessment.

Polyps can recur.

Chapter 12.4. Nabothian Follicle (Cyst)

This is the retention cyst of the columnar glands. The egress of fluid becomes blocked by overgrowth of squamous epithelium. Hence, the mucoid secretion of the columnar gland keeps accumulating. It can be microscopic or up to 15 mm in size. The larger ones may appear to be very prominent and sometimes project over the surface of the ectocervix.

It is almost always benign and asymptomatic, and it is often an incidental finding. It is also seen on transvaginal ultrasound scans as small, round, simple cysts in the lower half of the cervix.

No treatment is required. If the woman is anxious, the Nabothian follicle can be ablated by a diathermy needle.

Chapter 12.5. Ectropion

This used to be known as an erosion. It is the eversion of the endocervical columnar epithelium to the ectocervix. It appears as a dark-red area around the external cervical os.

It is commonly seen in adolescents, in women who are on the COC pill, or during pregnancy.

It may be asymptomatic, or it can cause intermenstrual and/or postcoital bleeding.

Treatment is only required when symptomatic. Treatment consists of ablation, either by cryotherapy or diathermy. Malignancy must be excluded by doing a Pap smear or cervical biopsy before any ablative procedure.

In some countries, a boric acid suppository 600 mg for two weeks or a deoxyribonucleic acid suppository 5 mg for two weeks is used. These agents are believed to acidify the vaginal pH.

Short-Answer Questions

Question 1

What are the advantages of HPV testing together with liquid-based cytology (LBC) over the conventional Pap smear?

Answer:

HPV testing with LBC has the following advantages over a Pap smear alone:

i.   Improved sensitivity of detection for CIN II or worse.

ii. Reduced incidence of high-grade CIN and cervical cancer in future.

   o   Early identification of high-risk HPV genotypes and the prompt treatment with LLETZ/cone biopsy will protect against future development of high-grade CIN and cervical cancer.

   o   HPV testing provides 60–70% greater protection against invasive cervical cancer compared with cervical cytology alone, with significantly reduced incidence of adenocarcinoma.

iii. Comparable specificity between the two modalities of screening.

iv. Partial HPV genotyping identifies women at the highest risk of cervical cancer.

   o   The identification of HPV 16 and 18 by partial HPV genotyping has shown to provide increased specificity for CIN II–III compared with HPV testing without partial genotyping.

v.   LBS has a distinct advantage over conventional Pap smear in terms of a reduced proportion of unsatisfactory samples and simplified logistics of screening.

vi. Two large RCTs have shown that HPV testing with LBC triage has a higher positive predictive value for high grade lesions compared with Pap smear alone.

vii. The combination of HPV testing with partial genotype and LBC triage will reduce referrals to colposcopy clinics.

viii. 5-yearly testing, starting at 25 years of age rather than 2-yearly testing starting at 18 years of age.

Question 2

You are seeing a 28-year-old G1P1 lady whose cervical smear persistently shows HSIL despite nothing abnormal being seen on colposcopy and a negative cervical biopsy.

Part a

Discuss your management, with rationale.

Answer:

From the information given above, it appears that at colposcopy, either:

- the TZ was not completely seen, or
- the lesion was in the endocervical canal and hence not seen, or
- the cervical biopsy was not appropriately colposcopically targeted.

Hence, I will perform an excisional surgery. Cone biopsy will have a slightly higher incidence of cervical stenosis and incompetence in any future pregnancy; hence, my first choice will be a LLETZ. The complication and success rates of the two procedures are similar.

Part b

If you decide to do surgery, how will you reduce intraoperative bleeding?

Answer:

Strategies to reduce intraoperative bleeding are the following:

- Exclude any coagulopathies preoperatively.
- Stop anticoagulation a week before surgery.
- Intra-operative measures:
  - Infiltrate vasopressin 20–30 mL (0.5 U/mL) or 1:200,000 adrenaline into the cervix before cutting.
  - Cutting cleanly in one pass with diathermy or knife using good surgical technique and ensuring there is no damage to the vagina, bowel, or bladder.
  - Ball diathermy the raw surface after cutting.
  - If bleeding continues, cervical suturing should be used. There are different techniques for suturing, but evidence is lacking to support one over another. According to some, suturing may adversely affect healing.
  - Using Monsel's paste (ferric subsulfate), a haemostatic agent, on the raw surface of the cervix.
  - Packing of the cervix with either oxidised cellulose (Surgicel®), or a vaginal pack soaked in Monsel's paste or diluted adrenaline solution.

Part c

If you decide to do a cone biopsy, how will you determine the size of the cone?

Answer:

The size of the cone in this young woman, who may be desirous of future pregnancy, is important for two reasons:

i) The cone should be of enough width and depth to cover the entire transformation zone (TZ) and the lesion. Hence, a colposcopy should be done just prior to surgery to demarcate the TZ. The cone should be narrower but deeper if the TZ and lesion are in the endocervical canal. However, the cone should be shallower and wider if the endocervical canal is free of disease. In postmenopausal women, the cone should be deeper, because the TZ is in the cervical canal.

ii) A larger cone (incision depth ≥ 10 mm) is associated with an increased incidence of cervical stenosis or incompetence.

Part d

If you decide to do a LLETZ procedure, how will you reduce thermal injury?

Answer:

Strategies to reduce thermal injury in LLETZ are the following:

- Use insulated speculums and lateral vaginal wall retractors.
- Use a smoke sucker to improve and maintain visibility.
- The diathermy generator is set to 30–40 watts of power and on blend 1. A well-blended electrical current mixes coagulating and cutting electrical currents, whereas with a higher-blend setting, there is increased coagulating current, which results in greater thermal damage.

Question 3

List the conditions where excision of the transformation zone is less likely to be complete.

Answer:

- TZ very wide on ectocervix or deep into the endocervical canal
- Lesion extending into vaginal fornices
- Lesion extending deep into the cervical stroma
- Not visualising the complete TZ or the upper limit of the lesion on colposcopy, immediately prior to excision

Question 4

Discuss the place of routine dilatation and curettage prior to any ablative or excisional procedure for HSIL.

Answer:

Endocervical curettage: It must be done just after (not before) any ablative or excisional procedure to ensure that there is no residual disease in the endocervical canal.

Endometrial curettage: There is no place for routine endometrial curettage. However, it may be needed in the following situations:

- When endometrial pathology is suspected, such as abnormal bleeding
- Abnormal glandular cytology
- Endometrial cells seen on cervical smear

Cervical dilatation: Although there are no studies to back it up, cervical dilatation after the procedure is believed to reduce the incidence of cervical stenosis.

Question 5

You are reviewing a 30-year-old woman, 6 weeks after a LLETZ for HSIL. The histology showed HSIL with margins of the lesion extending into the area of diathermy. How will you manage this woman?

Answer:

Management will be as follows:

Reassurance that there is no evidence of cervical cancer and that she does not need any immediate surgery again.

Colposcopy in 4–6 months from the initial surgery with evaluation of the endocervical margin. It is likely that the disease may not be present at that stage because the normal healing would have destroyed the disease. A cervical smear using the endocervical biopsy or endocervical curettage should be taken with the colposcopy at 4–6 months visit. If either the smear or the biopsy/curettage confirm the presence of HSIL, this woman will need a repeat LLETZ or cone biopsy. If, however, the smear or biopsy only shows LSIL, this could be followed up conservatively by another Pap smear in one year.

Question 6

Evaluate HPV screening.

Answer:

In the majority of cases, HPV is asymptomatic and self-limiting, and it does not progress to cervical cancer (Evidence Level III). The prevalence of HPV in cervical cancer is 99.7%. An estimated 70% of cervical cancers are caused by HPV type 16. HPV can be easily detected by PCR or hybrid capture test. Nearly 11% of CIN I progress to CIN III in 3 years, and 36% of CIN III progress to cervical cancer in 10–20 years. Progression of HPV to cervical cancer depends on the following:

- Integration into host cell genome
- Cofactors, such as smoking
- Presence of certain HLA
- Reduced cell-mediated immunity

From the data above, it is vitally important that HPV screening and detection take place in as large a population as possible, in an organised and systematic way. HPV detection and screening will have the following advantages over the conventional glass-slide cervical-smear method:

- It has higher sensitivity, specificity, and positive predictive value.
- The number of repeat cervical smears will be reduced.
- It is possible to detect high-risk strains of HPV.
- Due to its very high negative predictive value, the screening interval can be increased to up to 5 years.
- HPV screening for posttreatment follow-up is cost-effective (Evidence Level II).

Question 7

Discuss the HPV vaccine.

Answer:

The HPV vaccine has been developed to prevent the development of cervical cancers, because almost all cervical cancers are caused by high-risk HPV strains. HPV vaccine has been shown to reduce the lifetime risk of cervical cancer by 20–66%. The vaccine is administered in 3 doses to 12–13-year-old virginal schoolgirls. There are 2 types of vaccines.

i.   <u>Quadrivalent</u>: This HPV quadrivalent recombinant vaccine protects against HPV 6, 11, 16, and 18. As well as providing 100% protection against type-specific CIN (Evidence Level IA), it protects against vulvar and vaginal cancers and anogenital warts. It also protects against high-risk strains 31 and 45.

ii. <u>Bivalent</u>: This HPV bivalent recombinant vaccine only protects against types 16 and 18. It does not protect against anogenital warts.

<u>Mode of action</u>: The vaccine is manufactured in a way that the viral capsid protein, without its DNA, replicates in the host cell, maintaining its antigenic potential. In the absence of DNA, it is biologically inactive. These vaccines increase IgG, protect against type-specific viral infection and CIN.

<u>Uncertainties and limitations</u> are as follows:

- The duration of protection is uncertain.
- The need and frequency of a booster dose is uncertain.
- The vaccine does not provide significant immunity to those already exposed to the virus.
- Cost-effectiveness is uncertain.

Question 8

You are seeing a 30-year-old woman in the emergency department who had a LLETZ 7 days ago for HSIL. She is bleeding rather heavily vaginally and is worried. List the principles of your management.

Answer:

The following are the principles of my management:

- History
    - Duration and severity of bleeding
    - Any offensive discharge
    - Pain
    - Ensure normal bowel and bladder function
    - LMP
- General examination
    - Vital signs—temperature, heart rate, respiratory rate, blood pressure
    - Abdominal tenderness, mass

- Vaginal examination with a bivalve speculum
  - Evacuate any blood clot, if needed
  - Any vaginal trauma
  - Cervix: generalised ooze/active bleeding, cervical swab for microscopy, culture, and sensitivities
  - Any abnormal pelvic mass or tenderness
  - Any offensive discharge or pus

- Investigations
  - FBE, coagulation screen, CRP
  - Group and hold if indicated
  - β-hCG if possibility of pregnancy
  - Pelvic ultrasound scan to exclude any adnexal or pouch of Douglas haematoma
- Treatment
  - Reassurance
  - Resuscitate if haemodynamically compromised
  - If active bleeder seen, then cervical suturing under general anaesthetic in the operating theatre
  - If generalised ooze, then cauterise with either silver nitrate (AgNO₃) sticks or
    - Apply Monsel's paste
    - Pack the vagina with oxidised cellulose, Monsel's paste, or adrenaline-soaked vaginal pack.
  - Broad-spectrum IV or oral antibiotics, including anaerobic cover, for seven days
  - Admit for observation
  - Foley catheterisation if urinary retention develops
  - Remove vaginal pack after 24 hours
    - If still bleeding, cervical suturing
    - If bleeding has stopped, discharge on oral broad-spectrum antibiotic
  - Organise follow-up, check histology if available

Question 9

How will you counsel a woman who has been referred to your colposcopy clinic for HSIL on Pap smear?

Answer:

I will counsel her as follows:

- <u>Reassurance</u>: Pap smear has not shown that she has cervical cancer. It has only shown high-grade precancerous changes, 36% of which may turn into a cervical cancer in 10–20 years.
- <u>History</u>:
  - LMP, gravida, and parity; family complete/incomplete.
  - Contraception.
  - History of previous abnormal smear.
  - Vaccination against HPV.

- o   Use of any regular medication.
- o   Allergy especially to iodine, vinegar, or seafood.

- Colposcopy:
  - o   Explain that Pap smears have a false positive rate of 7–27% and false negative rate of 20–50%.
  - o   Colposcopy and directed biopsy are more definitive in diagnosis.
  - o   Explain the process of colposcopy and directed biopsy with special reference to pain, bleeding and postprocedure return to work.

- Subsequent follow-up: If the cervical biopsy showed HSIL, then she will require treatment with LLETZ, laser, cone (only for glandular abnormalities), or cryotherapy. Emphasise that no one treatment is better than another (Evidence Level IA), but excisional treatment affords the opportunity of histological confirmation of the diagnosis. These treatments will not affect her chances of conception, but the incidence of premature deliveries may increase slightly (Evidence Level IA). If however, the cervical biopsy showed LSIL, then she would need conservative follow-up as per the screening guideline of the country.

Question 10

Discuss this statement: "All women with abnormal Pap smears should have a colposcopy."

Answer:

The advantage of all women with abnormal Pap smear having colposcopy:

Since cervical smears have a false negative rate of 20–50%, many women with abnormalities are missed by Pap smear. A universal colposcopy will address this issue and such women will not be missed.

The disadvantage of all women with abnormal Pap smear having colposcopy:

This will considerably increase the demand for colposcopic services, which would not be cost-effective. Currently, colposcopy is only indicated for HSIL, persistent LSIL, follow-up of treatment, abnormal-looking cervix, and postcoital bleeding. With the planned changes of HPV-based cervical screening and liquid-based cytology, the sensitivity, specificity, and high positive and negative predictive values of screening will considerably improve in comparison to the current cervical screening program.

Hence, I am of the opinion that colposcopy for all women with abnormal Pap smears will not be cost-effective, nor will it increase the sensitivity and specificity more than the new screening program.

Question 11

Discuss the advantages and rationale of raising the age for starting cervical cancer screening from 18–20 years to 25 years with HPV screening.

Answer:

The rationale is as follows:

- It will reduce the risk of detecting transient HPV infection and regressive CIN.
- The analysis of data from the Australian Cervical Screening Program (ACSD) has shown that screening women from 20–24 years of age has not resulted in a decline in the incidence of cervical cancer in this age group (Sasieni P et al., 2009).

- Data from the UK has shown the screening of women between 22–24 years did not reduce the risk of cervical cancer for women 25–29 years of age (Sasieni P et al., 2009).
- Women in the 20–24-year age group will have a substantially lower risk of cervical cancer because of HPV vaccination. The uptake rate of vaccine in schoolgirls is about 70% (National HPV Vaccination Program Register 2015).
- The prevalence of HPV in this age group is very low.
- High-grade cytological abnormality rates have fallen in this group (Australian Institute of Health and Welfare, 2012–13).
- The participation rate of this group of women in the cervical screening program has been declining (Australian Institute of Health and Welfare, 2012–13).
- The combination of HPV vaccination in schoolgirls and HPV-based screening will reduce adenocarcinoma rates.

Question 12

Why has the routine cervical cancer screening program failed to reduce the rate of adenocarcinoma of cervix?

Answer:

There are 3 reasons for this:

i. Cells from precursor lesions in the endocervical canal are difficult to sample.

ii. Glandular cells are more difficult to interpret than squamous cells.

iii. The disease has satellite lesions in the cervical canal.

Question 13

Discuss the arguments for and against this statement: "All women with biopsy-proven CIN III whose childbearing is complete should have a hysterectomy as the primary treatment of CIN III."

Answer:

Arguments in favour of this statement:

- The failure rate of laser for CIN III was 17% after a single treatment and 12% after multiple treatments (Welcher S, 1984). Hence, laser treatment does not treat CIN III optimally. In addition, 6.4% women develop recurrent CIN after conisation.
- Hysterectomy could be considered in the following situations:
  o Positive margins after LLETZ/cone
  o Recurrent/persistent CIN III after a repeat LLETZ/cone
  o Scarred and short cervix from previous surgeries
  o Women who are not willing to submit to regular follow-up after LLETZ/cone

Arguments against this statement:

- Hysterectomy is a much bigger surgery than LLETZ/cone, in terms of cost, morbidity and mortality, and recovery time.

- According to Kesic V et al. (2003), the incidence of invasive cervical cancer was much higher in women who underwent a hysterectomy compared with the women who underwent a conisation. Hence, it was recommended by these authors that hysterectomy must be avoided as the primary treatment.

- An estimated 1–7% of women undergoing hysterectomy for CIN develop vaginal intraepithelial neoplasia (VAIN) in a few months to several years after surgery (Shockaert S et al., 2008).

- Occult vaginal invasion is more common in women who had hysterectomy as the primary treatment of CIN, compared with those who had LLETZ/cone. The possible reasons for this could be that the vaginal vault is more difficult to be examined colposcopically, and rates of vaginal cytological follow-up could also be lower (Ireland D, 1988).

Multiple-Choice Questions

Q1. Currently in Australia, a cervical smear is recommended every:

A. 1 year

B. 2 years

C. 3 years

D. 4 years

Answer: B

Q2. In a 45-year-old woman's routine cervical smear report, it is mentioned that the endocervical cells were not seen. What will you do?

A. Refer for a colposcopy

B. Refer for an endocervical curettage

C. Repeat the Pap smear immediately

D. Repeat the Pap smear in 4–6 months

E. Repeat the Pap smear in 4–6 months after a 2-week course of vaginal oestrogen

Answer: D

Q3. In a 65-year-old woman's routine cervical smear report, it is mentioned that the endocervical cells were not seen. What will you do?

A. Refer for a colposcopy

B. Refer for an endocervical curettage

C. Repeat the Pap smear immediately

D. Repeat the Pap smear in 4–6 months

E. Repeat the Pap smear in 4–6 months after a 2-week course of vaginal oestrogen

Answer: E

Q4. You are attempting to do a routine cervical smear in a 25-year-old, 6 weeks after a vaginal birth. She is completely breastfeeding. The woman finds it extremely uncomfortable and asks you to stop the procedure immediately. The vaginal walls look quite red and inflamed. What will you do?

A. Continue the procedure until completion, offering the patient to have someone present to support her

B. Stop and attempt a Pap smear in 2–3 weeks, after a 2-week course of vaginal oestrogen

C. Stop and attempt the Pap smear under general anaesthesia

D. Abandon the Pap smear and repeat it in 2 years when she is next due

Answer: B

Q5. A 35-year-old presents to you with postcoital bleeding. What will you do first?

A. Clinical examination with Pap smear

B. Refer for hysteroscopy and curettage

C. Colposcopy

D. Take vaginal swab to exclude any vaginal infection

Answer: A

Q6. Which of the following is incorrect with reference to the advantages of LBC over conventional glass-slide Pap smear?

A. LBC has improved sensitivity.

B. LBC has improved specificity.

C. HPV DNA can be diagnosed with LBC.

D. Certain STIs can be diagnosed with LBC.

Answer: B

Q7. A conventional Pap smear is useful in the diagnosis of all of the following, except:

A. Gonorrhoea

B. Trichomonas

C. Inflammatory changes

D. HPV

Answer: A

Q8. For the detection of persistent disease after treatment of HSIL, which of the following is a superior method?

A. Colposcopy alone

B. Colposcopy and cervical smear

C. Cervical smear alone

D. None of the above

Answer: D (There is no evidence that one method is superior to another.)

Q9. Which of the following statements is incorrect?

A. Nearly 75% of cervical cancers are related to HPV.

B. High-risk HPV testing detects 30% more CIN II and 22% more CIN III in women over 30 years of age.

C. A negative high-risk HPV test offers 50% better protection against CIN III in comparison to negative cytology.

D. Neither colposcopy nor cytology are dependable for detecting cervical glandular intraepithelial neoplasia.

Answer: A (Nearly all cervical cancers are related to HPV.)

Q10. Which of the following statements regarding cervical adenocarcinoma in situ is least correct?

A. HPV serotype 18 is most commonly associated with adenocarcinoma.

B. Cone-biopsy specimens with clear margins carry a greater than 20% risk of lesions higher up in the cervical canal.

C. Skip lesions are uncommon compared with squamous carcinoma in situ.

D. Extrafascial hysterectomy is the optimal treatment if childbearing is complete.

Answer: C

Chapter 13

Benign Diseases of the Ovary

Ovarian Cysts and Benign Neoplasms

Definitions

Cyst	Abnormal collection of fluid in a sac within the body, lined by an epithelium.
Ovarian cyst	A cyst in the ovary of at least 3 cm in diameter.
Follicle	A developing follicle in the ovary of less than 3 cm in diameter.
Simple cyst	It is a sonological term signifying a thin-walled, unilocular cyst containing only clear fluid with no septations or solid areas within. It is mostly benign. Approximately 20% of border-line ovarian tumours appear as simple cysts.
Complex cyst	It is a sonological term signifying a cyst with solid and cystic areas, with or without multiloculations. It could be either benign or malignant.
Functional cysts	These are physiological ovarian cysts largely due to an aberration of the normal physiology through abnormal gonadotropin or ovarian hormonal production.
Adnexal mass	An abnormal mass in the adnexa arising from the ovary, tubes, uterus, broad ligament, mesosalpinx, pouch of Douglas, or even bowel. It could be simple, complex cyst, or a completely solid mass.
Follicular cyst	An unruptured or nonatretic follicle greater than 3 cm in diameter.
Ovarian remnant	Ovarian tissue left behind unintentionally following an oophorectomy.
Papillary projection	Any protrusion of solid tissue in the cyst cavity with a height of 3 mm or greater.
Residual ovary	A symptomatic ovarian remnant.
Septation	A band of tissue traversing the cyst cavity, either completely or incompletely. A single, less than 3 mm thick septation is benign.
Tumour markers	Detectable chemicals in higher than normal amounts in body fluids or tissues of patients with specific malignancy.
Unilocular cyst	One cystic compartment, which may have incomplete thin septations, solid-wall irregularities of less than 3 mm in height, or internal echoes.

Table 13.1. Chapter 13. Definitions

Clinical Physiology

The ovaries develop from the germ cells. The ovarian cortex is a single-layered germinal epithelium. At about 13 weeks of gestation, meiosis occurs, and ova are formed.

The volume of a normal ovary in a premenopausal woman is less than 10 mL. The size, shape, and position of the ovary varies from person to person, and the consistency varies according to the stage of the menstrual cycle.

The blood supply of the ovaries is mainly from the ovarian arteries, which arise directly from the abdominal aorta, just below the renal arteries. Ovaries also receive blood supply from a small branch of the uterine artery. The plexus of ovarian veins, which lies mainly in the mesosalpinx, drains to the inferior vena cava on the right and to the left renal vein on the left. The lymphatic drainage is mostly to the periaortic lymph nodes but also to the superficial inguinal nodes in the groin.

Clinical Pathophysiology of an Ovarian Cyst

A dominant follicle, just before ovulation, measures 18–25 mm in diameter. The size varies in the same woman from cycle to cycle and between different women. The process of release of the oocyte from the dominant follicle takes about 10–12 minutes. If the dominant follicle fails to release the oocyte, or if the immature follicles fail to undergo atresia due to a yet poorly understood physiological aberration, then a follicular cyst results.

The cyst lining is made up of granulosa cells, and the theca interna cells lie deeper in the stroma. The granulosa cells, unless they have undergone pressure atrophy, secrete oestrogen, which may cause menstrual irregularity, such as prolonged intermenstrual interval followed by heavy menstrual bleeding; however, the majority of follicular cysts are asymptomatic and undergo spontaneous regression within 4–8 weeks. Occasionally, bleeding from the vascular theca cells fills the follicular cavity with blood, making it a haemorrhagic follicular cyst. A follicular cyst is the most common functional cyst.

A corpus luteum forms from the dominant follicle once the oocyte has been released. New, thin-walled capillaries reach the granulosa cells from the theca cells in 2–4 days after ovulation. Spontaneous bleeding from these thin-walled capillaries fills the space within the corpus luteum (occupied previously by antral fluid). With an enlarging corpus luteum, a corpus luteum cyst is formed with a diameter of 3–10 cm. Blood within the cyst slowly gets absorbed, and the space is occupied by fluid. A corpus luteum of pregnancy is 3–5 cm in diameter and occupies at least half of the ovarian volume. The corpus luteum cyst may continue to secrete progesterone, resulting in either delayed or absent menses.

With continued haemorrhage within the cyst, the pressure may rise, causing it to rupture and cause intraperitoneal bleeding between days 20–26 of the menstrual cycle. There has been reported right-sided predominance in the incidence of haemorrhage and cyst rupture due to a higher intracystic pressure because of the different right-ovarian venous drainage (Tany et al., 1985).

The theca leutin cyst, the least common among the functional ovarian cysts, results from prolonged or excessive ovarian stimulation by hCG or gonadotropins or is due to increased ovarian sensitivity to gonadotropins. They are almost always bilateral and may result in massive ovarian enlargement. They are usually asymptomatic when not too big.

Benign Ovarian Neoplasms

Up to 10% of women undergo surgery for some kind of ovarian neoplasm in their lifetime. An estimated 10% of suspected ovarian neoplasms turn out to be nonovarian in origin. The incidence of malignancy in a symptomatic ovarian mass in the premorbid menopausal age group is 1:500.

The benign ovarian neoplasms can arise from any type of ovarian cells—surface epithelia, germ cells, or stromal cells.

Benign neoplasms arising from surface epithelia (60%):

- Serous cystadenoma: do not transform into high-grade serous carcinoma.
- Mucinous cystadenoma.
- Endometrial cystadenoma—resembles endometrioma.
- Brenner tumour (transitional cell tumour):
    - Arises from the metaplasia of the coelomic epithelia into the transitional cell epithelia.
    - Luteinisation of the stromal cells may produce excessive oestrogen in a postmenopausal women, causing endometrial hyperplasia in 10–16% of women.
- Mixed epithelial tumour.

Benign neoplasms arising from germ cells (40%):

- Cystic teratoma (dermoid cyst, mature teratoma):
    - Arise from a single germ cell after the first meiotic division, which occurs at approximately 13 weeks of gestation.
    - Thus, the origin of ovarian dermoid cyst dates back to fetal life, no matter when it presents clinically.
    - The chromosomal makeup is 46XX. It has mature cells from all three germ layers.
    - The teeth are mainly molar and premolar, but the cyst may also have bone, hair, or fat.
    - Due to excessive fatty content, it usually floats in the peritoneal cavity and lies anterior to the uterus.
    - Due to predominance of one type of tissue, it can give rise to carcinoid or struma ovarri (thyroid).
    - It can be bilateral in 11% of women.
    - In women over 40 years, 2% are malignant, squamous carcinoma being the most common malignancy.

Benign neoplasms arising from stromal cells:

- Fibroma
    - The most common benign solid tumour of the ovaries.
    - Are composed of mature fibroblasts, stromal cells, and collagen fibres.
    - Fluid transudates from the fibroma, causing ascites. The transudation is proportional to the size of the fibroma.
    - The ascetic fluid can reach the pleural spaces through the lymphatics and cause hydrothorax.
    - The combination of fibroma, ascites, and hydrothorax is called Meigs syndrome. It affects postmenopausal age group and can slowly grow up to 30 cm.

- Thecoma
  - It is a solid ovarian neoplasm affecting women under 30 years of age.
  - It secretes oestrogen, which may cause abnormal uterine bleeding, endometrial hyperplasia, or even carcinoma.

- Cystadenofibroma

	Serous cystadenoma	Mucinous cystadenoma	Brenner tumour
Incidence	30%	20–25%	2–3%
Age distribution	Most common in reproductive years	Most common in 30–35 years age group	Most common in 50–70 years age group
Bilaterality	10%	5%	Rare
Loculi	Uni-/multiloculated	Multiloculated	Solid
Papillary projections	May be present	Rare	Absent
Epithelial lining	Columnar/cuboidal	Columnar mucin-producing	Transitional cell epithelium
Content	Thin, clear, yellowish fluid	Thick mucinous fluid	Solid tissue
Size	Variable	Can be very large	Small
Pseudomyxoma peritonei	Not possible	Possible if cyst ruptures	Not possible
Psammoma bodies (calcified circles)	Seen	Not seen	Not seen

Table 13.2. Comparison of benign neoplasms of ovarian origin arising from surface epithelia

History

The history should cover the following areas:

- Risk factors and protective factors for ovarian malignancy
- Abdominal distension of recent onset
- Change in appetite, including increased satiety
- Pelvic or abdominal pain
- Dysuria, urgency, or frequency
- Family history of ovarian, breast, bowel cancer

Symptoms of Benign Ovarian Growths

- Largely asymptomatic and discovered incidentally.
- Pain only occurs in the following cases:
  - Neoplasm undergoes torsion.
  - Cyst ruptures.
  - Infection occurs.
  - Haemorrhage occurs, either in the cyst or intraperitoneally.

When large, it may also cause pressure symptoms.

- Vomiting if torsion occurs.
- Uterine bleeding:
  - Oestrogen-secreting neoplasms such as a follicular cyst, thecoma, or a Brenner tumour can cause abnormal uterine bleeding or endometrial hyperplasia.
- Weight loss and anorexia are suggestive of malignancy.
- Dyspareunia and dysmenorrhoea are suggestive of endometrioma.

Examination

Clinical examination has a sensitivity of 15–51% for the detection of ovarian masses. Its true value is in the assessment of mobility, nodularity, tenderness, and ascites.

An abdominal, vaginal, and rectal examination should be done. Depending on the size of the ovarian mass, the woman's BMI, and the experience of the examiner, an ovarian mass may be palpated vaginally or, if large, abdominally. It may be mobile. A normal ovary is rarely palpable.

Ascites, if present, can be shown by a positive shifting dullness sign. If torsion is present, localised tenderness or guarding may be present. Inguinal lymph nodes should also be palpated.

Differential Diagnosis of Pelvic Mass

- Ovarian
  - Functional cysts
  - Ovarian neoplasms
  - Endometrioma
- Extraovarian
  - Paraovarian cyst
  - Peritoneal inclusion cyst
  - Broad ligament fibroid
- Tubal
  - Tubal pregnancy
  - Hydrosalpinx
  - Paratubal cyst
  - Fimbrial cyst (hydatid of Morgagni)
- Uterine
  - Pedunculated fibroid
  - Large subserous fibroid
- Gastrointestinal
  - Diverticular disease
  - Appendiceal abscess
  - Colorectal tumour

- Renal
  - o Pelvic kidney

Investigations

The aims of investigations are to do the following:

- Find out the nature, size, and site of the mass.
- Exclude malignancy, if a mass is present.
- Exclude torsion, if an adnexal mass and pain are present.
- Exclude any other pelvic pathology.

Ultrasound

A transvaginal ultrasound scan is the primary investigation. An abdominal ultrasound scan may be needed if the woman declines a transvaginal scan or the mass is very large and extends into the abdomen. Pattern recognition by an expert sonologist of sonographic morphologic characteristics with colour Doppler-flow assessment can accurately diagnose most adnexal masses (Levin D et al., 2010). Along with other features, Doppler-flow study and 3-D imaging will aid in the differentiation between benign and malignant neoplasms (Evidence Level III).

- A follicular cyst appears as a simple cyst, but when haemorrhagic, the cyst contains straight, hyperechoic lines almost in a geometrical pattern, mimicking a cobweb.
- A corpus luteal cyst may appear simple or complex, with surrounding vascularity in 30% of cases.
- A serous cystadenoma has 1–2 thin-walled loculi, a thin septum, and homogeneous water echogenicity. Papillary projections, when present, are very small.
- A mucinous cystadenoma has a regular wall, multiple loculi, and fluid of different echogenicities.
- A dermoid cyst has a thick wall and multiple hyperechoic lines and dots with posterior shadowing.

The benign ovarian masses have the following sonological features:

- Size less than 5 cm
- No solid areas or papillary projections less than 7 mm
- Thin-walled cyst
- Unilocular
- If multilocular, thin septations, less than 3 mm
- No ascites, lymphadenopathy, or metastases
- No blood flow

A hydrosalpinx has the following sonological features:

- Tubular, anechoic structure with thickened mucosal folds.
- Nodular projections into the lumen.

- The wall may be thick or thin.
- Presence of internal echoes in the distended lumen without any colour Doppler uptake indicates pyosalpinx.

Ultrasonic Appearance of a Torted Ovarian Cyst

The ultrasonic appearance of a torted ovarian cyst depends on the duration and degree of torsion and the presence of intraovarian mass or haemorrhage. Torsion is more common on the right side, because the sigmoid colon occupies the space in the left lower quadrant of the pelvis. Torsion is more frequent with ovarian dermoid cysts (16%), solid masses, and paraovarian cysts, although a normal ovary may also tort.

Torsion causes different degrees of lymphatic, venous, and arterial obstruction, in that chronological order. This results in oedema and haemorrhagic infarction.

Torsion of an adolescent ovary appears as several round, small cysts up to 25 mm in diameter placed at the periphery of an enlarged oedematous ovary.

Torsion of an ovarian mass shows as a complex mass, with or without pelvic fluid, thickened wall, and cystic haemorrhage, with a detection rate of only 46–74%. A twisted vascular ovarian pedicle can also be seen sonologically.

The diagnosis of torsion of an adnexal mass cannot be made with certainty, even when combined with Doppler assessment. Detection of flow using Doppler does not exclude ovarian torsion, because of different degrees of occlusion of vessels.

CT Scan

This is only needed when malignancy is suspected or any other abdominal organ also needs to be examined.

Tumour Markers

These are only needed when malignancy is suspected. When the ovarian mass is a simple cyst, tumour markers are not needed.

CA 125

This is a surface antigen on a high-molecular-weight glycoprotein that is detected by monoclonal antibodies. It is secreted by epithelial ovarian cancers, endometrial and pancreatic cancers, and in several benign conditions, such as menstruation, endometriosis, fibroids, pregnancy, peritoneal inflammation, heart failure, and chronic liver and kidney disease. It is also present in 1% of healthy women.

In epithelial ovarian cancer, its level is very high and keeps increasing; however, 50% of stage I epithelial cancer will have normal levels (Evidence Level IIA). It has a higher positive predictive value in postmenopausal women.

Other tumour markers:

Lactate dehydrogenase (LDH), alpha-fetoprotein (AFP), and hCG should be checked in women under the age of 40 with a complex ovarian mass. These are markers for germ cell tumours.

Human epididymis protein 4 (HE4) is a new marker but is not yet in clinical practice. It has a higher sensitivity and specificity than CA 125 for the detection of ovarian cancer.

CA 19–9 and carcinoembryonic antigen (CEA) should be done if a bowel tumour is suspected.

Risk of Malignancy Index (RMI)

RMI should be calculated if ovarian malignancy is suspected. There are many models of RMI, but RMI I is the most effective (Evidence Level IB).

RMI = U x M x CA 125

- "U" is the number of points given based on the following ultrasonic features: multilocular, solid areas, ascites, metastasis, bilaterality.
  - 0 points if none of the above features
  - 1 point if only one feature is present
  - 3 points if two or more features are present
- "M" refers to menopausal status. 1 point is given for premenopausal women and 3 points for postmenopausal women.
- CA 125 is the number of IU/mL.

An RMI I score of 200 has a sensitivity of 78% (95% CI 71–85%) and specificity of 87% (95% CI 83–91%) for the detection of ovarian cancers.

Other Investigations

- FBE, UEC, and LFT
- Group and hold
- β-hCG
- Midstream urine for microscopy, culture, and sensitivities (MSU MCS)

Management

An ovarian cyst with RMI score of less than 200 should be treated as follows:

- Asymptomatic simple cysts less than 5 cm in diameter require no intervention except reassurance. They resolve within 3 months (Evidence Level IV).
- Asymptomatic simple cysts between 5 and 7 cm are managed expectantly and should be followed up by yearly ultrasound scans (Evidence Level IV).
- Asymptomatic simple cysts larger than 7 cm should have an ovarian cystectomy (Evidence Level IV).
  - Absolute care should be taken to avoid spillage of cyst fluid into the peritoneal cavity because of the risk of spreading malignancy. A dermoid cyst's fluid is very irritant to the peritoneum, and copious peritoneal lavage should be done until clear fluid is aspirated.
- Cysts that persist or increase in size beyond 5 to 6 cm should be treated by a cystectomy because of the risk of torsion or rupture (Evidence Level IV).

- Cysts up to 7 cm could be treated by laparoscopy. The laparoscopic approach is cost-effective, causes less postoperative pain and febrile morbidity, and allows early discharge (Evidence Level IB). Removal of ovarian an cyst through the umbilical port causes less postoperative pain (Evidence Level I) compared with suprapubic or lateral ports. There is a lot of controversy about cyst size for which a laparotomy should be done in preference to laparoscopy.
- The local recurrence rate of an ovarian dermoid cyst is about 1%.
- Aspiration of cysts has a higher recurrence rate.
- Ovarian masses causing pain need emergency surgery, preferably by laparoscopy, to rule out torsion or rupture.
- A persistent complex cyst or a solid ovarian mass should be removed.
- In postmenopausal women, a bilateral salpingo-oophorectomy should be done instead of an ovarian cystectomy. In cases of suspicious ovarian masses, a full-staging laparotomy should be done instead of a laparoscopy (Evidence Level IV).

Chapter 13.2.   Ovarian Cysts in Pregnancy

The prevalence of ovarian cysts in pregnancy is 25%. It is 4 times higher in the first trimester than at term.

Common Types of Cysts in Pregnancy

i. Functional (most common):
  - times higher in first trimester than at term.
ii. Dermoid cysts:
  - The incidence is 24–40%.
  - Most common complex ovarian mass.
  - Pregnancy does not affect the growth of a dermoid cyst.
  - Complications: torsion, rupture, or dystocia, depending on the size and location.
  - Because dermoid cysts are heavy, they tort more often. There is more room to move in the second trimester when the cyst becomes an abdominal organ and in puerperium when the uterus is involuting. Hence, torsion of an ovarian dermoid cyst is common in these phases of pregnancy.
iii. Ovarian endometrioma:
  - Second most common complex cyst.
iv. Ovarian cancer:
  - Incidence in pregnancy: 0.004–0.04% (Evidence Level III).
  - Second most common gynaecological cancer diagnosed in pregnancy after cervical cancer. Usually of the borderline type or a germ-cell type.
  - Prognosis is relatively good because of early detection and lower stage of the cancer at diagnosis.

Management

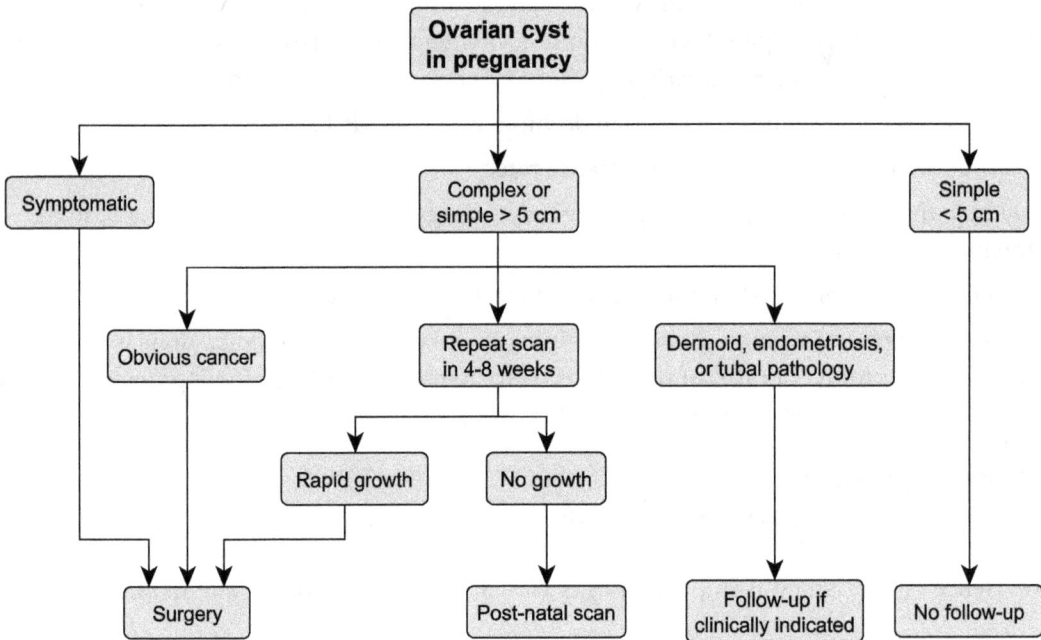

Figure 13.1. Flow chart of ovarian cyst management in pregnancy, developed at King's College Hospital, London

Laparotomy is the better choice if the cyst is very large, complex with suspicious features, or in advanced pregnancy. Emergency laparotomy increases the risks of miscarriage, premature labour, and thromboembolism (Evidence Level III). Laparoscopy can be performed if the cyst is simple, not large, and pregnancy is not advanced (relative).

Risks of laparoscopy in pregnancy are the following:

- Direct trauma to the uterus or fetus.
- Compromise of the uteroplacental perfusion due to increased intra-abdominal pressure.
- Effect of CO_2 pneumoperitoneum on fetal physiology and its teratogenic effect is uncertain.
- Fetal CO poisoning due to exposure of smoke from laser or diathermy.
- Significant increase in low-birth weight infants and delivery before 37 weeks of gestation. This applies to laparotomy as well.

The second trimester is the safest time to operate because of the following:

- Miscarriage rate is 5–6% as opposed to 12% in the first trimester.
- Rate of preterm labour in the second trimester is low. Prophylactic tocolytics are not beneficial.
- Uterus is still relatively small.
- Risk of teratogenicity is low.

For advanced disease, chemotherapy can be used with minimal fetal toxicity.

Short-Answer Questions

Question 1

A 19-year-old girl presents to the emergency department with intermittent lower abdominal pain for 3 days. The pain is now constant and radiates to her back. Her LMP was 10 days ago.

Part a

List your differential diagnoses.

Answer:

- Functional ovarian cyst, complicated by haemorrhage or torsion
- Germ-cell tumour (dermoid cyst) undergoing torsion or rupture
- PID
- Ectopic pregnancy
- Cystitis
- Appendicitis, if the pain is in the right iliac fossa

Part b

What investigations will you order?

Answer:

- FBE, group and hold, hCG.
- MSU.
- Transabdominal, perineal, and transvaginal ultrasound scan of the pelvis.
- Tumour markers, depending on the findings of the ultrasound scan. These may include CA 125, AFP, and/or LDH.
- Laparoscopy.

Question 2

A 28-year-old woman comes to see you with a viable pregnancy at 10 weeks. The ultrasound scan report from today mentions the presence of a left adnexal, complex mass of 6 cm in diameter.

Part a

List your differential diagnoses.

Answer:

- Corpus luteum
- Dermoid cyst
- Endometrioma
- Cystadenoma
- Germ cell tumour (usually stage 1 and low grade)
  - Incidence = 0.004–0.04% (Evidence Level III)

Part b

What further investigations will you carry out?

Answer:

1. Tertiary pelvic ultrasound scan (abdominal and transvaginal). Some adnexal masses have characteristic sonological appearance:
   - Corpus luteum: Complex mass with a surrounding "ring of fire" in 30% of cases. This will disappear in 2–3 weeks.
   - Endometrioma: Homogenous, ground-glass, hypoechoic contents with thick margins.
   - Dermoid cyst: Lines and dots with Rokitansky nodule.
   - Ovarian cancers: Larger than 5 cm; solid and cystic areas with increased low-resistance flow with neovascularisation; thick septa; presence of ascites/omental cakes.
2. MRI
3. Tumour markers, such as CA 125, hCG, α-fetoprotein, and inhibin, are of very limited value, because they are increased in pregnancy anyway.
4. Diagnostic laparoscopy after 14 weeks, if diagnosis is not clear.

Part c

Briefly discuss your management of the cyst and delivery of the baby.

Answer:

- If mild pain or ultrasound scan/MRI suggestive of cancer:
  - Laparoscopy/laparotomy after 14 weeks of gestation (Evidence Level IIA).
- If severe pain, cyst enlarging, or its nature changing:
  - Laparoscopy/laparotomy.
- If no pain or malignant features on ultrasound scan/MRI:
  - Conservative management with repeat imaging in 4 weeks.
  - Most benign cysts (not endometrioma or dermoid) will disappear in 4–6 weeks.
- If no pain or malignant feature on ultrasound scan/MRI and cyst not enlarging:
  - Continue with conservative management, and repeat imaging of the cyst with the morphology scan at 20 weeks and again in the third trimester.
- Delivery of the baby:
  - Ideally attempt a vaginal delivery.
  - Otherwise, caesarean section for obstetric indications. Cystectomy could be done at the time of caesarean section.
  - If the cyst diameter is > 6 cm and is placed low in the pelvis, then consider an elective caesarean because the cyst may obstruct the descent of the fetal head in the birth canal during labour.

Part d

What complications can be produced by this cyst?

Answer:

- Rupture of the cyst, causing intraperitoneal haemorrhage, peritonitis, and premature labour/ miscarriage, depending upon the gestation and thromboembolism (Evidence Level III).
- Torsion of cyst: common in first trimester or postpartum.
- Larger cysts in third trimester may cause fetal malpresentation or obstructed labour.

Question 3

You are about to do a laparoscopic right ovarian cystectomy in a 20-year-old who is 20 weeks pregnant. What precautions will you take to reduce the chances of maternal or fetal damage?

Answer:

I will use the following precautions:

- Woman in dorsal lithotomy position with a slight left lateral tilt to improve venous return.
- No cervical or uterine instrumentation to move the uterus.
- Veress needle pneumoperitoneum will be avoided.
- A Hasan technique may be used to create pneumoperitoneum/entry.
- The sites of ports will be higher than normal. The primary port should be supraumbilical or at Palmer's point. The lateral ports will also be higher and inserted under direct vision.
- If facilities exist, a gasless laparoscopy with mechanical wall lifting should be used to avoid the potential harmful effects of CO_2 pneumoperitoneum on the uteroplacental circulation.
- Keeping intra-abdominal pressure to 12 mm of Hg and reducing the length of the operative time will help in alleviating the risks of maternal hypercapnia and fetal acidosis.

Question 4

Justify this statement: "A transvaginal pelvic ultrasound scan is the single most effective way of evaluating ovarian cysts."

Answer:

Ultrasound scan is widely available and inexpensive. Transvaginal ultrasound scan, when carried out with a multifrequency transducer, has a much higher sensitivity (89%) than either abdominal ultrasound scan or clinical examination (15–51%). This is possible because a transvaginal transducer is able to achieve a much higher resolution and hence much clearer details of the internal structures of an adnexal mass. This enables an accurate calculation of RMI. It can show ascites and omental cake in addition to the ovarian cyst.

A transabdominal ultrasound scan may still be needed if the woman declines a transvaginal ultrasound scan, or the adnexal pathology extends into the abdomen, or you need to look for ascites or metastasis. A transabdominal transducer, on account of its lower frequency, gives a panoramic view with deeper penetration, at the cost of resolution. A transvaginal transducer on the other hand, due to its higher frequency, gives a much higher resolution at the cost of depth of penetration of the ultrasound beam.

Much of the triaging of an adnexal mass can be done on the basis of a transvaginal ultrasound scan.

Colour Doppler is not required for the initial assessment of an ovarian cyst in a postmenopausal woman (Evidence Level IIB). The value of spectral and pulse Doppler in differentiating benign from malignant ovarian cysts is very limited (Evidence Level IIA). The evidence is insufficient for the routine use of three-dimensional ultrasound scans in the investigation of an ovarian cyst.

A transvaginal ultrasound scan has similar sensitivity and specificity as MRI and better sensitivity and specificity than a CT scan, for the diagnosis of an ovarian cyst.

Question 5

A 64-year-old asymptomatic woman is found to have an ovarian cyst.

Part a

List the factors that will influence your management.

Answer:

- Size of the cyst
- Whether simple or complex cyst
- Sonological description of the cyst
- Risk of malignancy index
- Any associated abnormality, such as endometrial thickness and morphology or abnormality of the contralateral ovary
- Family history of breast or ovarian cancer
- Woman's general health and comorbidities

Part b

Justify the role of conservative management in this context.

Answer:

A simple ovarian cyst of less than 5 cm and normal CA 125 has a risk of malignancy of 1% (Evidence Level IIA) and hence can be justifiably managed conservatively. Such cysts resolve within 3 months (Evidence Level IV).

If the cyst resolves or persists unchanged after one year, no further follow-up is required.

A simple ovarian cyst of 5–7 cm is managed expectantly and is followed up with yearly, ultrasound scans, so long it remains asymptomatic (Evidence Level IV).

There is no role of conservative management for simple ovarian cysts larger than 7 cm, nonfunctional complex cysts, or symptomatic cysts.

Part c

Briefly discuss the principles of surgical management in this context.

Answer:

If the RMI is ≥ 200, she should be referred to a gynaecological oncologist for surgical staging. This will be done through a midline laparotomy and will include the following:

- Peritoneal or ascitic aspirate for cytology
- Biopsies from adhesions or abnormal-looking areas
- Total hysterectomy
- Bilateral salpingo-oopherectomy
- Infracolic omenectomy
- Pelvic and para-aortic lymphadenctomy

If the RMI is < 200, she could be managed with a laparoscopic bilateral salpingo-oopherectomy. Cyst aspiration is not recommended as it increases the risk of recurrence.

In the event of an unsuspected ovarian cancer seen either intraoperatively or on histology, a second surgery should be done as soon as possible by a gynaecological oncologist.

Question 6

You suspect an ovarian torsion in a 30-year-old.

Part a

What clinical features will support your diagnosis?

Answer:

Symptoms:

- Severe unilateral lower abdominal pain
- Pain that is intermittent to start with and later may become constant
- Nausea and vomiting in two-thirds of women

Signs:

- Fever if adnexal necrosis
- Presence of extremely tender, unilateral adnexal mass in 90% of women
- Peritonism in the lower abdomen on the affected side

Part b

Evaluate the investigations for ovarian torsion.

Answer:

Adnexal necrosis may cause leucocytosis. The ultrasound changes in a torted ovary depend on the duration and degree of torsion, presence of an intraovarian mass, and haemorrhage. The detection rate of ovarian torsion by ultrasound is 46–74%. The diagnosis of ovarian viability following torsion cannot be made with certainty, even when combined with Doppler assessment.

Detection of flow using Doppler does not exclude ovarian torsion because of different degrees of occlusion of vessels. The ovarian artery, which is last to be occluded, can still have some blood flow if the torsion of the infundibulopelvic ligament is incomplete. Nearly 50% of women with confirmed ovarian torsion will have a normal colour Doppler signal in the ovaries.

A transvaginal ultrasound scan has a higher sensitivity than a transabdominal scan.

CT and MRI scans do not improve sensitivity or specificity over transvaginal ultrasound scan.

Part c

Briefly outline the management of ovarian torsion in this woman.

Answer:

Differential diagnosis:

- Ruptured corpus luteum.
- Adnexal abscess.

Conservative surgery by laparoscopy or laparotomy:

- Early surgery.
- Untwisting of the ovary, followed by cystectomy and ovariopexy.
- Unilateral salpingo-oopherectomy if severe vascular compromise.
- The risk of pulmonary embolism is 2%.
- The ureter may be tented up in the torted infundibulopelvic ligament, and hence the ligament should be clamped with care.

Question 7

Discuss the mechanism of torsion of the ovary.

Answer:

Although an ovary of any size can tort, torsion usually occurs when it is at least 5 cm in diameter. Normal ovaries are known to tort more often in premenarchal girls, possibly because they have a longer ovarian ligament.

An ovarian mass, either physiological or pathological, is the main precipitating factor for torsion.

With torsion, the ovary rotates around both the infundibulopelvic and ovarian ligaments. The fallopian tube invariably undergoes torsion with the ovary.

With ongoing torsion, lymphatics and then veins get obstructed. This results in a cyanotic, oedematous ovary that is quite tender on palpation. With torsion progressing further, the ovarian artery is occluded, which results in ovarian ischaemia and necrosis. This causes fever and leucocytosis. Approximately 10% of women will have contralateral involvement as well.

Question 8

A 28-year-old presents with intermittent lower abdominal pain and gradual weight gain. On abdominal examination, you feel a full-term-pregnancy-sized mass. Her pregnancy test is negative.

Part a

List the clinical features that may indicate that the mass is possibly benign:

Answer:

- History of slow-growing mass.
- Relatively comfortable.
- No history of weight loss, anorexia, constipation, or dyspepsia.
- An absence of shortness of breath will suggest an absence of lung metastases.
- An absence of ascites also makes a benign diagnosis more likely.

Part b

What investigations will you do and why?

Answer:

- FBE—will reflect her general state of health, including anaemia and/or leucocytosis.
- UEC—abnormal renal function may indicate ureteric obstruction.
- LFT—as well as reflecting her general state of health, liver function tests may be deranged with liver metastases.
- Tumour marker (CA 125, AFP, hCG)—will be elevated if epithelial or germ-cell tumours.
    - CA 125 will be elevated with fibroids, pregnancy, or endometriosis.
    - CA 125 is elevated in stage I epithelial neoplasms in only 50% of women.
- Transabdominal and transvaginal ultrasound scan:
    - Size.
    - Side of origin.
    - Bilateral or unilateral involvement.
    - Unilocular or multilocular.
    - Solid or cystic areas.
    - Presence of ascites.
- MRI—if suspicion of malignancy, MRI will show lymphadenopathy if present.

Part c

How will you plan her treatment?

Answer:

Treatment will be surgery.

If the RMI is < 200:

- Treated by a general gynaecologist.
- Midline vertical incision.
- If contralateral ovary is normal, then a salpingo-oophorectomy should be done.
- If the contralateral ovary is absent or diseased, then an ovarian cystectomy is more appropriate.

If the RMI is > 200:

- Treated by a gynaecological oncologist.
- Will require a midline staging laparotomy.

Question 9

A 53-year-old lady presents with a history of pelvic pain and pressure in the pelvis. A transvaginal ultrasound scan has shown an 8-cm multilocular right ovarian cyst and no ascites. List the principles of your management.

Answer:

- A full gynaecological history, including any comorbidities.
- Physical examination, including vital signs, abdominal palpation checking for peritonism, and vaginal examination.
- Order CA 125, and then calculate RMI.
- If RMI < 200, a laparoscopic bilateral salpingo-oophorectomy should be performed.
- If RMI > 200, then refer to a gynaecological oncologist for surgery.
- If peritonism is present, then organise urgent surgery to exclude torsion.

Multiple-Choice Questions

Q1. A 55-year-old complained of abdominal pain. Ultrasound scan showed a 4 cm bilateral ovarian mass with increased vascularity. What is your management?

A. Ultrasound-guided ovarian-cyst aspiration

B. Observe

C Surgery

D. Combined oral contraceptive pill

Answer: C

Q2. Dermoid cysts:

    A. Often have a 46XY chromosomal composition

    B. Are bilateral in 40% of cases

    C. Are the most common ovarian neoplasm in pregnancy

    D. Are malignant in 10% of cases

Answer: C

Q3. A 35-year-old woman has a 3x4-cm right-sided simple ovarian cyst. What is the first line of management?

    A. Laparoscopy

    B. Combined oral contraceptive pill

    C. Observe

    D. CA 125

Answer: C

Q4. What is the most common ovarian neoplasm to undergo torsion?

    A. Mature cystic teratoma

    B. Serous adenoma

    C. Dysgerminoma

    D. Brenner tumour

Answer: A

Q5. What is the most common functional ovarian cyst?

    A. Corpus luteum

    B. Haemorrhagic cyst

    C. Follicular cyst

    D. Theca lutein cyst

Answer: C

Q6. In which of the following will you consider a laparoscopic aspiration of an ovarian simple cyst?

    A. In a 15-year-old

    B. In a 35-year-old

    C. In a 65-year-old

    D. In a 20-year-old at 20 weeks' gestation with a twin pregnancy

Answer: D

Q7. Which of the following patterns of uterine bleeding is **not** consistent with a corpus luteum?

    A. Intermenstrual bleeding

    B. Normal menstrual bleeding

    C. Delayed menstruation

    D. Amenorrhoea

Answer: A

Q8. Why does a corpus luteum commonly rupture between day 20–26 of the menstrual cycle?

A. Increased transudation of fluid within the cyst

B. Increased intracystic pressure due to increased bleeding within the cyst

C. Increased proteolytic activity in the cyst wall

D. Because of increased progestogenic activity during that period, the cyst wall degenerates

Answer: B

Q9. Which of the following should **not** be in the differential diagnosis of severe right-sided acute pain in a 22-year-old female with suspected ruptured corpus luteum?

A. Ectopic pregnancy

B. Ruptured endometrioma

C. Diverticulitis

D. Adnexal torsion

Answer: C

Q10. Which of the following is **not** correct about a dermoid cyst?

A. It arises in fetal life.

B. It arises from a single germ cell.

C. It is 46XX in karyotype.

D. It is bilateral in 25% of cases.

Answer: D

Q11. Which is the most common feature of a dermoid cyst?

A. Asymptomatic

B. Torsion

C. Rupture

D. Malignant transformation

Answer: A

Q12. Which is the most common benign solid neoplasm of the ovary?

A. Thecoma

B. Fibroma

C. Luteoma

D. Brenner tumour

Answer: B

Q13. What percentage of women will have ascites if they have a 7-cm fibroma of the right ovary?

A. 30%

B. 40%

C. 50%

D. 60%

Answer: C

Q14. The most common age of ovarian-cyst torsion is:

A. Midtwenties

B. Midthirties

C. Midforties

D. No common age

Answer: A

Q15. Which of the following statements is **not** correct?

A. The incidence of simple cysts in postmenopausal women is 5–17%.

B. Ovarian cysts 5 cm or less in postmenopausal women are rarely malignant.

C. An estimated 10% of suspected ovarian masses are ultimately found to be nonovarian.

D. The sonographic appearance of a mucinous cystadenoma and a hydrosalpinx are identical.

Answer: D

Q16. The level of which of the following is **not** affected by pregnancy?

A. CA 125

B. β-hCG

C. Inhibin

D. LDH

Answer: D

Q17. Which of the following is secreted by the decidual cells in pregnancy?

A. β-hCG

B. CA 125

C. Inhibin

D. LDH

Answer: B

Q18. When is an ovarian dermoid least likely to tort?

A. 1st trimester of pregnancy

B. 2nd trimester of pregnancy

C. 3rd trimester of pregnancy

D. Puerperium

Answer: C

Q19. Regarding ovarian thecoma (OT), which of the following statements is incorrect?

A. OT are typically benign.

B. OT are characteristically unilateral.

C. OT have a recognised association with endometrial hyperplasia.

D. OT characteristically occur before puberty.

Answer: D

Q20. Which of the following statements is **not** correct regarding the right ovary?

A. Most pregnancies originate from the ovum of the right ovary.

B. Ovarian torsion is more common on the right side.

C. A haemorrhagic cyst is more common in the right ovary.

D. Most haemorrhagic cysts rupture around day 10–14.

Answer: D

Q21. Which of the following has the highest incidence of torsion?

A. Mucinous cystadenoma

B. Mature cystic teratoma

C. Brenner tumour

D. Haemorrhagic cyst

Answer: B

Chapter 14
Benign Diseases of the Vulva

The vulva is the area bounded by the superior border of mons pubis, genitocrural folds laterally, and posteriorly by the anus. Medially, it is bound by the hymenal ring. It contains labia majora and minora, clitoris, vestibule, and perineum. The vulvar area forms 1% of the total body surface area.

Histology

The skin has two layers: superficial epidermis and deeper dermis.

Epidermis: This has 3 types of cells:

- Keratinocytes: These are the cells derived and differentiating from the basal cells that form the stratum corneum layer of the epidermis. These cells synthesise keratin and cornified cell envelopes. Adhesion between the adjacent cells is facilitated by a molecule in the cell wall known as desmosomes.
- Melanocytes: These cells transfer melanin to keratinocytes and are responsible for the skin colour.
- Langerhan's cells: These cells originate from the monocyte-macrophages and constitute nearly 5% of the epidermal cells. These cells are immunocompetent.

Dermis: This has 2 layers of cells:

- The upper layer is rich in capillaries, lymphatics, and nerve endings, and it supplies oxygen and blood to the epidermis.
- The deeper layer is made up of collagen, elastin, and ground substance secreted by fibroblasts. This layer provides support to the skin layers and contains the pain fibres and sweat glands.

Nerve supply: Vulvar innervation is by the anterior labial branches of the ilioinguinal nerve (L1), genitofemoral nerve (L1–2), and branches of the pudendal nerves (S2–4).

History

History-taking for vulvar diseases requires attention to more than issues affecting the vulvar skin. Explore symptoms from other skin areas, and take a thorough medical, drug, and family history (Evidence Level IV).

Encourage the woman to narrate the course of the disease since it started, such as since pregnancy or menopause. Certain diseases follow a specific event, such as atrophic vaginitis, which starts around one year after the ovaries have ceased to function. Recurrent candidiasis may start after a course of antibiotic or from puberty. If the complaint is related to sexual intercourse, the disease process may be due to an organic or psychosexual origin.

Pruritus (itching) is the most common vulvar disease presentation. Burning, stinging, soreness, and vulvodynia fall within the spectrum. It is multifactorial.

Vestibular inflammation may present with dysuria.

Splitting of the vulvar skin is usually seen in the fourchette and perineal area. It results from the intraepidermal oedema secondary to inflammation; splitting exposes the nerve endings and hence is very painful. Candidiasis is the most common cause.

A general obstetric and gynaecological history is taken as usual.

Anxiety and depression can manifest into vulvar complaints and dyspareunia.

The presence of intercurrent diseases should be inquired about. For example, atopic dermatitis may be related to hay fever and asthma. Lichen planus affects the mouth in some women (Evidence Level III).

A detailed history of past medical and surgical treatment to the area should be obtained. Diathermy, cryotherapy, and laser may have unintended consequences.

Examination

The vulvar examination is done in the dorsal position with a good light source at the foot end. The woman may point to the area of maximum discomfort with the end of a swab-stick. Biopsy, if needed, should be taken from this area. Examine the whole skin and mouth (Evidence Level IV).

Investigations

- Thyroid function
- Diabetes mellitus
- STI screen
- Iron studies, looking at ferritin
- Biopsy, if not responding to treatment or cancer is suspected

Management

- Provide rest to the severely inflamed skin, even by hospitalisation.
- Saline soaks for 2–4 times a day for 15 minutes each can relieve skin inflammation.
- Corticosteroid creams, applied twice daily, exert anti-inflammatory and immunosuppressive effects by changing lymphocyte differentiation and inhibition of cytokine production.
- Skin atrophy due to prolonged use of potent corticosteroids is treated by its cessation and use of oral tetracycline and emollients.
- Potent steroids should not be used for more than 4–6 weeks.
- Use of nightly sedation may be required if the pruritus is very severe.
- A biopsy from the point of maximum pain, pruritus, or inflammation may be needed.

Potency of Corticosteroids

Potency depends on the actual chemical, its strength, and the vehicle in which it is administered.

- Most potent
  - Clobetasol propionate 0.05%
  - Betamethasone dipropionate 0.05% (in propylene glycol vehicle)

- Potent
  - Mometasone furoate 0.1%
  - Betamethasone valerate 0.1%
  - Betamethasone dipropionate 0.05%
  - Methyl prednisolone aceponate 0.1%
  - Triamcinolone acetonide 0.1%

- Less potent
  - Betamethasone valerate 0.02%
  - Triamcinolone acetonide 0.02%

- Least potent
  - Hydrocortisone acetate 1%

Chapter 14.1.   Lichen Sclerosus

Lichen sclerosus is a chronic dermatitis that could be seen at any age, in both men and women, and on any skin surface. However, it is most common in postmenopausal women and prepubertal girls, and it is seen predominantly on vulvar skin. It features a thin epithelium, with loss of subcutaneous fat, hyalinisation, and lymphocytic infiltration of the dermis.

Causes

The aetiology of lichen sclerosus is unclear. An autoimmune basis is suggested, especially thyroid disease.

History

- Pruritus
- Vulvar discomfort
- Some women may be asymptomatic

Examination

- Affects labial skin, perineal, and perianal skin
- The skin appears white, parchmentlike, and lichenified, and there may be skin splitting.
- Adhesion of labia

Diagnosis

- By appearance and palpation.
- Occasionally, biopsy may be needed.
- Lichen planus and squamous cell carcinoma may coexist in 1–4% of women.

Management

- Avoid chemical and mechanical insult to the affected skin.
- Prepubertal lichen sclerosus often corrects at puberty.
- Initially, most potent corticosteroid cream, followed by less potent corticosteroid cream for long-term maintenance is used.
- Resolution of symptoms occurs in 54–96% of women.
- Improvement in skin colour and texture happens less commonly.
- In women in whom the above treatment fails, the second-line treatment includes tacrolimus and pimicrolimus topical creams, which act as immunosuppressive agents (Evidence Level III).
- Since squamous cell carcinoma may develop or coexist, regular 6-monthly review is essential.
- The most common cause of the failure of the above treatments is candida infection.
- The disease tends to recur at the same place if excised. Its relapse rate is 84% after 4 years.
- Lichen sclerosus is unaffected by pregnancy. Vaginal delivery is not contraindicated.
- The role of surgery and CO_2 laser vaporisation is limited to adhesiolysis of the labia to restore urinary or sexual function (Evidence Level III).

Prognosis

Lichen sclerosus is an incurable disease, but symptoms can be controlled with proper treatment. Regular surveillance is needed to detect the onset of squamous cell carcinoma.

Chapter 14.2. Lichen Planus

Lichen planus is an uncommon dermatosis that has predilection for vulvovaginal skin and oral mucosa. Usually women between 30–60 years of age are affected.

Causes

The cause is unknown. An autoimmune basis is suspected. It is associated with other autoimmune diseases, such as ulcerative colitis, vitiligo, and alopecia. It is also associated with hepatitis B and C, low iron store, and stress. It may occur as a reaction to some drugs, such as beta-blockers and ACE inhibitors.

History

- Pruritus
- Pain
- Burning sensation
- Dyspareunia and vaginal stenosis
- Discomfort with eating if oral lesions present

Examination

- Patchy erosion on the medial surface of labia minora, which may extend into the vagina.
- Eroded areas are red, moist, well-defined, and vary in size from a pinhead to many centimetres.

Diagnosis

- By appearance and palpation
- Biopsy will confirm the diagnosis

Treatment

- Initially, use a highly potent corticosteroid cream, followed by less potent corticosteroid creams.
- Treat the oral lesion too, if present.
- In chronic resistant cases, use dapsone for many months.
- Six-monthly surveillance is needed because of an association with vulvar carcinoma.

Prognosis

Lichen planus may undergo spontaneous remission. Oral lichen planus may be more resistant to treatment. Vaginal lichen planus may be difficult to treat because the creams do not adhere well to the surface.

Chapter 14.3.   Lichen Simplex

Lichen simplex is a common, chronic, inflammatory condition that often starts in response to some other pruritic condition, such as atopic dermatitis or candidiasis.

Causes

The cause is unknown.

History

- Severe pruritus, especially at night and of long duration.
- Exacerbation by stress and sleep disorders.
- Sexual dysfunction may be present.

Examination

- Inflamed, thickened skin involving labia majora, mons pubis, perineum, and inner thighs.
- Scratch marks.
- Hair may be absent or distorted.
- If moist, skin may look white and macerated, with splitting.

Diagnosis

- By appearance and palpation.
- By excluding other conditions.
- Biopsy, if there has been no improvement with treatment. Unfortunately, correlation between clinical and histological features is not high.

Treatment

- Avoid irritants and use emollients.
- Antihistamines or night sedation.
- Potent or less potent corticosteroid creams.

Chapter 14.4. Psoriasis Vulvitis

Psoriasis is an autoimmune disease that waxes and wanes. It affects nearly 3% of adult women. Approximately 20% of such women will have psoriatic vulvitis. Approximately 25% of women with psoriasis will have an affected family member. Like candidiasis, it may be the first indication of HIV infection.

History

- Asymptomatic
- Pruritus
- Anxiety and depression

Examination

- Usually affects intertriginous (genitofemoral fold) areas
- Vagina not affected
- Discrete, well-defined, red papules with white scales (variable amount)

Differential Diagnosis

- Candidiasis
- Seborrheic dermatitis
- Eczema

Management

- Mild disease: 1% hydrocortisone cream
- Severe disease: fluorinated corticosteroid cream

Chapter 14.5.   Candida Vulvovaginitis

Pathophysiology

The pathogen is *Candida albicans*. Nonalbicans *Candida* species are either not pathological or of uncertain significance.

Candida vulvovaginitis can be transmitted by oral ingestion or perineal contamination.

Women in their reproductive age are most likely to be affected.

Precipitating Factors

- Glycogen in the vaginal cells
    - Forms due to oestrogenic action.
    - Acts as a substrate for *Candida*.
    - The metabolite (which contains alcohol) is an irritant to the sensitive vulvar skin after exiting from the vagina.
    - Usually, the pathogen is found in the vagina and not where pruritus is felt.
    - In long-standing cases, *Candida* may be found in the superficial layer of the vulvar skin.
- Hyperoestrogenic states, such as obesity or women on HRT.
- Diabetes mellitus
    - Hyperglycaemic state predisposes to *Candida* infection.
- Immunosuppressive conditions, such as HIV.
    - Vulvovaginitis may be the first indication of HIV.
- Antibiotic use promotes fungal growth.

History

- Pruritus
- Thick, whitish, curdlike vaginal discharge
- Dyspareunia
- Premenstrual exacerbation of symptoms because of increase in vaginal glycogen

Examination

Examination findings vary from normal to severe inflammation.

- Mild-to-moderate erythema around the vaginal introitus.
- Blisters and ulcers may be present on the vulva.
- Vaginal mucosa usually is not inflamed.
- Curdlike, whitish discharge in the vagina, which does not stick to the vaginal wall.

Diagnosis

Diagnosis is suspected by clinical features and is confirmed by the microbiological test of vaginal discharge, which has a detection rate of 80%. Histology of the affected tissues has a 50% sensitivity.

Management

- Vaginal imidazole cream every night for a week.
- Eliminate predisposing factors as far as possible.
- Nonalbicans *Candida* do not respond to imidazoles.
  - o Local application of boric acid helps in such cases.

Recurrent Vulvovaginal Candidiasis

When the second episode of candidiasis happens within six months of the primary episode, it is labelled as recurrent. Each episode of candidiasis needs to be confirmed by a microbiological examination of a vaginal swab. Management involves:

- Substitute oestrogen-based contraception to depot medroxyprogesterone acetate to create a hypoestrogenic state in the vagina.
- Vaginal imidazole cream, nightly, for a week.
- Prophylaxis:
  - o Nystatin 100,000 units pessary nightly for up to 6 months. It can be used in pregnancy also.
  - o Fluconazole 100 mg orally twice weekly. It is the most effective and least toxic oral antifungal agent.
  - o Ketoconazole, 200 mg, orally, daily for six months. Hepatotoxicity is a side effect.

Chapter 14.6. Vulvodynia

Vulvodynia is defined as vulvar pain of at least 3 months' duration without a clear identifiable cause. The most common age group affected is between 18 and 25 years. The prevalence is 3–7% in the reproductive age group, but it can occur in any age group. This disease is more common in Hispanics.

Pain may be at a localised spot in the vulva or generalised. It may start unprovoked, or provoked by touch or contact. Pain may be intermittent or persistent.

Pathophysiology

The pathophysiology is poorly understood, but other chronic pain conditions, such as painful bladder syndrome, fibromyalgia, and irritable bowel syndrome may predispose to this condition. Pelvic-floor overactivity is common. An increased number of mast cells in the affected vulva suggests an inflammatory origin. Subepithelial and intraepithelial nerve fibres have been detected in affected women. Higher sensitivity to touch in nongenital areas has also been observed. In some women, there is a history of psychiatric disorders and sexual abuse. In some women, use of the COC has been found to be associated with vulvodynia, possibly because the COC increases sensitivity of vestibular mucosa. Vaginal-prolapse repair has been seen to ameliorate the condition.

Diagnosis is by exclusion of other causes of vulvar pain, such as inflammatory, infectious, neoplastic, or neurogenic.

Management

- Good perineal hygiene. Avoid perineal irritants.
- Manage predisposing factors if identified.
- Pharmacotherapy:
  - o Tricyclic antidepressants or gabapentin.
  - o Topical agents have not been found to be useful.
  - o Nerve blocks have been used with varying success.
- Pelvic-floor-muscle training including biofeedback has also been used with varying degree of success.

Remission occurs in 26% to 38% of cases, depending upon the duration of pain.

Chapter 14.7.   Vulvar Intraepithelial Neoplasia

Vulvar intraepithelial neoplasia (VIN) is a premalignant condition of the vulvar skin, characterised by marked loss of maturation of the squamous epithelium, increase in nuclear-cytoplasmic ratio, and mitotic activity. Its natural history is not as well understood as CIN.

Grading

It is based on severity of cell maturation and depth of epithelial involvement.

- VIN I (mild dysplasia): Atypical changes are confined to the lower one-third of the epithelium.
- VIN II (moderate dysplasia): Atypical changes are confined to the lower two-thirds of the epithelium.
- VIN III (severe dysplasia; carcinoma-in-situ): Atypical changes affect the full thickness of the epithelium.

Clinical Pathophysiology

HPV infection is incriminated in some VIN, especially in younger women. The most common HPV types associated with VIN are HPV 16 and HPV 33. Multiple types may be present in the severe lesions.

The incidence of HPV-associated VIN is increasing, possibly because of the following:

- Improved detection measures
- More younger women smoking
- Changing sexual attitudes leading to more HPV infections

Cytological screening of the vulva is not helpful because, the vulvar skin is:

- Thick
- Keratinised
- Does not shed cells readily

As opposed to CIN, a much smaller proportion of HPV infections progress to VIN, and a much smaller proportion of VIN III progress to any invasive cancer, especially in younger women. VIN III may even regress. The premalignant potential to VIN is about 10%. Because some VIN III lesions will progress to invasive cancer, all VIN III must be treated. VIN could also be multifocal.

History

- Asymptomatic
- Itching, soreness, and burning in up to 60% of women

Examination

The lesions are usually seen on:

- Whitish/pigmented patch on the vulva especially
- Labia minora
- Perineum
- Perianal areas and mucosa

Diagnosis

- By clinical features as in symptoms and appearance
- Colposcopy (vulvoscopy): In contrast to the colposcopy of the cervix, colposcopy of the vulva is difficult and different because of the following:
  o Skin surface is larger, uneven, and with folds.
  o There are no characteristic colposcopic changes as in the cervix.

- The colposcope with low magnification and with the use of 3% acetic acid allows identification of the whitish/pigmented area, from which a punch biopsy can be taken.

Differential Diagnosis

The differentials for whitish vulvar lesions are as follows:

- Lichen sclerosus, planus, and simplex
- Squamous hyperplasia (hyperplastic dystrophy without atypia)
- Condylomata
- Vitiligo
- Squamous cell carcinoma

3.4% of VIN lesions progress to invasive cancer, based on the following features:

- Lesions with aneuploid chromosomal pattern
- Older women
- Immunosuppressed women
- Raised lesions with irregular surface pattern

Management

Asymptomatic HPV vulvar infections and VIN I require no treatment. VIN II and VIN III must be treated. The following treatment modalities are available:

- Wide local excision
    - "Skinning vulvectomy," which involved excision of the entire vulvar skin except the clitoris and replacing the area with a split-thickness skin graft is less commonly practiced.
    - Wide local excision of the VIN lesion now suffices. This treatment suits older women with raised lesions.
    - The risks of surgery are infection, scarring, cosmetically unpleasant vulva, and dyspareunia.
- Carbon dioxide laser
    - Laser treatment is done to a depth of 1–3 mm, with deeper depth at hair follicles.
    - Tissue up to upper reticular dermis is destroyed.
    - More than one treatment cycle may be needed.
    - This treatment modality is particularly suited for younger women.
    - Invasive cancer must be excluded before his treatment is commenced.
- Imiquimod
    - It is a topical immunomodulator that has been used to treat VIN in experimental settings.
- Cidofovir:
    - This drug has also shown benefit in the treatment of VIN.

Long-term surveillance is essential.

Prognosis

The recurrence after treatment is as follows:

- 50% if VIN extended to the cut margin
- 17% if VIN did not extend to the cut margin
- 70% after laser ablation

Causes of recurrence are as follows:

- VIN is a multifocal disease.
- The HPV reservoir from the skin is not able to be removed.

Short-Answer Questions

Question 1

How will you manage a nonspecific vulvar pruritus in a 35-year-old?

Answer:

- Avoid synthetic underwear, strong soaps, detergents, and perfumes in the perineal area.
- Twice-daily perineal application of the following creams is particularly helpful for itching:
  o Fluorinated corticosteroids—0.1% triamcinolone acetonide, fluorocinolone acetonide, or betamethasone valerate 1%
- Replenish iron stores.
- It takes 1–2 weeks for the itching to improve.
- Prolonged use will cause corticosteroid-induced vulvar atrophy.
- A biopsy should precede any pharmacological treatment.

Question 2

List the risk factors for vulvar dermatitis.

Answer:

The risk factors for vulvar dermatitis are as follows:

- Dermatitis at other areas in the body (e.g., mouth)
- Relevant family history
- History of atopy (e.g., asthma, eczema, hay fever)
- Iron deficiency
- Hepatitis B or C
- Use of certain drugs (e.g., antibiotics, sulphonylurea, β-blockers, ACE inhibitors)
- Use of perineal irritants (e.g., soaps, perfumes, deodorants, tight and synthetic underwear)
- Dry skin
- Heat and moisture cycle
- Past treatments (e.g., laser cryotherapy and diathermy to the vulvar area)

Question 3

List the differences between lichen scleorsus, planus, and simplex.

Answer:

Features	Lichen sclerosus	Lichen planus	Lichen simplex
Age	Any age, but usually prepubertal or postmenopausal	30–60 years	Any age
Precipitating factors	Autoimmune disease	Autoimmune disease, hepatitis B and C, drug reaction	Atopic condition, use of certain drugs, perfumes, deodorants
Main presenting symptoms	Pruritus and burning	Pain, especially at night	Pruritus, irritation
Examination	• Affects labial, perianal and perineal areas • White, parchment-like skin with/out splitting	• Medial surface of labia minora, which may extend into the vagina • Patchy erosions, which are red, well-defined, and vary in size from a pin-head to many centimetres • May have lesions in mouth or on flexor surfaces	• Labia majora, mons, inner thighs, and perineum • Inflamed, thickened kin with splitting and loss of hair • Scratch marks may be present
Vagina involved	No	Yes	No
Histological features	Hyalinisation and lymphocyte infiltration of deeper layer of dermis	Acanthosis, degeneration of basal cell layer, lymphocytic infiltration of upper dermis	Hyperkeratosis, distorted rete ridges, no distinct features
Treatment	• Perineal hygiene and support • Remove irritants • High potency corticosteroids for 4–6 weeks, followed by low potency for a prolonged period • Biopsy surveillance because of risk of squamous cell carcinoma	• Same as lichen sclerosus • Treat mouth lesions, if present • Use night sedation	• Perineal hygiene and support • Remove irritants • Use emollients and night sedation • Potent or less potent corticosteroid cream
Risk of vulvar cancer	Yes	Yes	No

Table 14.1. Differences between lichen sclerosus, planus, and simplex

Question 4

Compare and contrast CIN with VIN.

Answer:

	CIN	VIN
Natural history	Well understood	Poorly understood
Associated with HPV	Nearly 100%	Only a small percentage of VIN
Screening program	Well established program present	No screening possible
Lesions adjacent to malignancy	90%	25%
Stage III progressing to invasive cancer	36%	3.4%
Interval between Stage III and invasive disease	10-20 years	20-30 years
Spontaneous regression	30% of CIN III 40% of CIN II 60% of CIN I	Up to 40% Regression more common in women under 35 years

Table 14.2. Comparison between CIN and VIN

Question 5

A 62-year-old woman presents with a 5-year history of vulvar itch and soreness.

Part a

What macroscopic features will indicate a diagnosis of lichen sclerosus?

Answer:

The following features will indicate a diagnosis of lichen sclerosus:

- Affected skin appears white, parchmentlike, lichenified, and may have splitting.
- Evidence of scratching.
- Labial and perianal skin are usually affected.
- Skin lateral to the labia majora, vagina, and cervix are not affected.
- In severe cases, skin atrophy, loss of architecture of labia and clitoris, vaginal stenosis.
- Extragenital lesions may be present.

Part b

How will you counsel this woman?

Answer:

The counselling will involve the following:

- That it is an incurable autoimmune disease.

- It is a benign disease, and squamous cell carcinoma may coexist in up to 4% of cases.
- Symptoms can be successfully treated, and the disease requires long-term surveillance.
- The disease responds to better perineal hygiene and pharmacological treatment.
- Role of surgery is limited to adhesiolysis and restoring urinary and sexual functions.

Question 6

List principles of treatment of VIN III.

Answer:

Principles of treatment of VIN III are as follows:

- Address behaviour that promotes HPV infection.
- Advice regarding good perineal hygiene.
- Treatment to relieve symptoms, restore anatomy and function, and prevent progression to invasive disease.
- Wide local excision, especially if the woman is older and the lesion is raised.
- CO_2 laser in younger woman.

Question 7

You are consulting a 65-year-old with vulvar ulceration.

Part a

What questions will you ask on history? Justify these questions.

Answer:

Question	Justification
Severe vulvar pruritus present?	Will indicate vulvar candidiasis, dermatoses, and VIN.
Does she use strong soaps, perfumes, tight synthetic underwear?	Can lead to inflammatory dermatoses (Evidence Level III).
Presence of pain?	Vulvar cancer and VIN are painless.
Is the woman sexually active?	Will indicate the possibility of STI.
Any history of CIN?	CIN may be associated with VIN.
History of any systemic disease?	Will help to identify diseases, such as lichen planus, Behcet's disease, and Crohn's disease.
Drug history, allergy?	Will indicate drug allergic manifestations or contact dermatitis.

Table 14.3. Questions to ask on history for vulvar ulceration

Part b

What signs in the clinical examination will be relevant and why?

Answer:

Features	Why
Site, size, number, and depth of ulcer(s)	Solitary ulcer: syphilis, lymphogranuloma venereum, cancer. Multiple ulcers: Herpes, Behcet's or Crohn's disease.
Tenderness	Herpetic, Behcet's, or Crohn's disease ulcers. Cancerous ulcers are nontender.
Whitish lesion	Lichen sclerosus, planus, and VIN.
Presence of ulcers in the mouth	Lichen planus, systemic disease.
Labial fusion, resorption of clitoral hood	Lichen sclerosus.
Inguinal or supraclavicular lymphadenopathy	Vulvar cancer, chancroid.

Table 14.4. Signs on examination for vulvar ulceration

Part c

What investigations will you do to make a diagnosis?

Answer:

- Swab from the ulcer for bacterial culture and viral PCR
- Colposcopy for VIN
- Biopsy of the ulcer from the edge for vulvar cancer

Multiple-Choice Questions

Q1. The primary group of lymph nodes that drain the vulva is:

A. Deep inguinal
B. Superficial inguinal
C. Deep femoral
D. Obturator

Answer: B

Q2. A 67-year-old presents with a long history of vulvar irritation that has been treated for thrush. Examination shows thickened white areas with labial resorption. What is the most likely diagnosis?

    A. Chronic keratinised *Candida*

    B. Epidermolysis bullae

    C. Lichen sclerosus

    D. Lichen simplex chronicus

Answer: C

Q3. What is the most characteristic histological feature of lichen sclerosus?

    A. Plasma cell infiltration in the dermis

    B. Acanthosis and dermal fibrosis

    C. Thinning and effacement of squamous epithelium

    D. Hyalinisation of upper dermis

Answer: D

Q4. A 60-year-old complains of incessant vulvar itching. Her skin is fragile with defined plaques. No other site is involved. Which of the following could be most correct diagnosis?

    A. Lichen sclerosus

    B. Lichen planus

    C. Lichen simplex

    D. Vulvar psoriasis

Answer: A

Q5. A woman with lichen sclerosus is not responding to clobetasol cream 0.05%, twice daily. What else can you offer her?

    A. Local emollient creams

    B. Local imiquimod cream

    C. Topical tacrolimus

    D. Laser vaporisation

Answer: C (Evidence Level III)

Q6. How will you treat lichen sclerosus in a 45-year-old?

A. Wide local excision

B. Skinning vulvectomy

C. Corticosteroid injection into the lesion

D. Topical corticosteroid

Answer: D

Q7. Which of the following statements regarding Paget's disease of the vulva is incorrect?

    A. It has raised lesions.

    B. It recurs despite free excisional margins.

    C. Coexistent carcinoma is present in approximately 25% of cases.

    D. Immunocytochemistry suggests an eccrine-gland origin of the cells.

Answer: D

Q8. The photobiopic basis for action of the CO_2 laser on tissue is absorption of CO_2 laser energy by:

A. Intracellular water

B. Intracellular proteins

C. Mitochondria

D. Cell wall

Answer: A

Q9. You find a cystic structure at the fourchette in the midline. What is the most likely diagnosis?

A. Sebaceous cyst

B. Skene's gland cyst

C. Gartner's duct cyst

D. Epidermoid cyst

Answer: D

Q10. Vulvar Paget's disease is best treated by:

A. Radiotherapy

B. Simple vulvectomy

C. Topical 5-FU cream

D. Local excision

Answer: D

Q11. The most appropriate treatment for VIN III in a 37-year-old is:

A. Wide local excision

B. Simple vulvectomy

C. Laser ablation

D. Reassessment in 3 months

Answer: A

Q12. Lichen sclerosus is best diagnosed by:

A. Basal-cell antibodies

B. Skin biopsy

C. Parietal-cell antibodies

D. Skin mycology culture

Answer: B

Q13. Which of the following drugs is most potent?

A. Betamethasone dipropionate 0.05% in propylene glycol vehicle

B. Betamethasone dipropionate 0.05%

C. Betamethasone valerate 1%

D. Betamethasone valerate 0.2%

Answer: A

Chapter 15
Malignant Diseases of the Uterus

Chapter 15.1.	Endometrial Cancer

Definitions

Adenocarcinoma	Malignant tumour of glandular epithelium.
Brachytherapy	A type of radiotherapy in which the source of radiation, such as a needle, rod, or tandem, is placed very close to the tumour.
Cancer (Latin: crab)	Refers to a malignant tumour.
Carcinoma	Malignant neoplasm arising from epithelial cells. They are named after the cells of their origin.
Carcinoma-in-situ	Refers to an epithelial neoplasm with malignant features that has not yet invaded through the epithelial basement membrane and hence has no access to routes of metastasis.
Carcinomatosis	The widespread metastasis of a carcinoma.
Carcinosarcoma (mixed Müllerian tumour)	A combination of uterine adenocarcinoma and sarcoma.
Clear cell carcinoma	Aggressive form of uterine adenocarcinoma that is histologically similar to clear cell carcinomas arising from other organs.
Extrafascial hysterectomy (Class I hysterectomy)	Same as simple hysterectomy, it involves removal of the fascia of the cervix and lower half of the uterus, which is rich in lymphatics. Uterus and cervix are also removed.
Grading	An assessment of the degree of aggressiveness of a tumour. It is determined histologically by mitotic activity, nuclear features, and degree of differentiation.
Invasion	The erosion of the basement membrane by tumour cells and thereby gaining access to the routes of metastasis. It is the most important criterion of malignancy and is due to decreased cellular cohesion, abnormal cell motility, and synthesis of proteolytic enzymes.
Malignant tumour	An uncircumscribed, rapidly growing cell mass with altered nuclear features that partially resembles the parent cells and metastasises locally (invasion) or distally.
Metastasis	The spread of malignant cells either locally by direct contact or distally via lymphatics, blood vessels, or peritoneal spread.
Modified radical hysterectomy (Class II hysterectomy)	A surgery involving removal of the uterus and cervix with some adjoining paracervical tissues. The ureter is not dissected below the uterine artery.

Poorly differentiated tumour	Cells of the tumour and the organisation of the tumour's tissue do not resemble the parent tissue.
Radical hysterectomy	A surgery involving removal of the uterus, cervix, upper third of vagina, and some parametrial and paracervical tissue. The ureter is dissected up to the uterovesical junction. When combined with pelvic lymphadenectomy, it is called Class III hysterectomy.
Sarcoma	Malignant neoplasm arising from connective tissues.
Staging	The extent of spread of the tumour. It is determined by clinical examination, imaging, and histological examination of the tumour.
Teletherapy	A type of radiotherapy in which the source of radiation is at a distance from the patient.
Tumour (neoplasm)	A lesion arising due to uncontrolled proliferation of cells that persists even when the initiating stimulus has been removed. It can be benign or malignant.
Well-differentiated tumour	Cells of the tumour and the organisation of the tumour's tissue closely resemble the parent tissue.

Table 15.1. Definitions of terms used in this chapter

Epidemiology

Endometrial cancer is the most common cancer of the female genital tract and is the fourth most common cancer in females.

The incidence of endometrial cancer is rising. This rise is most marked in the 60-year to 79-year age group.

Survival rate from endometrial cancer is also improving. The five-year age-standardised relative survival is 77% (i.e., net survival measure over 5 years representing cancer survival in the absence of other causes of death). The overall survival rate for Stage I disease is 85%, and for stage IV disease, it is 25%.

Risk Factors

Type I Cancers (Grade I and II)

Women with prolonged or higher-dose exposure to oestrogen fall under this category. This type of cancer is more common, with better prognosis than Type II cancer. Risk factors include the following:

- Unopposed oestrogen exposure—relative risk increase (RRI) of 4–8 times
  - Interrupted use does not lower the risk compared with daily use.
- Late menopause, after 52 years—RRI of 2.4
- BMI > 30—RRI of 3
- Nulliparity—RRI of 2
- Diabetes—RRI of 3
- Oestrogen-secreting ovarian tumour

- PCOS
- Tamoxifen therapy—RRI of 2–3
- Lynch syndrome (hereditary nonpolyposis colorectal cancer syndrome), which affects relatively young women < 45 years old

The following are factors that decrease the risk of type I endometrial cancer:

- Regular ovulatory cycles
- Progestin treatment (cyclical or sequential)
- Combined oral contraceptive pill
- Menopause before 49 years of age
- Multiparity
- Normal BMI

Type II Cancers (Grade III)

They are mostly seen in the postmenopausal age group, in women with a background of endometrial atrophy. They are more aggressive than type I endometrial cancers. This group of cancers includes clear cell carcinoma, papillary serous carcinoma, and grade III endometrioid adenocarcinoma.

Clinical Anatomy

Blood Supply to the Uterus

- Uterine artery, a branch of the anterior division of the internal iliac artery
- Tubal artery, a branch of the ovarian artery originating directly from the aorta

Lymphatic Drainage of the Uterus

- Lymphatics along the infundibulopelvic ligament drain to para-aortic nodes. They cover the fundal area.
- Broad-ligament lymphatics drain to pelvic nodes (internal, external, and common iliac nodes). They cover the uterine body.
- Small lymphatics along the round ligament drain to inguinal and femoral nodes.

The following factors affect lymph node metastasis:

- Tumour grade
- Depth of myometrial invasion
- Lymphovascular invasion
- Nonendometrial tumours

Clinical Pathology

Grading

A tumour's grade reflects the aggressiveness of the tumour. The prognosis worsens with advancing grade.

- Grade I: well differentiated
- Grade II: intermediate differentiation
- Grade III: poorly differentiated

Staging

Stage		A	B	C
I	Confined to uterine body	No or less than half thickness myometrial invasion	Half, or more than half, thickness myometrial invasion	—
II	Invades cervical stroma but does not extend beyond the uterus	—	—	—
III	Local/regional spread	Invades uterine serosa or adnexa	Vaginal/parametrial involvement	Lymph node involvement
IV	Rectum or bladder spread, or distant metastasis	Rectum or bladder involved	Distant metastasis, inguinal lymph node involvement	—

Table 15.2. FIGO staging for endometrial cancer (2009)

Classification

An estimated 95% of uterine cancers are adenocarcinomas originating from the endometrium. The WHO classification of endometrial carcinoma (2003) is as follows:

- Adenocarcinoma
- Endometrioid
- Mucinous
- Serous
- Clear cell
- Mixed cell
- Squamous cell
- Transitional
- Small cell
- Papillary serous
- Undifferentiated
- Carcinosarcoma

History

Symptoms of uterine cancer include the following:

- Postmenopausal bleeding
- Abnormal premenopausal bleeding
- Abnormal perimenopausal bleeding
- Delayed menopause

A detailed history should include the following:

- Age
- Parity
- Duration, type, and severity of vaginal bleeding, with or without pain
- Past gynaecological history: age at menarche and menopause, regularity of menstrual cycle
- Comorbidities: diabetes, hypertension, obesity
- Medications: unopposed or high-dose oestrogen, tamoxifen
- Family history: Lynch syndrome

Examination

The examination follows the same principles as those discussed in the "Dysfunctional Uterine Bleeding" and "Postmenopausal Bleeding" chapters.

Investigations

The diagnosis of endometrial carcinoma is made by endometrial biopsy, either by Pipelle or by dilatation and curettage.

Endocervical curettage rules out any cervical extension.

A routine Pap smear of the cervix detects endometrial carcinoma in about 50% of women with the disease.

If the diagnosis is unclear, an endocervical curettage is done, followed by a hysteroscopy and endometrial curettage.

Staging

Staging determines the extent of spread of a tumour, treatment modality, and whether surgery should be done by a general gynaecologist or a gynaecological oncologist. For endometrial cancers, staging is done surgically and pathologically. This involves the following:

- Transvaginal ultrasound scan or MRI to assess depth of myometrial invasion
  - MRI has higher accuracy and specificity for assessing depth of myometrial and cervical invasion compared with ultrasound or CT scans.
- Hysterectomy
- Bilateral salpingo-oophorectomy

- Pelvic and para-aortic lymphadenectomy
- Cytology of peritoneal fluid
- Chest X-ray
- Intravenous pyelogram
- CT scan of abdomen and pelvis
  - The positive predictive value of a CT scan for nodal disease is only 50%.
  - Postoperative monitoring with CT scan does not improve survival.
- Cancer Antigen (CA) 125
  - If elevated before surgery, it indicates stage III (extrauterine) disease and hence indicates the need for lymphadenectomy.
  - It is useful for serous endometrial cancer.

Differential Diagnosis

- Endometrial hyperplasia
- Endometrial polyp
- Degenerating submucous leiomyoma

Management

The management is always determined after a multidisciplinary consultation.

Stage I, Grade I

Extrafascial total abdominal/laparoscopic hysterectomy and bilateral salpingo-oophorectomy. Peritoneal fluid cytology is taken. Postoperative radiotherapy is only done if there is deep myometrial invasion.

Stage I, Grades II and III

In addition to the above, pelvic and para-aortic lymphadenectomy and postoperative radiotherapy for all patients.

Stage II

Modified radical or radical hysterectomy with pelvic lymphadenectomy, followed by postoperative radiotherapy.

Role of Lymphadenectomy

The MRC ASTEC trial (2008) has shown that lymphadenectomy did not improve recurrence-free, disease-free, or overall survival rates (Evidence Level IB). The evidence does not support routine lymphadenectomy in early-stage endometrial cancer.

Role of Radiotherapy

Vault brachytherapy is used to prevent recurrence of cancer in the vault. External beam radiotherapy is used to prevent recurrence in the parametrium and pelvic side walls. The evidence does not support the use of radiotherapy in an unselected population. Radiation as the sole treatment has worse outcomes.

The survival rate is reduced by 20% where primary surgery is not possible.

Role of Progesterone or Tamoxifen Therapy

There is no benefit from either, as the survival rate is not improved.

Oestrogen-Replacement Therapy

Oestrogen-replacement therapy (ERT) is not usually prescribed for up to 2 years after surgery. ERT is not prescribed in a case of endometrial stromal sarcomas, although this practice is not supported by evidence. Ovarian preservation in younger women with treated early stage disease does not improve survival.

Stage III

Surgery as per stage II and radiotherapy, or radiotherapy alone, when surgery is inappropriate.

Stage IV

Chemotherapy followed by radiotherapy.

Early-Stage Papillary Serous Carcinoma

These tumours have metastatic disease even at presentation. Treatment consists of full staging surgery, followed by chemotherapy and radiotherapy.

Recurrent Disease

An estimated 10% of recurrences happen after 5 years of treatment. Pelvic recurrence is treated by radiotherapy, with a 5-year survival rate of 25–50%. Vault recurrence could be treated by pelvic exenteration (complete removal of all organs in the pelvis, leaving the patient with a permanent colostomy and urinary diversion).

Prognosis

- Clinical indicators of prognosis:
    - Age: older age carries a worse prognosis.
    - Race: Caucasians have better prognosis than women of African origin.
    - Associated comorbidities: worse prognosis.

- Pathological indicators of prognosis:
    - Tumour stage and grade: higher stage and grade carries a worse prognosis.
    - Histological type: adenocarcinoma has a good prognosis; papillary serous carcinoma has a worse prognosis.
    - Myometrial invasion: this corresponds with the risk of extrauterine spread
    - Tumour size:
        - ≤ 2 cm — 4% chance of lymph node involvement.
        - > 2 cm — 15% chance of lymph node involvement.
        - Entire endometrial cavity involved — 35% chance of lymph node involvement.
    - Peritoneal fluid cytology: conflicting evidence as a prognostic indicator.

Chapter 15.2.   Uterine Sarcoma

Uterine sarcomas make up less than 5% of uterine cancers.

- Homologous sarcomas: Sarcomas arising from native uterine tissues, such as leiomyosarcoma and angiosarcoma
- Heterologous sarcomas: Sarcomas arising from nonnative uterine tissues, such as chondrosarcoma, osteosarcoma, and liposarcoma
- Carcinosarcoma (mixed malignant Müllerian tumour): When sarcomas are admixed with adenocarcinoma

Risk factors and staging criteria for uterine sarcomas are similar to those for adenocarcinomas. Operative staging is the most important predictor of survival in sarcomas.

Leiomyosarcoma

Uterine leiomyosarcomas make up to 1–2% of uterine cancers. The exact aetiology is unknown, but they are now not thought to arise from a leiomyoma. The incidence increases with increasing age.

A histological diagnosis is made by the presence of the following:

- Number of mitoses in 10 hpf
- Cytological atypia
- Abnormal mitotic figures
- Nuclear pleomorphism

An increase in mitotic count in leiomyomas occurs in pregnancy and combined oral contraceptive use. Vascular invasion and extrauterine disease extension worsens the prognosis.

Symptoms

The cardinal symptoms of a leiomyosarcoma are a rapidly enlarging uterine mass in a postmenopausal/perimenopausal woman with vaginal bleeding and pain. An estimated 85% of women with this disease are diagnosed when the disease is in stage I and II.

Management

This is determined by the multidisciplinary oncology team. It consists of total abdominal hysterectomy, bilateral salpingo-oophorectomy, and staging. An estimated 50% of cases recur within 2 years. Recurrences are mostly outside the pelvis. Adjuvant radiotherapy has not been shown to improve survival rate or disease-free interval.

Carcinosarcoma

It has a much worse prognosis than high-grade endometrial carcinoma. It affects a much older age group, women older than 62 years. Previous pelvic irradiation is a risk factor. The mode of spread is similar to other endometrial carcinomas.

Clinical Features

Postmenopausal bleeding with a large uterus.

Management

The diagnosis is established on histological examination of the uterine curettings, or of the whole uterus. The depth of myometrial invasion and extent of the tumour are primary determinants of prognosis.

Treatment

Total abdominal hysterectomy, bilateral salpingo-oophorectomy, and staging. The 5-year survival rate of 58% has been reported when the tumour is confined to the uterus. The overall survival rate after 2 years for high-stage carcinosarcomas after the use of adjuvant chemotherapy was 82%.

Short-Answer Questions

Question 1

Justify the preoperative investigations in a 50-year-old with endometrial cancer.

Answer:

A. The preoperative investigations help partially in staging the endometrial cancer. Staging determines the extent of spread of the disease, type of surgery, and prognosis after treatment. The following investigations are done:

- FBE, UEC, LFT: These reflect the woman's state of health and ability to cope with anaesthesia and surgery.
- Chest X-ray or CT chest: Will show any lung metastasis.
- Transvaginal ultrasound scan: Shows size, site of tumour, and depth of myometrial invasion. It may also show any cervical spread.
- MRI abdomen and pelvis: The best investigation for showing size and site of tumour, depth of myometrial invasion, cervical extension, and lymph node involvement. If the MRI showed cervical extension, then the following investigations should be done:
  o Colposcopy and cervical biopsy
  o Intravenous pyelogram
  o Sigmoidoscopy
  o Cystoscopy

- CA 125: If elevated (> 35 U/mL), indicates extrauterine spread of the disease.

B. The preoperative investigations also determine who should be performing surgery. If the endometrial cancer is of low risk and limited to the uterus, a general gynaecologist can perform surgery. If, however, the disease is high risk or with extrauterine extension, then a gynaecological oncologist should ideally be performing surgery.

Question 2

List the possible complications of lymphadenectomy.

Answer:

The possible complications of lymphadenectomy are as follows:

- Increased operative time.
- Increased incidence of DVT and postoperative infection.
- Increased incidence of ureteric, nervous, and vascular trauma.
- Increased incidence of pelvic abscess, lymphoedema, and pseudocyst formation.
- May increase complications due to subsequent radiation, such as oedema of lower abdominal wall and leg.
- The MRC ASTEC trial of 2008 showed an increased incidence of ileus, DVT, lymphocyst, and major wound dehiscence in the group of women who were randomised for lymphadenectomy.

Question 3

List the survival rates for different stages of endometrial cancer.

Answer:

Stage	Survival rate (%)
IA	90
IB	85
II	65
III	50
IVA	25
IVB	20

Table 15.3. Survival rates of different stages of endometrial cancer

Question 4

List the incidence of lymph node metastasis with different degrees of myometrial invasion.

Answer:

Myometrial invasion	Pelvic lymph node (%)		Para-aortic lymph node (%)	
	Grade I	Grade III	Grade I	Grade III
Endometrium only	0	0	0	0
Inner third	3	9	1	4
Middle third	0	4	5	0
Outer third	11	34	6	23

Table 15.4. Incidence of lymph node metastasis based on myometrial invasion

Question 5

Justify radiotherapy for endometrial cancer.

Answer:

75% of women with endometrial cancer present with stage I disease and respond well to surgical treatment alone. No trial has compared surgical treatment with radiotherapy alone.

Endometrial adenocarcinomas are radiosensitive (Evidence Level III). For early-stage disease, radiotherapy is only used where the risk of recurrence is estimated to be higher, such as high-grade tumour or higher depth of myometrial invasion. Radiotherapy does reduce the rate of recurrence of the tumour, but it does not improve the rate of survival (Evidence Level IA).

Palliative radiotherapy for stage IV disease treats vaginal bleeding and bony pain.

Question 6

Discuss the complications secondary to radiotherapy for gynaecological malignancies. How will you manage them?

Answer:

The complications from radiotherapy could be early or late.

Early complications: They occur within days to weeks and are due to the necrosis of a large population of cells. The total dose, and to some extent the dose per fraction, determines the severity of complications. Most early complications can be managed medically without interrupting radiotherapy.

Late complications: They occur after months or years and are due to parenchymal-connective-tissue loss and vascular damage. The dose per fraction primarily determines the severity of complications. The Prospective Radiation Therapy in Endometrial Cancer trial (PORTEC) showed a 25% incidence of complications. In half of these women, symptoms resolved after some years.

Complications	Management
Skin erythema at the site. Loss of hair. Skin breakdown due to loss of basal layer of the epidermis.	Non-metal-containing creams and emollients.
Bladder damage due to loss of diploid cells. Radiation cystitis causing dysuria, frequency, and haematuria. Bladder fibrosis.	Analgesia with pyridium. Use of sclerosing solution or fulguration through a cystoscope.
Ureteric stricture is rare and may appear even after 20 years. Seen following radiotherapy for stage I carcinoma cervix.	Urinary diversion.
Bowel damage: Renewing stem cells get depleted within 2–4 days after the start of radiotherapy, causing sigmoiditis, enteritis, manifesting as cramps, bleeding, and diarrhoea. Radiation proctitis: a late complication due to vascular damage and is dose related. Decreased vitamin B12 and bile acid absorption.	Minor cases treated with antispasmodics and low-roughage diet. Severe cases may need bowel resection or a stoma. Bowel stenosis or fistula will require appropriate surgery.
Haemopoietic complications: due to loss of bone marrow stem cells, manifests as pancytopaenia.	Growth factor support. Erythropoietin and/or granulocyte colony stimulating factor.
Vesicovaginal and rectovaginal fistula: due to extensive damage of intervening tissues. Occur 6–24 months after treatment.	Resection of the fistula, exclusion of recurrence of malignancy in the fistulous tract. May need urinary diversion.

Table 15.5. Complications of radiotherapy

Question 7

How will you prevent the side effects of radiotherapy?

Answer:

A balanced diet and optimisation of comorbidities, such as anaemia, vitamin deficiency, and inflammatory bowel disease, will help the woman in better coping with the side effects of radiotherapy.

Radiation, when given in multiple fractions, allows time for normal tissue to regenerate in between the fractions. External beam radiation should be given 2–3 weeks after brachytherapy.

Bowel and bladder should be frequently emptied during treatment. The perineum should be shielded to avoid radiation burns.

Vaginal dilators or early commencement of regular coitus will avoid vaginal stricture.

Constant support by the treating team and family goes a long way in alleviating side effects.

Question 8

You are seeing a 50-year-old who underwent an abdominal hysterectomy for abnormal uterine bleeding. The histology has shown endometrial cancer. How will you give prognostic information to this woman?

Answer:

The prognostic indicators can be found from the following sources:

- Operation report
  - o Whether the uterus and adnexal organs looked normal.
  - o Any palpable lymphadenopathy.
  - o Whether concurrent salpingo-oophorectomy was done.

- Histology report
  - o Type of tumour: adenocarcinoma, sarcoma.
  - o Depth of myometrial invasion, less or more than 50%.
  - o Degree of differentiation.
  - o Whether the cervix is involved.

- Arrange a chest X-ray to check for lung metastasis.
- Arrange an MRI of the abdomen and pelvis to check for lymph node metastasis.
- CA 125

On the basis of the above information, staging and grading of the endometrial cancer can easily be done. The stage and grade will determine the prognosis. For stage I grade I endometrial cancers, the survival rate is 90%. This woman will require no further treatment except regular surveillance for recurrence.

Higher stage cancers and/or grade II or III cancers will require radiotherapy. Adenocarcinomas carry a very good prognosis.

Her prognosis will also depend on her race and comorbidities.

Question 9

How will you manage a 55-year-old woman with abnormal uterine bleeding with atypical endometrial hyperplasia? Justify your answer.

Answer:

By obtaining a history, I will first explore any risk factors for endometrial hyperplasia, such as the following:

- Unopposed or high-dose oestrogen
- Obesity
- Tamoxifen use
- Oestrogen-secreting ovarian neoplasms

I will address any issues identified in the history. Atypical endometrial hyperplasia has a 29% chance of progression to endometrial cancer. In 25–50% of cases, an endometrial carcinoma may coexist. Hence, I will arrange the following investigations, in case there was a coexistent endometrial cancer:

- Chest X-ray—lung metastasis
- MRI abdomen and pelvis—depth of myometrial invasion, cervical involvement, nodal involvement
- CA 125—if > 35 U/mL, there is a higher chance of extrauterine spread

Management:

Because of the higher risk of malignant transformation or of a coexistent endometrial cancer, expectant management is not an option. The woman will have the following options for her treatment:

- Total abdominal or laparoscopic hysterectomy and bilateral salpingo-oophorectomy. This is the best option due to the following:
  - Endometrial pathology is removed.
  - The ovaries, which could be a possible source of oestrogen, are also removed.
  - Removes any occult carcinoma, which is so far undiagnosed.
  - No further follow-up needed if the histology showed only hyperplasia.
  - If histology showed endometrial cancer, it is usually of stage IA, and hence no further adjuvant therapy will be needed.
- Progestogens—high-dose progestogens systemically for 3–6 months or through an intrauterine device.
  - Such treatment requires long-term follow-up because the hyperplasia and/or carcinoma may recur.
  - This treatment is only an option if the woman is unfit to have surgery or does not want it.
- Brachytherapy
  - If the above treatments are not options, then brachytherapy could be an option. It induces endometrial atrophy.
  - It can cause complications associated with radiotherapy.
  - Recurrence of disease may not be easily diagnosed following this treatment.

Question 10

You are operating on a 50-year-old with endometrial cancer. You see intraoperatively that the cancer has spread to the cervix. What will you do?

Answer:

Intraoperatively:

Once I see that the cancer has extended to the cervix, I will treat the woman as having a cervical cancer.

Involve a gynaecological oncologist, if possible.

- Explore the extent of spread of the disease.
- Perform cystoscopy and sigmoidoscopy.
- Perform a radical hysterectomy and bilateral pelvic lymphadenectomy.

Postoperatively:

I will counsel the woman and the family at the earliest opportunity available. I will await the histology report and arrange the case to be discussed in the multidisciplinary oncology meeting.

I will arrange a chest X-ray and MRI of the abdomen and pelvis to detect metastasis. I will also perform FBE and UEC, and anticoagulate.

Question 11

A 42-year-old woman is scheduled for a total abdominal hysterectomy. What are the early and late complications of this surgery? What are the advantages and disadvantages of a subtotal hysterectomy?

Answer:

Early complications:

Complication	Incidence (%)
Bladder/ureteric trauma	0.7
Bowel trauma	0.04
Bleeding necessitating blood transfusion	1.5
Return to theatre	0.6
Pelvic abscess	0.2
Thromboembolism	0.4

Table 15.6. Incidence of complications post total abdominal hysterectomy

The following comorbidities, if present, could alter the incidence of complications:

- Bleeding disorders
- Use of anticoagulation
- Presence of serious cardiorespiratory problems
- Obesity
- Previous abdominal surgery

Late complications:

- Bladder dysfunction—conflicting evidence (Evidence Level III)
- Sexual dysfunction—inconclusive evidence
- Earlier menopause (Evidence Level IIB)
- Vault/cervical prolapse

<u>Advantages and disadvantages of a subtotal hysterectomy</u>:

- Advantages
  - ○ Shorter operative time
  - ○ Quicker recovery
  - ○ Reduced incidence of bleeding and bladder/ureteric trauma (Evidence Level IA)

- Disadvantages
  - ○ Continued cyclical bleeding (Evidence Level IA)
  - ○ Need for ongoing cervical cytological surveillance
  - ○ Incidence of cancer in the cervical stump—0.1%
  - ○ Removal of cervical stump is not always easy

There is no difference in the incidence of urinary, bowel, or sexual dysfunction between total and subtotal hysterectomy (Evidence Level IA).

Question 12

A 40-year-old woman complains of postcoital bleeding. What will you ask in the history? How will you assess this lady?

Answer:

<u>History</u>:

My history will cover the following areas:

- Duration and frequency of symptoms
- Any associated pain
- Bowel, bladder, and sexual dysfunction
- LMP, regular or irregular cycle
- Last cervical smear and its outcome
- Gravida and parity
- Use of any contraception
- Sexual history:
  - ○ Age of first sexual intercourse
  - ○ Number of sexual partners
  - ○ Number of partners' partners
  - ○ History of STI
- Any medical or surgical active problems
- Drug use and allergies

Assessment:

- General examination—vital signs, any lymphadenopathy, dependent oedema
- Abdominal examination
    - Any palpable mass
    - Ascites
    - Renal angle tenderness
- Speculum examination
    - Bleeding or contact bleeding
    - Condition of vaginal walls
    - Any foreign body, e.g., forgotten tampon
    - Appearance of cervix—ulcer, exophytic growth
- Bimanual examination
    - Consistency of cervix
    - Nodularity or induration affecting paracervical area
    - Uterine size
    - Any adnexal mass
- Rectal examination—parametrial infiltration

Investigation:

- Colposcopy and targeted biopsy
- If a cervical cancer is suspected:
    - IVP
    - MRI abdomen and pelvis
    - Chest X-ray

Multiple-Choice Questions

Q1. The lifetime risk of endometrial cancer in the general population is:

A. 3%

B. 6%

C. 9%

D. 12%

Answer: A

Q2. The lifetime risk of developing endometrial cancer in a woman with Lynch syndrome is:

A. 10–20%

B. 20–40%

C. 40–60%

D. 60–80%

Answer: C

Q3. The lifetime risk of developing colon cancer in a woman with Lynch syndrome is:

    A. 10–20%

    B. 20–40%

    C. 40–60%

    D. 60–80%

Answer: C

Q4. Which malignancy is most associated with obesity?

    A. Breast cancer

    B. Ovarian cancer

    C. Cervical cancer

    D. Endometrial cancer

Answer: D

Q5. What percentage of women with stage I endometrial cancer will have lymph node involvement?

    A. 6%

    B. 12%

    C. 18%

    D. 24%

Answer: B

Q6. What percentage of women with stage III endometrial cancer will have lymph node involvement?

    A. 6%

    B. 12%

    C. 18%

    D. 24%

Answer: C

Q7. What percentage of women with endometrial cancer present with stage I disease?

    A. 75%

    B. 60%

    C. 45%

    D. 30%

Answer: A

Q8. What percentage of women present with stage IV endometrial cancer?

    A. 3%

    B. 6%

    C. 9%

    D. 12%

Answer: A

Q9. Which of the following is **not** a common site of endometrial cancer metastasis?

A. Brain

B. Bone

C. Lung

D. Vagina

Answer: A

Q10. Why does papillary serous carcinoma of the endometrium have a worse prognosis compared with the other endometrial cancer?

A. It is diagnosed late.

B. Women with this disease have many comorbidities.

C. It metastasises early.

D. Excess oestrogen leads to thromboembolic complications.

Answer: C

Q11. Which of the following is **not** an important determinant of survival following stage IV-B endometrial cancer?

A. Optimum debulking surgery

B. Residual disease after surgery

C. Age

D. Depth of myometrial invasion at presentation

Answer: D

Q12. A woman with stage I-A, grade I endometrial cancer will need which of the following adjuvant treatments?

A. Chemotherapy

B. Radiotherapy

C. Chemotherapy followed by radiotherapy

D. No treatment

Answer: D

Q13. Which of the following cancers of the uterus has the worst prognosis?

A. Papillary serous carcinoma

B. Endometrioid adenocarcinoma

C. Adenocarcinoma with cervical extension

D. Clear cell carcinoma

Answer: D

Q14. What is the stage of an endometrial carcinoma that involves > 50% of the myometrium with extension into the vagina, negative peritoneal cytology, and no lymph node involvement?

A. IIIa

B. IIIb

C. IIIc

D. IVb

Answer: B

Q15. In a leiomyoma of the uterus, what is the least likely change to occur?

A. Calcification

B. Hyaline degeneration

C. Red degeneration

D. Sarcomatous change

Answer: D

Q16. Tamoxifen use increases the incidence of endometrial cancer by:

A. 2-to 3-fold

B. 3-to 6-fold

C. 6- to 9-fold

D. Does not increase the incidence

Answer: A

Q17. Complex hyperplasia will develop into endometrial cancer in:

A. 19% of patients

B. 29% of patients

C. 39% of patients

D. 49% of patients

Answer: B

Q18. CT scans may miss up to what percentage of nodal disease?

A. 20%

B. 30%

C. 40%

D. 50%

Answer: D

Q19. An estimated 90% of recurrences of adenocarcinoma of the endometrium occur within:

A. 2 years

B. 3 years

C. 4 years

D. 5 years

Answer: D

Q20. What are the most frequent sites of distant metastasis of adenocarcinoma of the endometrium?

A. Vagina, bone, and brain

B. Lung, retroperitoneal nodes, and abdomen

C. Cervix, vagina, and bladder

D. Cervix, iliac crest, and rectum

Answer: B

Q21. A woman's father and paternal grandmother had bowel cancer, and her paternal uncle had bowel and renal cancers. The women herself has been diagnosed with endometrial cancer. Genetic study will show the presence of which of the following gene mutations?

A. C-myc gene mutation

B. BRCA–2 gene mutation

C. HNPCC gene mutation

D. P53 gene mutation

Answer: C

Chapter 16
Malignant Diseases of the Cervix

Chapter 16.1. Cervical Cancer

Incidence

Cervical cancer is the most common cancer in women in developing nations and sixth most common in developed nations.

The incidence of cervical cancer peaks at two age groups: 30 to 40 years and over 80 years of age. The incidence of adenocarcinoma of the cervix has increased in most developing nations in the younger age group.

Risk Factors

- Squamous carcinoma of the cervix
    - HPV infection
    - Early and frequent coitus
    - Multiple sexual partners
    - Immunosuppression
    - Smoking
    - High parity
    - Low socioeconomic status

- Adenocarcinoma of the cervix
    - Oral contraceptive use
    - Lack of cervical cytological screening
    - HPV infection

Pathology

There are 4 types of cervical cancer:

- Squamous cell carcinoma (80–85%)
    - Large cell (keratinising/nonkeratinising)
    - Small cell (< 5%); in younger women, very aggressive
    - Verrucous

- Adenocarcinoma (15–20%)
  - Endocervical type (80%) with mucin production stains positive for carcinoma-embryonic antigen
  - Endometroid: little mucin production
  - Clear cell: identical to ovarian clear cell carcinoma
  - Adenoma malignum: extremely virulent; invades and metastasises early
- Mixed carcinoma: common in pregnant women
- Sarcoma and melanoma: extremely rare

Routes of Metastasis

- Direct spread into cervical stroma and parametrium.
- By lymphatics to parametrial and para-aortic lymph nodes, pelvic side walls, and the obturator fossa.
- Haematogenous spread is rare, occurs late, and metastasises to the lungs, liver, and rarely to bone.

History

Symptoms of cervical cancer may include:

- Abnormal vaginal bleeding or discharge, usually postcoital.
- Intermenstrual bleeding.
- Back pain and loss of weight and appetite.
- Haematuria.
- Urinary incontinence.
- A history of not having regular cervical screening.

Examination

The tumour may appear as an ulcer on the cervix or an exophytic growth with vaginal extension. If the growth is endophytic, the cervix may look normal, and the woman may be asymptomatic.

- General examination
  - Pallor
  - Palpable supraclavicular (Virchow's node) and inguinal lymph nodes
- Chest examination
  - Auscultation of the lungs for any metastasis
- Abdominal examination
  - Ascites
  - Hepatomegaly
  - Enlarged uterus
- Rectal examination
  - May show involvement of rectal mucosa, rectovaginal septum, or parametrial infiltration

Diagnosis

Diagnosis of cervical cancer is made by biopsy of the following:

- The tumour
- The nodularity or induration in the area close to the cervix
- Endocervical curettage or cone biopsy

Staging

Staging is done primarily by the following:

- Clinical pelvic examination
- General physical examination
- Chest X-ray
- Intravenous pyelogram
- CT and MRI of pelvis and abdomen
- Positron Emission Tomography (PET)
  - o   Findings from a PET scan are a better predictor of survival than CT or MRI scan alone.

As opposed to endometrial cancer, staging of the cervical cancer is not based on operative findings. These imaging modalities have poor sensitivity and false negative rates. MRI has better sensitivity than CT, especially in detecting parametrial spread, tumour location, size, and stromal invasion.

FIGO Staging of Cervical Carcinoma

Stage		Pathological findings
I		Carcinoma confined to cervix, irrespective of its extension to uterus.
	IA	Invasive cancer identified only microscopically. All gross lesions are IB carcinomas.
	IA1	Stromal invasion ≤ 3 mm in depth. Stromal invasion ≤ 7 mm in width.
	IA2	Stromal invasion ≥ 3 mm in depth. Stromal invasion ≤ 7 mm in width.
	IB	Clinical lesions confined to cervix or preclinical lesions greater than IA.
	IB1	Clinical lesions ≤ 4 cm.
	IB2	Clinical lesions > 4 cm.
II		Carcinoma extending to outside the cervix but not reaching pelvic walls or lower third of the vagina.
	IIA	No clear parametrial involvement.
	IIB	Clear parametrial involvement.
III		Carcinoma extending to the pelvic wall and/or involving the lower third of the vagina and/or hydronephrosis or nonfunctioning kidney.
	IIIA	Carcinoma extending to the lower third of the vagina with no extension to the pelvic wall.
	IIIB	Carcinoma extending to the pelvic wall and/or hydronephrosis or a nonfunctioning kidney.
IV		Carcinoma extending beyond the true pelvis or clinically involving vaginal or rectal mucosa.
	IVA	Carcinoma extending to adjacent organs.
	IVB	Carcinoma extending to distant organs.

Table 16.1. FIGO staging of cervical carcinoma (1994)

Five-Year Survival Rates of Different Stages

IA	95%
IB	80%
II	64%
III	38%
IV	14%

Table 16.2. Five-year survival rates of different stages of cervical cancer

Prognostic Indicators

- FIGO staging is the most important prognostic indicator.
- Tumour size: prognosis worsens with increasing size.
- Involvement of lymph nodes. Women with positive pelvic or para-aortic lymph nodes have a 35–40% worse survival rate than women who have negative results in these nodes. Factors affecting lymph node involvement are lymphovascular space invasion, increasing tumour size, and depth of stromal invasion.

Stage	Pelvic lymph nodes (%)	Para-aortic lymph nodes (%)
IA1	0	0
IA2	5	< 1
IB	15	2.2
IIA	25	10
IIB	30	20
III	45	30
IVA	55	40

Table 16.3. Lymph node involvement in different stages of cervical cancer, by prevalence

- Histological indicators—the following are indicators of worse prognosis:
  - Evidence of spread ≥ 10 mm beyond cervix.
  - Deep stromal invasion (> 70%).
  - Lymphovascular space invasion.
  - Adenocarcinoma cervix, compared with squamous cell carcinoma.
  - The value of tumour grade as a prognostic indicator for squamous cell carcinoma is disputed.
- Serum squamous cell carcinoma antigen
  - It predicts disease progression and outcome with or without treatment.
  - Elevated levels of this antigen predict a poor survival rate.

Management

The aims of management are as follows:

- To stage the disease
- To treat the primary lesion and metastasis

The management plan is decided following a multidisciplinary consultation. The factors that influence the treatment modality are:

- Age and comorbidities
- Stage of the disease
- Tumour size

Radiotherapy could be used to treat all stages of cervical carcinoma. Surgery is only an option for stage I and IIA disease. Five-year disease-free survival rate is similar for both treatment modalities for stage I and IIA.

- Advantages of surgery:
    - Ovarian conservation possible in premenopausal women.
    - Lymphadenectomy possible, and hence it enables the extent of metastatic disease to be ascertained.
    - Chronic bowel, bladder, and sexual dysfunction, which are common sequelae of radiotherapy, are avoided.
- Disadvantages of surgery:
    - Small bowel obstruction: 5%.
    - Renal tract fistulae, more commonly ureterovaginal fistula: 1%.
    - Intraoperative haemorrhage and visceral trauma.
    - Lymphocyst formation.
    - Chronic bowel and bladder dysfunction are possible due to parasympathetic denervation.

Treatment of Disease by Stage

- IA1 (invasion ≤ 3 mm)
    - Cone biopsy or loop excision with endocervical curettage.
    - If the margin is free of disease, no further treatment is required.
    - If the disease is present at the margin, a total abdominal hysterectomy is done.
    - These women must have a long-term follow-up with clinical examination and vault cytology.
- IA2 (invasion 3–5 mm)
    - Total abdominal hysterectomy and pelvic lymphadenectomy.
- IB-IIA disease
    - Radical hysterectomy and pelvic lymphadenectomy (obturator, external, internal, and common iliac nodes).
    - If the lymph nodes are involved, adjuvant chemoradiation will be needed.
- IIB and above
    - Radical radiotherapy

Recurrent Cervical Cancer

If the initial treatment was surgical, then radiotherapy is carried out. If the initial treatment was radiotherapy, then pelvic exenteration is done.

Cervical Stump Cancer

Because of the shorter length of the cervix and absence of the uterus, brachytherapy is not possible. These cancers are treatment by external radiation.

Cervical Cancer during Pregnancy

It is the most common cancer in pregnancy. The treatment during pregnancy depends upon the following:

- Stage of the disease
- Gestational age at diagnosis of the cancer
- Woman's desire in terms of continuation of the pregnancy

Cervical cancer diagnosed before 20 weeks of gestation:

- Treatment should be given without delay.
- Treatment is radical hysterectomy and pelvic lymphadenectomy for stage IB and IIA. The risk of blood loss is increased.
- For higher-stage disease, teletherapy is given over a period of 4–6 weeks. This will cause spontaneous pregnancy loss, following which brachytherapy is given.
- In the event of the lack of spontaneous pregnancy loss, pregnancy is terminated, either medically or surgically, and then brachytherapy is started.

Cervical cancer diagnosed after 20 weeks of gestation:

- Treatment is delayed until fetal viability.
- The fetus is delivered by a caesarean section, and then appropriate therapy is given for the stage of the disease.

Outcomes of treatment in pregnancy are similar to those in the nonpregnant state.

Early-Stage Cervical Cancer in Women Wishing to Maintain Fertility

Premenopausal women with early-stage disease (stage IA and IB1) with a lesion size ≤ 2 cm and no lymph node metastasis can be treated with either conisation or excision of the entire cervix (radical trachelectomy). Radical trachelectomy can be performed either vaginally or abdominally. Following conisation, if the margin is clear of disease, no further treatment is required. Lymphovascular space invasion within the tumour alone is not a contraindication for trachelectomy. Approximately 33% of women will fall pregnant, and 75% of them will carry the pregnancy to term. Women wishing to receive radiotherapy should undergo ovarian transposition prior to radiotherapy, to move the ovaries away from the field of radiation.

HRT for Severe Menopausal Symptoms in Women Undergoing Treatment for Cervical Cancer

The available evidence shows that hormone replacement therapy (HRT) does not increase the risk of recurrence of cervical cancer or the replication of HPV. Hence, HRT could be prescribed to a woman experiencing severe menopausal symptoms as she undergoes treatment for cervical cancer, provided there are no other contraindications to HRT.

Adenocarcinoma of Cervix

The incidence of adenocarcinoma of the cervix is 15–20%.

It originates from the endocervical glandular epithelium. It is usually endophytic with a normal-looking ectocervix. Occasionally, it can be exophytic.

Adenocarcinoma has skip lesions and hence is treated by hysterectomy. The outcome posttreatment is the same as squamous cell carcinoma, stage for stage.

Short-Answer Questions

Question 1

How can the incidence of cervical cancer be reduced?

Answer:

Cervical cancer is a preventable cancer due to the long latency period of its precancerous stage. Cervical cancer screening has reduced the incidence of cervical cancer by 50%. The incidence could be further reduced by the following:

- HPV testing and liquid-based cytology triage of HPV-positive women. This will further reduce the incidence by 15%.
- In-built tools within the national screening program to encourage noncompliant women to join screening.
- Defined and accessible pathways for managing all abnormal Pap smears, even in remote areas.
- Easy access to accredited colposcopists.
- HPV vaccination of school girls with an effort to further improve the participation rate in the vaccination program.
- Educating adolescents and teenagers about the risks of an early start to their sex lives, promiscuity, and having many partners.
- Giving up smoking.
- Using barrier contraception.

Question 2

A 28-year-old nulliparous woman consults you with cervical cancer. Justify the investigations you will do. What factors will affect the proposed treatment for this woman?

Answer:

The investigations that I will do are listed below with their justifications:

- Preoperative—this set of investigations will determine the woman's state of health and fitness to undergo treatment.
  - FBE: this will show anaemia if present. Surgery will be risky in an anaemic woman, and response to radiotherapy will be poor.
  - UEC: abnormal kidney function may be due to advanced disease.

- o   Group and hold: for giving blood transfusion either preoperatively, intraoperatively or postoperatively.
- o   Chest X-ray: to assess fitness for surgery and staging.

- Staging
  - o   Chest X-ray: as above.
  - o   MRI: for detecting stromal invasion, parametrial spread, tumour size, and location.
  - o   IVP: to detect signs of hydroureter or hydronephrosis.
  - o   PET scan: detects spread of disease and correlates better with survival rate.

Factors affecting proposed treatment are as follows:

- The prognostic indicators as mentioned in the main text.
- The woman's desire for future fertility.
  - o   If the woman has stage IA disease and she is desirous of maintaining her fertility, then she could be easily treated with a radical trachelectomy. An estimated 33% of such women will conceive, and 75% will be able to carry the pregnancy to term.
  - o   For higher stage disease, either oocyte cryopreservation or ovarian transposition could be considered to keep the ovaries away from the field of radiation.
- Presence of severe comorbidities: radical radiotherapy is the preferred option in the presence of severe comorbidities.

Question 3

What role does radiotherapy play in the management of cervical cancer? Or Evaluate the role of radiotherapy in cervical cancer management.

Answer:

The evidence is lacking to support preoperative radiotherapy in the management of cervical cancer. For early-stage disease (IA), radiotherapy is only used when there is metastatic lymph node disease or when the disease extends to within 5 mm of the resected vaginal margin. Still, the survival rate following radiotherapy in early-stage disease does not improve (Evidence Level II).

Radical radiotherapy is used for advanced-stage disease and/or in the presence of serious comorbidities. The dose, duration, and frequency affect the outcome and complications.

Chemoradiation (cisplatin concurrent with radiotherapy) offers improved survival rates for stage IB2-IVA disease (Evidence Level IA). This modality of treatment does increase the complication rate but reduces the risk of death by 30%.

Question 4

Compare and contrast radical surgery with radiotherapy in the treatment of cervical cancer.

Answer:

	Radical surgery	**Radiotherapy**
Indication	For early stage disease	Advanced stage disease
Cost	Cheaper	More expensive
Duration	Shorter	Prolonged
Ovarian preservation	Possible	Not possible, but ovaries could be transposed
Sexual function	Possible	Not possible due to vaginal narrowing and dyspareunia
Early complications	Haemorrhage Visceral trauma Thromboembolism Lymphocyst formation Infection Fistula formation	Nausea and vomiting Diarrhoea Loss of hair
Late complications	Uncommon Small bowel obstruction Bladder dysfunction	Proctitis Cystitis Vaginal stenosis Fistula formation
Presence of comorbidities	Makes surgery and recovery more difficult	Does not affect recovery
Survival rate	85%	85%
Mortality	1%	1%

Table 16.4. Comparison of radical surgery to radiotherapy for the treatment of cervical cancer

Question 5

List the potential long-term complications in a woman undergoing radical hysterectomy and pelvic lymphadenectomy for cervical cancer.

Answer:

- Incidence of small bowel obstruction—5%.
- Incidence of ureterovaginal fistula—1%.
    - The incidence of fistula could be lowered by the following:
        - Use of antibiotics.
        - Prevention of retroperitoneal collection.
        - Avoiding direct handling and devascularisation of the ureter.

- Bladder dysfunction:
  - o Due to disruption of autonomic innervation.
  - o Complete resection of cardinal ligaments delays urinary voiding.
- Sexual dysfunction:
  - o Decreased libido and lubrication, and vaginal shortening causes dyspareunia.
- Lower-leg oedema.

Multiple-Choice Questions

Q1. Which of the following statements is **not** correct in reference to a cervical carcinoma?

A. Pregnancy does not adversely affect the survival rate.

B.. Recurrences after 3 years of treatment have a better prognosis than an earlier recurrence.

C. Pelvic exenteration can have a 5-year survival of 50%.

D. Large increments in radiation dose will increase the cure rate.

Answer: D

Q2. Which of the following is the most common method of spread of cervical cancer?

A. Local spread by direct contact

B. Through lymphatics

C. Through blood vessels

D. Transperitoneal

Answer: A

Q3. The risk of spread of cervical carcinoma to pelvic nodes for stage I disease is:

A. 15%

B. 20%

C. 25%

D. 30%

Answer: A

Q4. Which of the following statements is **not** correct?

A. A normal cervix is resistant to radiation.

B. Radiation complications of the intestine are more frequent within the first 2 years of treatment.

C. Radiation complications of the bladder are more frequent than intestinal complications.

D. Bladder complications of radiation can occur even after 20 years of treatment.

Answer: C

Q5. In a woman who has been treated for cervical cancer, leg pain or unilateral leg oedema is an indicator of:

    A. Lymphoedema

    B. DVT

    C. Recurrence of carcinoma cervix

    D. Anaemia

Answer: C

Q6. The treatment of choice of stage IIIB cervical cancer is:

    A. Chemotherapy.

    B. Radiotherapy.

    C. Extended radical hysterectomy and pelvic lymphadenectomy.

    D. C followed by B.

Answer: B

Q7. The diagnosis of microinvasive carcinoma of the cervix is made by:

    A. Cervical biopsy

    B. Cone biopsy

    C. Large loop excision of the transformation zone (LLETZ)

    D. Cervical smear

Answer: B

Q8. Which of the following will have a better prognosis in a case of cervical cancer?

    A. Older woman

    B. Higher-stage disease

    C. HPV-positive younger woman

    D. Larger tumour size

Answer: C

Q9. Which of the following does **not** affect the prognosis of adenocarcinoma of cervix?

    A. Stage of tumour

    B. Grade of tumour

    C. Depth of invasion

    D. HPV status

Answer: D

Q10. Which of the following does **not** correlate with metastasis to regional lymph nodes in stage I squamous cervical cancer?

    A. Age of the woman

    B. Lesion size

    C. Depth of invasion

    D. Lymphovascular space invasion

Answer: A

Q11. Which group of lymph nodes would be first to be involved in a 50-year-old woman with cervical cancer?

A. Internal iliac

B. External iliac

C. Obturator

D. Paracervical

Answer: D

Q12. For stage IB cervical cancer, which of the following will **not** need to be removed in a 35-year-old with cervical cancer?

A. Uterosacral ligament

B. Pelvic lymph nodes

C. Parametrium

D. Ovaries

Answer: D

Q13. Which of the following is **not** an advantage of surgical treatment of cervical cancer over radiotherapy?

A. Preservation of ovaries

B. Preservation of vaginal function

C. Better survival rate

D. None of the above

Answer: D

Q14. Therapeutic conisation is indicated in:

A. Microinvasive carcinoma of cervix

B. CIN III

C. Abnormal-looking cervix

D. Cervical metaplasia

Answer: A

Q15. A 55-year-old lady presents with postmenopausal bleeding and a 1-cm ulcer on the cervix. What will be your next step?

A. Pap smear

B. Punch biopsy

C. Endocervical curettage

D. Colposcopy and targeted biopsy

Answer: D

Q16. Advantages of surgery over radiotherapy for cervical carcinoma include all of the following except:

    A. Emotional satisfaction

    B. Higher cure rate

    C. Accuracy of surgical staging

    D. Complications more readily corrected

Answer: B

Q17. The incidence of lymph node involvement in microinvasive carcinoma of the cervix is:

    A. 1%

    B. 5%

    C. 10%

    D. 15%

Answer: A

Q18. Intraoperative findings that are indications for abandoning radical hysterectomy for cervical cancer include all of the following except:

    A. Stage IIA disease with a unilateral 3-cm ovarian cyst

    B. Intraperitoneal metastasis

    C. Pelvic side wall disease

    D. Unresectable pelvic lymph node disease

Answer: A

Chapter 17

Malignant Diseases of the Ovary

Chapter 17.1.   Ovarian Cancer

Ovarian cancer is less common than endometrial cancer but more common than cervical cancer. More women die of ovarian cancer than any other gynaecological cancers because of its presentation at an advanced stage.

Definitions

Borderline tumours	Also referred to as tumours of low malignant potential; epithelial ovarian cancers in which the cancerous cells do not invade the stroma
Cytoreductive surgery	The surgery for ovarian cancer in which the gross disease is removed as far as possible
FIGO	International Federation of Gynaecology and Obstetrics
Germ cell tumour	Tumours that contain ectodermal, mesodermal, or endometrial embryonic tissue
Immature teratoma	Malignant dermoid tumour
Interval cytoreduction	Cytoreductive surgery preceded by chemotherapy
Krukenberg tumour	Metastatic solid, bilateral ovarian cancers, the primary tumour being in the gastrointestinal tract or breast
Neoadjuvant chemotherapy	Primary chemotherapy that is followed by cytoreductive surgery
Second-look surgery	A surgery in which extensive biopsy and cytological specimens are taken from the peritoneal cavity when the woman is in remission

Table 17.1. Chapter 17. Definitions

Incidence

The lifetime risk of ovarian cancer is 1: 54. The incidence increases with age, with the maximum incidence in the 50 to 70 year age group. An estimated 80% of women present at the advanced stage of disease. Women with BRCA tumour suppressor gene on chromosome 17q mutation have the disease at an early age. With one first-degree affected relative, the risk of ovarian cancer increases by 1.5 to 5% over and above the lifetime risk. With two first-degree affected relatives, the risk increases to 7% over and above the lifetime risk.

Risk Factors

Factors that increase the risk of ovarian cancer are as follows:

- Frequent ovulation
  - Nulliparity
- Family history of breast or ovarian cancer
- Personal history of breast cancer
- Advancing age
- Industrialised country
- Use of talcum powder in the perineum
- Nonvegetarian diet
- Caucasian race
- Clomiphene use for more than one year

Factors that decrease the risk of ovarian cancer:

- Oral contraceptives: decreases the risk up to 50% after 5 years of use
  The protective effect improves with the duration of use and persists up to 15 years after the pill has been stopped.
- Breastfeeding
- Pregnancies
- Tubal ligation with hysterectomy

Types

A. Epithelial tumours: An estimated 90% of ovarian cancers are epithelial. They may be bilateral and sometimes secrete hormones.

- Serous carcinoma—An estimated 70% originate in the fimbrial end of the fallopian tube and disseminate in the peritoneal cavity with an overexpression of the mutant p53 protein.
- Endometrial carcinoma, 10%.
- Clear cell carcinoma, 10%.
- Mucinous carcinoma, 3%.
- Low-grade serous carcinoma, < 5%.

B. Sex cord stromal tumours: These consist of different proportions of the following:

- Granulosa cell (most common).
- Theca cell.
- Sertoli cell.
- Leydig cell.
- Fibroblast.

C. Germ cell tumour: This is the most common ovarian cancer in the first two decades of life. Overall, germ cell tumours constitute 5% of all ovarian cancers.

- Dysgerminoma: most common germ cell cancer, 10–15% bilateral.
- Immature teratoma: second most common germ cell malignancy, usually unilateral.

D. Embryonic tumours: very rare

- Yolk sac tumour—raised AFP
- Embryonal carcinoma —raised AFP and hCG
- Ovarian choriocarcinoma—secretes hCG
- Polyembryoma—secretes AFP and hCG

E. Gonadoblastoma: consists of a mixture of germ cell and sex cord tumours. It occurs in abnormal ovaries, mostly in the second decade of life. The most common karyotype is 46XY and 45X0/46XY (mosaic).

F. Secondary ovarian cancers: the most common sites of primary cancers are the colon, stomach, breast, and female genital tract. These tumours are bilateral, solid, and contain signet ring cells (Krukenberg tumour).

G. Primary peritoneal carcinoma:

- Highly malignant.
- Arises from peritoneum and mimics epithelial ovarian cancer.
- A woman with bilateral oophorectomy can develop primary peritoneal carcinoma, which will mimic an epithelial cancer.

Aetiology

Environmental factors: There are racial and geographical differences in the prevalence of ovarian cancer. It is more common in Caucasian women in affluent and industrialised countries. The frequency of ovulation (use of oral contraceptive pill) is also an important factor.

Genetic factors: Family history of ovarian cancer increases the relative risk of developing ovarian cancer. Hereditary ovarian cancers form about 20% of all ovarian cancers. The following genes/mutations are involved in the genesis of ovarian cancers:

- Breast cancer (BRCA 1–2) gene was cloned in 1994. It resides on chromosome 17q and acts as a tumour suppressor gene, which is highly expressed in borderline ovarian cancers and high-grade serous cancers (17%). Mutations of BRCA 1 and 2 genes are strongly associated with a higher risk of breast and ovarian cancers. Mutation of BRCA 1 is strongly associated with 5% of ovarian cancers below the age of 40 years.
- The gene for Lynch II syndrome has been identified, and the carriers of this gene are believed to have a seven times higher risk of ovarian cancers.
- Other genes, such as RAD51C and RAD51D, are also known to increase the risk of ovarian cancer, although testing for them is not in clinical practice yet.

Blood supply to the ovaries:

- Mainly through the ovarian artery, a direct branch of the abdominal aorta. It runs in the infundibulopelvic ligament.
- A small branch of the uterine artery.

Venous drainage of the ovaries:

- The left ovary drains through a set of veins known as the pampiniform plexus, which drains into the left renal vein.
- The right ovarian pampiniform plexus drains directly into the inferior vena cava.

Nerve supply: the nerve supply comes from the ovarian and uterovaginal plexus of nerves.

Lymphatic drainage: The lymphatics from the ovary run into the infundibulopelvic, ovarian, and round ligaments and drain into the para-aortic, paracaval, obturator, iliac, and inguinal lymph nodes.

Routes of metastasis:

- Transcoelemic to viscera and peritoneal surfaces
- Lymphatic spread to para-aortic nodes, up to renal vessels, iliac, obturator, and inguinal lymph nodes
- Direct spread to the uterus, tubes, and sigmoid colon
- Haematogenous spread to liver, lung, and brain

History

Symptoms of ovarian cancer are nonspecific and hence lead to delayed presentation.

- Pressure symptoms: urinary frequency, constipation, pelvic pain, dyspareunia
- Advanced-stage disease: bloating, constipation, early satiety, loss of appetite, increased abdominal girth
- Abnormal vaginal bleeding

Examination

- General: vital signs, pallor
- Lymph nodes: supraclavicular, axillary, and inguinal
- Breast
- Chest for pleural effusion
- Abdomen: liver, spleen, mass (ovarian, omental cake), ascites
- Vagina: vagina/cervix, Pap smear (occasionally ovarian cancer cells may be seen), palpable adnexal mass, uterine size
- Rectal: pelvic mass

Investigations

Investigations aimed at:

- Establishing a diagnosis of ovarian cancer
- Determining the extent of surgery
- Determining the fitness to undergo surgery

Investigations include:

- Ultrasound scans of the pelvis, kidneys, and liver.
    - o   Advanced ovarian cancer can cause hydronephrosis.
    - o   Liver metastases suggest a nonovarian primary.
    - o   Ultrasound features of a malignant ovary are as follows:
        - ▪   Size greater than 10 cm
        - ▪   Irregular solid or multilocular
        - ▪   Prominent blood flow on colour Doppler
        - ▪   Ascites
- Chest X-ray for effusion and metastasis.
- CA 125, CEA (to identify a GIT primary).
- AFP, β-hCG in women under 40 years to exclude germ cell and embryonal tumours.
- FBE, UEC, and LFT to assess general health and any renal or hepatic compromise.
- CT scan/MRI of abdomen and pelvis:
    - o   To show extent of disease.
    - o   To assist in surgical planning.
    - o   Will show lymphadenopathy.
- Colonoscopy or barium enema to exclude gastrointestinal pathology.
- RMI: sensitivity of 78% and specificity of 87% for the prediction of ovarian malignancy, when RMI is > 200 (Evidence Level IA).

Diagnosis

Diagnosis of ovarian cancer can be made by the following:

- Histology of ovarian tissue removed at surgery.
- Frozen section is known for its underdiagnosis in many women and hence can't be relied on. If it shows a definitive diagnosis of malignancy, that may be valuable information.
- Demonstrating ovarian cancer cells found in cytology of an ascitic tap.

Staging

Staging determines

- extraperitoneal spread,
- prognosis, and
- the need for adjuvant treatment.

The investigations listed above indicate the extent of extraperitoneal spread. Staging is determined by the surgical findings. A staging laparotomy is done by the following:

- A midline vertical incision extending above the umbilicus
- Arranging cytological examination of ascitic fluid

- Doing a total abdominal hysterectomy and bilateral salpingo-oophorectomy (TAHBSO)
- Omentectomy
- Biopsy of suspicious-looking areas in the peritoneal cavity
- Assessment and resection of para-aortic and pelvic lymph nodes
- Assessment of upper abdominal viscera and surfaces

Staging according to FIGO (2013)

- Stage I: tumour confined to ovaries/tubes
- Stage II: tumour has pelvic extension below pelvic brim
- Stage III: Stage II + extension to pelvic and abdominal peritoneum and/or metastasis to retroperitoneal lymph nodes
- Stage IV: stage III + distant metastasis to liver/spleen and extra abdominal organs and lymph nodes

Stage I–III are further divided into A, B, and C categories. Stage IV is divided into A and B.

Prognostic Indicators

- FIGO staging
- Histological type, grade, and ploidy
- Size of the tumour
- Residual disease after surgery
- Intraperitoneal rupture/spill of the tumour
- Presence of ascites
- Age and performance status of the woman

Management

The emphasis in early-stage epithelial cancer is to identify occult metastases by meticulous exploration, whereas in advanced-stage epithelial cancer, it is tumour reduction. The surgical procedure has been described in the Staging section above. The tumour should be removed as completely as possible (cytoreduction). If not, residual disease of < 1 cm should be achieved. Optimal cytoreduction may be difficult in the liver, porta hepatis, and root of the small bowel mesentery.

After neoadjuvant chemotherapy, both primary surgery and interval debulking surgery have similar survival outcomes. The latter has been shown to have less morbidity.

Women with low-grade stage IA and IB disease do not need adjuvant chemotherapy unless the women have significant risk factors. All women with advanced-stage disease require chemotherapy. Combination chemotherapy with carboplatin and paclitaxel has a better survival rate than monotherapy. The role of intraperitoneal chemotherapy is not yet clear.

Women with recurrent or persistent disease after primary treatment have a lower survival rate. Women with a disease-free interval of 6 months, no ascites, and local recurrence will benefit from secondary cytoreductive surgery.

Some women with recurrent disease will develop small-bowel obstruction or, less commonly, large-bowel obstruction. There could be multiple sites of obstruction, and so such women will benefit from stoma formation. The median survival of such women is about 3–12 months.

The treatment of germ cell tumours involves surgical staging, excision of the primary tumour, and then three or more cycles of combination chemotherapy. Most such women have normal survival afterward.

The treatment of sex cord tumours in younger women involves excision of the ovary and endometrial biopsy to exclude endometrial adenocarcinoma. In older women, complete surgical staging should be done. Later recurrence of these tumours is very common.

Fertility-sparing surgery: Younger women who would like to maintain fertility should have surgical staging, but the uterus and contralateral ovary, if looking normal, should be preserved. The decision regarding chemotherapy should be made in consultation with the woman and the oncological multidisciplinary team. Women with stage IA dysgerminoma and stage I grade I immature teratoma do not require any further treatment. Sex cord tumours in younger women could also be similarly managed. Sex cord tumours, because of their oestrogen production, can cause endometrial hyperplasia (40%) and adenocarcinoma. Hence, a simultaneous endometrial biopsy is always advised.

Younger women with borderline ovarian tumours could be treated by unilateral oophorectomy. They could have TAHBSO after childbearing is completed. The recurrence rate of these tumours after surgery is 7%.

Chapter 17.2.   Borderline Malignant Ovarian Tumours

These are also referred to as tumours of low malignant potential. These are epithelial tumours with cellular characteristics of malignancy without stromal invasion. They form 10–15% of all the epithelial tumours. They are common in premenopausal women, are asymptomatic, slow-growing, and can be very large. They are mostly of serous and mucinous types. Borderline mucinous ovarian tumours are usually at least 10 cm in diameter with more than 10 loculi (Fruscella E et al., 2005). CA 125 does not rise in borderline malignant tumours. They are managed by laparotomy and surgical staging. Prognosis is very good. Late recurrence does occur, and hence long-term follow-up is justified. Borderline mucinous tumours can lead to pseudomyxoma peritonei.

Short-Answer Questions

Question 1

Why is total abdominal hysterectomy and bilateral salpingo-oophorectomy a part of surgical staging of ovarian cancer?

Answer:

Total abdominal hysterectomy and bilateral salpingo-oophorectomy is part of surgical staging because of the following:

- There is a high incidence of tumour in the contralateral ovary and metastasis in the uterus.
- There may be a coincidental primary endometrial cancer, especially if the ovarian cancer is of endometrioid type.
- There may be a coincidental endometrial adenocarcinoma in the presence of a sex cord tumour.

Question 2

A 44-year-old complains of pelvic pain, bloating, and urinary frequency. Clinical examination shows an adnexal mass. A transvaginal ultrasound scan shows a 10-cm complex left adnexal mass. An MRI of the abdomen and pelvis confirms the finding. There is no lymphadenopathy. CA 125 is 160 U/mL. The woman does not have a history of cancer in the family.

Part a

How will you ascertain that this mass is malignant?

Answer:

- Focused history.
- Thorough gynaecological examination.
- Ultrasound features of malignant ovary:
  - Multiple thick septae.
  - 4 papillary projections.
  - Solid areas > 7 mm.
  - Size ≥ 10 cm.
  - Presence of ascites (PPV 95% for malignancy; however, the incidence of ascites in early-stage disease is 20%).
- Increased CA 125: could be increased due to benign reasons as well.
- Calculate RMI = U x M x CA 125:
  - "U" is the number of points given based on the following ultrasonic features: multilocular, solid areas, ascites, metastasis, bilaterality.
    - 0 points if none of the above features is present.
    - 1 point if only one feature is present.
    - 3 points if two or more features are present.

- ○ "M" refers to menopausal status. 1 point is given for premenopausal women and 3 points for postmenopausal women.
- ○ CA 125 is the number of IU/mL.
- ○ An RMI I score of 200 has a sensitivity of 78% (95% confidence interval 71–85%) and specificity of 87% (95% CI 83–91%) for the detection of ovarian cancers.

Part b

Briefly discuss the role of laparoscopic staging in ovarian cancer.

Answer:

An optimal staging of ovarian cancer includes the following:

- Inspection and palpation of all peritoneal surfaces
- Peritoneal washings
- TAHBSO
- Omentectomy
- Biopsies from any suspicious lesions
- Biopsies of pelvic and para-aortic lymph nodes

These things will not be possible laparoscopically by even the most experienced gynaecological oncologist. The rate of optimal surgical staging by laparotomy is 97%, if performed by a gynaecological oncologist.

Part c

What is the treatment for an apparent early-stage ovarian cancer?

Answer:

A midline laparotomy and full surgical staging, as described above.

Part d

What will you do if you find ovarian cancer unexpectedly during a laparotomy?

Answer:

- Request a gynaecological oncologist to take over the procedure.
- If a gynaecological oncologist is not available to come, then take advice.
- Take biopsies for confirmation of the diagnosis.
- Manage the acute situation, e.g., bowel obstruction.
- Perform minimal additional surgery.
- Refer to a gynaecological oncologist postoperatively.

Question 3

A 30-year-old lady is having a laparotomy for an ovarian mass. You suspect ovarian malignancy intra-operatively and so collect peritoneal fluid for cytological examination, inspect and palpate the mass, take a frozen section, and biopsy the other ovary.

She undergoes a unilateral salpingo-oopherectomy. The histology shows borderline ovarian carcinoma. How will you follow her up?

Answer:

- If childbearing is desired, offer TAHBSO when childbearing has been completed.
- Follow up with 6-monthly clinical examination, looking for signs such as hepatomegaly, abdominal mass, ascites, lung secondaries, and any abnormal pelvic mass.
- Transvaginal ultrasound scan for any abnormal pelvic mass every 6 months.
- Vault smear once a year.
- Although CA 125 does not rise in borderline carcinomas, it may rise if there is progression to frank epithelial cancer. This will be done every 6 months.
- Total follow-up for 5 years.

Question 4

Discuss the constraints in ovarian cancer screening.

Answer:

The screening modalities for ovarian cancers are insensitive, have poor predictive value, and are not cost-effective. Ovarian cancers also do not have a premalignant stage, like cervical cancers. The available modalities are discussed below:

<u>Family history</u>: The incidence of ovarian cancer in the general population is 1.8%. With one first-degree affected relative, this incidence increases to 5%, and with two first-degree affected relatives, it goes up to 7%. An estimated 90% of women with ovarian cancer do not have an affected family member.

<u>Clinical pelvic examination</u>: The anatomical position of the ovaries within the pelvis makes them relatively inaccessible to a bimanual clinical examination. Bimanual pelvic examination has a low sensitivity and specificity. It is also operator-dependent.

<u>Genetic testing</u>: Mutations of BRCA 1 and 2 and Lynch II genes increase the incidence of ovarian cancer in the family members. Some other gene mutations, such as RAD51C and RAD51D, are still not used in clinical practice. BRCA 1 and 2 gene mutations have a 40% and 20% lifetime risk of ovarian cancer in carriers, respectively. Carriers of Lynch 2 gene mutation have a 7 times higher lifetime risk of ovarian cancer. Testing for these genes is only done when there are one or two affected family members with either breast or ovarian cancers. Prophylactic interventions are limited to oophorectomy.

<u>Transvaginal ultrasound scan</u>: It has poor specificity; however, this has improved with the use of colour Doppler. It identifies features within the ovary that are believed to represent malignancy.

<u>Serum CA 125</u>: It is nonspecific and cannot be recommended for the entire population. CA 125 is raised in only 50% of early-stage epithelial cancers and not raised in nonepithelial cancers. It is also raised in

many benign conditions and endometrial cancer.

If used separately, none of the modalities listed above reach the required sensitivity and specificity for a screening test. Sequential multimodal screening with CA 125, followed by transvaginal ultrasound scan if CA 125 is raised, will have a higher positive predictive value (Evidence Level IB).

Question 5

Compare the screening of cervical and ovarian cancers.

Answer:

Screening for cervical cancer: The anatomical position of the cervix makes it easily accessible. Cervical cancer has a long precancerous stage. Because of these reasons, cervical cancer screening has been successful in reducing cervical cancer incidence by 32% and mortality by 60% over the past 30 years. Due to these reductions, cost-effectiveness of cervical cancer screening is well established.

Screening for ovarian cancer: In contrast to the cervix, the ovary is neither clinically easily accessible nor does it have a precancerous stage. The modalities used for ovarian cancer screening, such as CA 125, ultrasound scan, and bimanual pelvic examination, have low specificity. An estimated 90% of women with ovarian cancer do not have a family history of the disease. These limitations have prevented an effective screening program for ovarian cancer.

Question 6

Discuss the role of prophylactic bilateral salpingo-oophorectomy (PBSO) in women who are positive for BRCA 1 and 2 gene mutations.

Answer:

Women with BRCA 1 and 2 mutations have a 40% and nearly 20% lifetime risk, respectively, of developing ovarian cancer. In women who are positive for these mutations, PBSO decreases the risk of ovarian cancer to almost zero (Evidence Level IIA). It also decreases the risk of breast cancer by 50% in these women. The risk of primary peritoneal cancer remains unaffected. Removing the fallopian tubes eliminates the risk of fallopian tube cancer in the future. The ideal age for performing PBSO is after childbearing has been completed. PBSO could be done either by a laparoscopy or by laparotomy. Women with these mutations who are also on tamoxifen for breast cancer should undergo a hysterectomy as well, because of the small risk of endometrial cancer.

Question 7

What is the benefit of early detection of ovarian cancer.

Answer:

At present, early screening methods for ovarian cancers are ineffective. However, ovarian cancer, when diagnosed early, has an overall 5-year survival rate of 80%. Currently, the overall 5-year survival rate of ovarian cancer is 23%, because 80% of women with ovarian cancer present at an advanced stage.

Question 8

Briefly discuss the new treatments for ovarian cancer.

Answer:

Immunotherapy: It targets those proteins that stimulate malignant change in the cells. When combined with chemotherapy, it improves the survival rate of advanced-stage ovarian cancer.

Gene therapy: It is being used in research settings to supplement chemotherapy.

Viral therapy: It is also getting popular.

Question 9

A 31-year-old woman with one previous full-term caesarean section complains of a pelvic mass equivalent to a 14-week-sized pregnancy.

Part a

Discuss the clinical features of this woman and their significance.

Answer:

History:

- Symptoms:
    o Duration of symptoms
    o Urinary frequency
    o Constipation
    o Pelvic pain
    o Dyspareunia
    o Bloating
    o Increase in abdominal girth
- Significance: these are nonspecific symptoms and may suggest a pregnancy, pelvic mass, or an ovarian cancer.
- LMP: a recent LMP will suggest that the woman is not pregnant.
- Family history of breast or ovarian cancer: with a positive family history, this lady will also have a higher chance of an ovarian cancer.

Examination:

- Vital signs: indicate general state of health.
- Fever: indicates infection, pelvic abscess, or adnexal necrosis due to torsion.
- Lymphadenopathy: indicates metastasis secondary to a cancer, possibly originating from the pelvis.
- Chest: a pleural effusion may indicate lung metastasis.
- Abdomen:
    o Tenderness may indicate torsion, abscess, or red degeneration of a fibroid.
    o Palpable mass: hepatosplenomegaly, omental cake, may suggest ovarian cancer.

- o Ascites: indicates ovarian cancer, chronic liver disease, peritoneal metastasis from any intraperitoneal neoplasm.
- o Mobility, regularity, consistency of the 14-week-sized mass: differentiates between pregnancy, fibroid, pelvic endometrioma, ovarian neoplasm.
- Rectal examination: palpable mass will suggest a pelvic neoplasm.

Part b

An ultrasound scan shows features of left ovarian cancer. Justify your investigations.

Answer:

- FBE, UEC, LFT, coagulation studies—indicate the general state of health and suitability for surgery.
- Group and hold—in case the woman needs a blood transfusion preoperatively, intra-operatively, or postoperatively.
- CA 125, AFP, hCG, LDH—can be used to track progress.
- CEA—raised CEA may indicate a gastrointestinal malignancy.
- Abdominal ultrasound scan—may show ascites, liver and kidney metastasis, or hydronephrosis.
- Chest X-ray (erect PA view)—for pleural effusion, lung metastasis.
- MRI abdomen and pelvis—looking for lymphadenopathy and omental caking, which will assist in surgical planning.

Part c

Investigations suggests early-stage dysgerminoma of the left ovary. How will you manage this woman?

Answer:

- Referral to a gynaecological oncologist.
- Counselling.
- Left salpingo-oophorectomy.
- With accurate staging, if the disease is of stage IA, there is no need for adjuvant chemotherapy. However, she will require regular follow-up.
- Recurrence rate of early-stage dysgerminoma: 15–20%
- Overall 5-year survival rate: 90%

Question 10

A 34-year-old nulliparous woman's grandmother and mother had ovarian cancer, and her sister has breast cancer. What are her management options?

Answer:

- She is at a high risk of developing breast and ovarian cancer.
- BRCA 1 and 2 mutation seem very likely.
- Arrange psychological and genetic counselling for her and her family members. Advise genetic testing (BRCA 1 and 2) for all consenting family members, including her.
- Advise that in the presence of BRCA 1 and 2 mutations, the lifetime risk of breast cancer increases tenfold.
- If the woman's test for BRCA 1 and 2 is negative, her lifetime risk of ovarian cancer is 7% and of breast cancer is 8%. There is variable penetrance of mutated genes.
- If she refuses genetic testing, or is positive for BRCA 1 and 2 mutations:
  - Breast self-examination every month and by her doctor every 6 months.
  - Mammograms every year.
  - Yearly transvaginal ultrasound scan and CA 125.
  - She should be advised that these interventions do not reduce her mortality from ovarian cancer.
  - Combined oral contraceptive pill reduces ovarian cancer by 50%.
  - Tamoxifen will reduce breast cancer, but its risk-benefit ratio is not yet established.
  - Offer bilateral mastectomy with reconstruction. Prophylactic mastectomy reduces breast cancer incidence by 1–19%.
  - Offer prophylactic laparoscopic bilateral salpingo-oophorectomy (PBSO), although it will not prevent primary peritoneal cancer.
  - Discuss the need for HRT if she undergoes PBSO.

Question 11

Discuss the role of MRI and Doppler in the diagnosis of ovarian cancer.

Answer:

MRI is highly sensitive (96.6%) and specific (83.7%–94%) for the diagnosis of ovarian cancer (Iyer V et al., 2010). A meta-analysis has concluded that MRI with contrast enhancement provides higher posttest probability of ovarian cancer confirmation (Anthoulakis C et al., 2014) than sonography or PET for the evaluation of ovarian masses that are difficult to evaluate on sonography alone.

On Doppler, usually increased central vascularity correlates with increased malignant potential. However, the absence or presence of colour flow cannot be used in isolation to determine the risk of malignancy. Malignancy can occur even without measurable colour flow. Spectral Doppler characteristics alone do not effectively discriminate malignant from benign lesions (Levine D et al., 2010).

Multiple-Choice Questions

Q1. Signet ring cells are characteristic of:

A. Brenner tumour

B. Krukenberg tumour

C. Sex-cord tumour

D. Dysgerminoma

Answer: B

Q2. Which of the following is the leading cause of death in women?

A. Cervical cancer

B. Uterine cancer

C. Ovarian cancer

D. Vaginal cancer

Answer: C

Q3. Which of the following does **not** decrease the incidence of ovarian cancer?

A. Combined oral contraceptive pill

B. Progesterone-only pill

C. Salpingectomy

D. Hysterectomy

Answer: B

Q4. Which of the following is correct regarding genetic testing for breast and ovarian cancer?

A. Genetic testing should begin with the woman who has ovarian cancer or early-stage breast cancer.

B. All female relatives of a woman with breast and ovarian cancer should have genetic testing.

C. Genetic testing is only done for women with affected relatives on the maternal side of her family.

D. In a woman with the BRCA 2 mutation, the risk of ovarian cancer is 40%.

Answer: A

Q5. A 35-year-old pregnant woman is at risk of developing which of the following cancers?

A. Vaginal

B. Cervical

C. Endometrial

D. Ovarian

Answer: B

Q6. A cystic adnexal mass of 8 cm diameter in a menstruating female is (choose the most appropriate answer):

A. Pathological

B. Functional

C. Borderline tumour

D. Neoplastic

Answer: B

Q7. The risk of para-aortic lymph node involvement:

A. Increases with high-stage disease

B. Is greater for well-differentiated carcinoma

C. Is nearly 40% for poorly differentiated carcinoma

D. Is greater for immature teratoma

Answer: A

Q8. Which one of the following is not a good prognostic indicator for ovarian carcinoma?

A. Tumour size

B. Tumour grade

C. Residual disease after surgery

D. Parity

Answer: D

Q9. The overall 5-year survival rate of stage I grade I ovarian cancer is:

A. 60%

B. 70%

C. 80%

D. 90%

Answer: C

Q10. The 5-year survival rate after negative second-look surgery is:

A. 20%

B. 30%

C. 40%

D. 50%

Answer: D

Q11. A woman with an uneventful hysterectomy and bilateral salpingo-oopherectomy, in which a self-retaining retractor was used, complains of weakness and inability to weight bear on day 1. There is numbness and decreased sensation over the anterior left thigh. The patellar reflex is absent. What is this injury caused by?

A. Haematoma pressing on a nerve

B. Stress resulting from Trendelenberg position

C. Pressure from the self-retaining retractor on the psoas muscle and underlying nerves

D. Pressure from the tight restraining strap across the upper thighs

Answer: C

Q12. Which artery is ligated while performing an omentectomy?

A. Middle colic

B. Gastroepiploic

C. Middle sacral

D. Epigastric

Answer: A

Q13. During surgery on a 14-year-old, a stage IA grade I, 10-cm immature teratoma is found on the right ovary. Initial treatment will include:

A. Right salpingo-oopherectomy

B. Bilateral salpingo-oopherectomy

C. Bilateral salpingo-oopherectomy and omentectomy

D. Bilateral salpingo-oopherectomy, omentectomy, and hysterectomy

Answer: C

Q14. A 28-year-old woman had a left salpingo-oopherectomy for a left-sided ovarian germ cell tumour. She completed chemotherapy 6 months earlier. When can she try to get pregnant?

A. She has a high risk of fetal congenital malformation whenever she tries.

B. She should wait until the effects of chemotherapy on the right ovary have worn off.

C. She is unlikely to get pregnant as the chemotherapy causes premature ovarian failure.

D. Chemotherapy has a variable effect on a woman's reproductive function.

Answer: D

Q15. Endodermal sinus tumours of the ovary are characteristically associated with higher concentrations of:

A. AFP

B. CEA

C. CA 125

D. β-hCG

Answer: A

Q16. Which of the following statements is **least** correct?

A. The lifetime risk of breast cancer is approximately 9%.

B. The lifetime risk of breast cancer is approximately 50% in BRCA 1 and 2 gene carriers.

C. Hereditary nonpolyposis colorectal cancer (HNPCC) is associated with an increased risk of endometrial cancer.

D. HNPCC is associated with an increased risk of ovarian cancer.

Answer: B

Q17. A 24-year-old woman complains of acute right iliac fossa pain. You palpate an enlarged right adnexal mass. Which sonographic feature of this mass will indicate the need for urgent surgery?

A. Lack of ascites

B. Unilocularity

C. Multiple papillary vegetations

D. Diameter of the mass is 8 cm

Answer: C

Q18. A 54-year-old undergoes a laparotomy for a right ovarian neoplasm. A large omental cake is seen. Frozen section confirms metastatic serous cystadenocarcinoma. What surgery will be most appropriate in this situation?

A. Excision of omental metastasis and right ovarian cystectomy

B. Excision of omental metastasis and right oophorectomy

C. Omentectomy and bilateral salpingo-oophorectomy

D. Total abdominal hysterectomy, bilateral salpingo-oophorectomy, and omentectomy

Answer: D

Q19. Which is **not** true for Krukenberg tumours?

A. Enlarged ovaries

B. Bilateral

C. The stomach is the most common site of primary tumour

D. None of the above

Answer: D

Q20. In a 56-year-old woman with lower abdominal pain, an ultrasound scan shows a 4-cm bilateral ovarian mass with increased vascularity. What will you do next?

A. Ultrasound-guided ovarian biopsy

B. Observation

C. CA 125

D. Combined oral contraceptive pills for 3 cycles

Answer: C

Q21. Which one of the following is a feature of a borderline ovarian cancer?

A. Presence of prominent nucleoli

B. Presence of mitotic figures

C. Presence of extraovarian implants

D. None of the above

Answer: D

Chapter

18

Malignant Diseases of the Vulva

Definitions

Cream	Preparation of a drug for topical use that contains a water base. It is a preparation of oil in water.
Ointment	Preparation of a drug for topical use that contains an oil base. It is a preparation of water in oil.
Lichenification	Thickened, pigment part of the skin due to constant rubbing and scratching.
Corticosteroid	Steroid hormone produced from the adrenal cortex. They can be glucocorticoid or mineralocorticoid.
Hydrocortisone	It is a less potent corticosteroid.
Differentiated VIN	A virulent form of VIN that quickly changes into invasive carcinoma. "Differentiated" applies to keratin production.

Table 18.1. Chapter 18. Definitions

Chapter 18.1.　　Vulvar Cancer

Vulvar cancer is a rare cancer. The age group most affected is between 60 and 75 years. However, it is becoming more common in younger populations due to the increasing prevalence of HPV in younger populations.

Risk Factors

- HPV: 30% of patients with vulvar cancer have HPV infection.
- VIN, especially differentiated variety (DVIN).
- Vulvar dermatoses such as lichen sclerosus.
- Extramammary Paget's disease—occasionally associated with cancer of the apocrine gland.
- Alteration in protein p53 expression, which is seen in 30% of vulvar cancer.
- Smoking works as a cofactor in HPV-related vulvar cancers.

Pathology

The following types of vulvar cancer are seen:

- Squamous cell cancer (SCC) (86%)—3 types
  - o Keratinising SCC: associated with an increased extracellular and intracellular keratin, DVIN, and not associated with HPV
  - o Warty basaloid SCC: associated with HPV-related VIN
  - o Verrucous carcinoma: rare, appears as a slow-growing wart
- Melanoma (6%)
- Adenocarcinoma of Bartholin's gland (4%)
- Basal cell carcinoma (2%)
- Sarcoma (2%)

Routes of Metastasis

- Local spread to vulva, vagina, and perianal area.
- Lymphatic spread to inguinal and femoral nodes and then to pelvic nodes. This form of spread starts early.
  - o Tumours at the clitoris, urethra, and perineum can metastasise to lymph nodes on either side.
- Haematogenous spread (rare) to the lungs, liver, and bone.

History

- Asymptomatic
- Bloody discharge
- Painful lump in the vulva
- Vulvar itch
- Foul odour
- Groin mass
- Leg oedema

Examination

Common sites of vulvar cancer:

- Labia majora (50%)
- Labia minora (15–20%)
- Clitoris
- Bartholin's gland
- May extend to the vagina and perianal area

Morphological characteristics of vulvar cancer:

- Raised, flat, ulcerated, indurated
- Plaquelike
- Polypoidal
- May mimic a florid warty VIN if very early

The maximum tumour diameter should be measured. Entire vulva, vagina, and perianal area should be inspected and palpated. Inguinal and femoral group of lymph nodes must be palpated. A cervical smear and colposcopy should also be done.

Investigations

Diagnosis is made by a full-thickness biopsy including part of the normal-looking adjoining skin. This is essential for accurate histological and depth-of-invasion assessment. CT or MRI scans may be performed if there is a clinical suspicion of lymph node involvement.

Staging

Staging is done surgically (FIGO staging 2009):

Stage	Features
IA	Lesion ≤ 2 cm Confined to vulva and perineum Stromal invasion < 1 mm No lymph node involvement
IB	Lesion > 2 cm Confined to vulva and perineum Stromal invasion > 1 mm No lymph node involvement
II	Lesion extending to adjoining structures, such as lower one-third urethra, anus, and vagina Irrespective of its size No lymph node involvement
IIIA	Lesion extending to adjoining structures, such as lower one-third urethra, anus, and vagina Positive inguinofemoral lymph nodes are follows: i) 1 lymph node ≥ 5 mm ii) 1–2 lymph nodes < 5 mm
IIIB	As Stage IIIA, except for the following: i) ≥ 2 lymph nodes ≥ 5 mm ii) ≥ 3 lymph nodes < 5 mm
IIIC	Lymph node involvement with extracapsular spread
IVA	Lesion extending to upper urethra or vagina
IVB	As IVA, plus distant metastasis, including pelvic lymph nodes

Table 18.2. FIGO staging of vulvar cancer, 2009

Prognostic Indications

- Stage of the cancer
- Cancer size (maximal diameter)
- Involvement of lymph nodes. Predictors of lymph node involvement are:
  - Depth of invasion
  - Tumour grade
  - Fixed or ulcerated nodes
  - Lymphovascular space involvement
  - Older age

Management

These cancers should be managed by a gynaecological oncologist after a multidisciplinary consultation.

- The cancer should be excised with at least 10 mm of normal surrounding skin and subcutaneous tissue. A 10-mm surrounding disease-free margin ensures zero local recurrence and also allows for tissue shrinkage during fixation in the histological laboratory.
- Inguinofemoral lymphadenectomy is needed for all cancers, except the superficially invasive (≤ 1 mm) squamous cell cancers. This is not needed for melanomas, basal cell, and verrucous cancers. Laterally situated cancers will only need ipsilateral lymphadenectomy, whereas midline cancers will need bilateral lymphadenectomy. Pelvic lymphadenectomy is usually not needed.
- Advanced vulvar cancers are managed by a multimodal approach. Neoadjuvant chemotherapy and radiotherapy, prior to surgery, is used, which helps in preserving bowel and bladder function.

Prognosis

The 5-year survival rate, according to the 25th FIGO Annual Report (2003), is as follows:

- Stage I—76.9%
- Stage II—54.8%
- Stage III—30.8%
- Stage IV—8.3%

Multiple-Choice Questions

Q1. Which of the following is the best predictor of risk of nodal metastasis in vulvar cancer?

A. Depth of invasion

B. Lesion size

C. Tumour grade

D. Ulcerated lymph node

Answer: A

Q2. Inguinal lymph node excision is mandatory when the depth of invasion of a squamous cell vulvar cancer is:

 A. > 1 mm

 B. > 2 mm

 C. > 3 mm

 D. > 4 mm

Answer: A

Q3. Vulvar cancer accounts for what percentage of cancers of the lower genital tract?

 A. 2%

 B. 4%

 C. 6%

 D. 8%

Answer: B

Q4. The cancers that develop as a result of lichen sclerosus mostly affect:

 A. Urethral area

 B. Perianal area

 C. Labia majora

 D. Clitoris

Answer: D

Q5. Laser treatment for VIN is most suitable for:

 A. Older women

 B. Younger women

 C. Younger women who do not have a raised lesion

 D. HPV-associated VIN

Answer: C

Q6. Which one of the following is **not** a prognostic indicator for vulvar cancer?

 A. Tumour size

 B. Tumour grade

 C. Bilaterality

 D. Presence of lymphovascular space involvement

Answer: C

Q7. Which of the following statements is incorrect regarding nodal involvement and survival rate of vulvar cancer?

 A. 95% survival rate with negative nodes

 B. 94% survival rate with one positive node

 C. 80% survival rate with two positive nodes

 D. 50% survival rate with three positive nodes

Answer: D (12% survival rate)

Q8. Which of the following statements is incorrect regarding verrucous carcinoma?

    A. It is a type of squamous cell cancer.

    B. Radiotherapy is contraindicated.

    C. It metastasises to regional lymph nodes.

    D. Local surgical excision is the treatment.

Answer: C

Q9. Which of the following statements is correct regarding basal cell vulvar cancer?

    A. It metastasises early.

    B. It is treated by wide local excision.

    C. It is treated by local excision.

    D. Local recurrence occurs in about 50% of cases.

Answer: B

Q10. Which of the following is correct about HPV?

    A. HPV DNA is found in some squamous cell vulvar cancers.

    B. HPV replication in the cytoplasm causes koilocytosis.

    C. Dysplasia associated with HPV infection is not a true precursor of cancer.

    D. HPV–16 is associated with condylomata.

Answer: A

Q11. Which of the following statements is **not** true?

    A. The vulvar skin forms 1% of the total body skin surface.

    B. An estimated 5–10% of melanomas occur in the vulva.

    C. A routine lymphadenectomy is not required in the treatment of a vulvar melanoma.

    D. The overall 5-year survival rate of women with vulvar melanoma is nearly 25%.

Answer: D (50%)

Chapter 19

Drugs Used in Gynaecological Surgery

Chapter 19.1. Antibiotics in Gynaecological Surgery

Up to 5% of women develop surgical-site infection. In gynaecology, the sources of pathogens are as follows:

- Abdominal skin incision: *Staphylococcus aureus* and *Staphylococcus epidermidis*
- Perineum and groin incisions: faecal flora, such as Gram negative and anaerobic bacteria

When the vagina is opened during surgery, polymicrobial aerobic and anaerobic vaginal flora are possible sources of infection. In surgeries, such as laparotomy or laparoscopy, where the vagina is not opened, infection is mostly caused by skin flora.

The following are the risk factors for surgical-site infection:

- Immunosuppression
- Smoking
- Obesity
- Diabetes
- Previous or current PID
- Duration of surgery > 3 hours
- Intraoperative bleeding > 1.5 L
- Use of foreign bodies, such as sutures, clips, mesh

Role of Prophylactic Antibiotics in Surgery

Antibiotics augment natural immune defenses in-vivo and kill the pathogens that are inoculated in the surgical site. Prophylactic antibiotic should be administered at induction of anaesthesia. For prolonged surgery, the antibiotic should be repeated at intervals of one or two times the half-life of the antibiotic. A delay of only 3–4 hours can make the prophylaxis ineffective. In the presence of multiple risk factors, antibiotic should be continued postsurgery.

Choice of Antibiotic

Cephalosporins are most widely used, largely because of their broad-spectrum cover profile, low incidence of allergic manifestations, and side effects. Cefazolin is the most commonly used antibiotic, because of its long half-life (1.8 hours) and low cost. The dose is 1 g for women < 80 kg and 2 g for women > 80 kg in body weight. The rate of adverse reaction from cephalosporins ranges from 1–10%, with an anaphylaxis rate of < 0.2%. Women with a history of an immediate hypersensitivity reaction to penicillin should not be administered cephalosporins.

In general, antibiotic prophylaxis is not required for low-risk procedures, such as insertion of intrauterine devices, hysteroscopy, medical termination of pregnancy, and laparoscopy. Sonohysterography, hysterosalpingogram, and chromotubation also do not need any prophylaxis in a healthy woman without risk factors. If risk is increased, such as immunosuppressed conditions, valvular heart disease, septic abortion, or PID, the appropriate antibiotics should be administered.

Termination of Pregnancy

In surgical termination of pregnancy, screening should be performed to rule out or treat chlamydia and bacterial vaginosis prior to the termination. The most appropriate antibiotic is oral doxycycline, either a single 400-mg dose an hour before the procedure, or 100 mg an hour before the procedure and 200 mg 90 minutes after it. Evidence is lacking that adding metronidazole to this regime has any impact on outcomes.

For a hysterosalpingogram in a patient with a history of PID or with dilated fallopian tubes, 100 mg doxycycline can be given prophylactically.

Hysterectomy

The appropriate antibiotics before a vaginal hysterectomy are

- cephazolin 2 g IV before the incision, and
- metronidazole 500 mg IV before the incision.

For an abdominal hysterectomy, the above dose of cephazolin can be given without metronidazole.

Patients should be screened and treated for bacterial vaginosis before the operation to reduce BV-associated cuff infection.

Hair at the incision site should be removed immediately prior to surgery by a depilatory or clipping method rather than by shaving. This reduces the pathogenic contamination of the surgical site and infection risk.

Chapter 19.2. Thromboprophylaxis in Gynaecological Surgery

Women undergoing major gynaecological surgery (laparotomy and any other surgery, including laparoscopy, lasting more than 45 minutes) require thromboprophylaxis for prevention of venous thromboembolism (VTE).

Risk factors for VTE are the following:

- Active inflammation
- Reduced mobility
- Age > 60 years
- Malignancy

- BMI > 30
- Concurrent oestrogen and SERM therapy
- Pregnancy or puerperium
- Strong family history of VTE
- Thrombophilia
- Varicose veins

Low molecular weight heparin (LMWH) or unfractionated heparin (UFH) can be used for 1 week after the operation or stopped earlier if the patient becomes fully mobile before then. In practice, as LWMH is equally effective at preventing VTE when compared with UFH, LMWH is the preferred option as it is easily given as a once-a-day subcutaneous injection. Because of its more predictable anticoagulant and pharmacokinetic response, frequent monitoring and dose adjustments are not required.

The prophylactic doses in patients with preserved renal function (creatinine clearance > 30 mL/min) are as follows:

- LMWH: 40 mg, subcutaneous, daily
- UFH: 5000 units, subcutaneous, 8- or 12-hourly

During the time of pharmacological thromboprophylaxis, women should also use graduated compression stockings or other mechanical prophylaxis, such as intermittent pneumatic compression devices or venous foot pumps. The mechanical thromboprophylaxis should be especially used with high-risk women or where pharmacological thromboprophylaxis is contraindicated.

Contraindications to mechanical thromboprophylaxis are the following:

- Severe peripheral arterial disease
- Recent skin graft to legs
- Severe peripheral neuropathy
- Severe leg deformity or morbid obesity preventing correct fit
- Severe lower-limb oedema

Cancer-Related Surgery

Active cancer is an independent risk factor for VTE, increasing the risk by at least 4 times. Women undergoing major abdominal or pelvic surgery to remove a cancer should have at least 7 days of LMWH or UFH. Consideration of risk of VTE needs to be carefully made, and it may be appropriate to give up to 28 days of LMWH in certain cases.

The decision to anticoagulate also depends upon the patient's bleeding risk. It is possible to reverse UFH with protamine sulphate if bleeding occurs, while it is much more difficult to do this with LMWH.

Multiple-Choice Questions

Q1. The reversal agent for enoxaparin is:

    A. Calcium gluconate

    B. Vitamin K

    C. Protamine zinc sulphate

    D. None of the above

Answer: D

Q2. Which of the following statements is **not** correct regarding LMWH?

    A. This is a diverse group of chemically different compounds.

    B. The available products have similar mean molecular weights.

    C. They have predictable pharmacokinetic profiles and ease of use.

    D. They have higher anti-Xa/anti-IIa ratios, compared with UFH.

Answer: B

Index

A

Ablation 2, 7, 20, 24, 25, 26, 28, 42, 137, 172, 173, 174, 176, 201, 257, 266, 268, 347, 350, 362, 364, 410, 416
Abortion 47, 67, 96, 99, 105, 121, 127, 223, 235, 482
Acetowhite 361
Adenocarcinoma 358, 361, 362, 417, 420, 435, 439, 440, 443, 446, 474
Adenomyosis 6, 8, 22, 23, 27, 28, 162, 166, 167, 198, 203, 343, 345, 346, 347
Adjuvant Therapy 430
Adnexal Mass 6, 12, 72, 100, 107, 110, 111, 114, 164, 177, 195, 198, 266, 294, 295, 382, 383, 389, 390, 391, 433, 456, 460, 468, 470
Adrenarche 13, 54, 63, 64
Androgen 32, 40, 44, 189
Androstenedione 185, 188
Anorexia Nervosa 15, 43, 46, 199, 229
Anovulation 15, 17, 24, 179, 180, 181, 182, 183, 184, 185, 186, 190, 194, 196, 199, 219
Antifibrinolytic 19
Anti-Müllerian Hormone (AMH) 41, 170, 197, 215, 216
Apical Prolapse 284, 288, 289
Arachidonic Acid 6
Arcus Tendineus 276, 316, 326
Aromatase 60, 181
Asherman Syndrome 45
Atypia 265, 267, 268, 273, 274, 356, 409, 424

B

Bacterial Vaginosis 146, 241, 482
Behcet's Disease 413
Bethesda System 358
Bivalve Speculum 18, 107, 109, 146, 243, 361, 370
BMI 44, 48, 86, 107, 109, 190, 194, 195, 196, 199, 219, 220, 223, 262, 266, 273, 311, 344, 381, 418, 419, 483
Body Mass Index 246
Brachytherapy 417, 430
BRCA, BRCA Gene 353, 437, 453, 455, 462, 463, 466, 467, 470
Brenner Tumour 379, 380, 381, 395, 396, 398, 467

C

CA 125 170, 174, 383, 384, 387, 388, 390, 393, 394, 395, 397, 425, 429, 430, 457, 459, 460, 461, 462, 463, 465, 466, 470, 471
Cabergoline 210

Candida 147, 150, 402
Carcinoma 136, 182, 262, 263, 264, 265, 268, 353, 356, 358, 359, 375, 379, 380, 402, 403, 407, 409, 411, 413, 415, 417, 419, 420, 421, 423, 424, 428, 430, 435, 436, 439, 440, 442, 443, 444, 446, 449, 452, 454, 455, 462, 468, 473, 474, 479
Carneous Degeneration *See also* Red Degeneration 343, 344, 436
Cervicitis 82, 98, 149, 264, 266, 364
Chancroid 139, 148
Chemotherapy 122, 123, 194, 254, 423, 435, 450, 469
Chlamydia 8, 134, 138, 139, 140, 147, 149, 150, 151, 152, 156, 196, 243, 305
Choriocarcinoma 59, 120, 123, 125, 129, 455
Climacteric 254, 256
Clomiphene 454
CO2 Laser 84, 362, 402, 413, 416
Colour Doppler 382, 383, 392, 457, 462
Colpocleisis 285, 287, 289, 295
Colpoperineorrhaphy 284, 285, 289, 295, 299
Colpopexy 280, 287, 289, 291, 295, 296, 298, 299
Colporraphy 327
Colposcopy 359, 361, 362, 363, 365, 366, 367, 368, 370, 371, 373, 375, 408, 475
Colposuspension 280, 295, 309, 320, 321, 327
Combined Oral Contraceptive (COC) 9, 12, 64, 24, 115, 123, 126, 168, 208, 210, 216, 231, 232, 233, 234, 235, 236, 237, 238, 243, 244, 245, 246, 248, 249, 250, 252, 331, 334, 335, 338, 339, 342, 364, 394, 395, 407, 419, 466, 467, 471
Complex Cyst 377
Condylomata Acuminata 136
Conisation 362, 372, 373, 445, 451
Cornual Pregnancy 96
Corpus Luteum 6, 10, 11, 14, 17, 30, 70, 94, 98, 100, 124, 194, 203, 208, 378, 392, 395, 396
Cream 40, 62, 137, 143, 147, 181, 402, 403, 405, 406, 411, 415, 416
Cryotherapy 137, 362, 363
Cryptomenorrhoea 29
Curettage 24, 27, 47, 80, 83, 101, 115, 121, 127, 265, 267, 345, 349, 350, 351, 367, 368, 373, 374, 421, 441, 444, 451
Cyproterone 171, 181
Cyst 116, 117, 129, 141, 164, 168, 170, 172, 173, 364, 377, 378, 379, 380, 381, 382, 383, 384, 385, 386, 387, 388, 389, 390, 394, 395, 396, 397, 398, 416, 452
Cystadenoma 379, 380, 382, 397, 398

Cystocoele 276, 278, 282, 299
Cytoreduction 453, 458
Cytoreductive Surgery 453

D

Danazol 17, 171, 227, 335, 338
Decidua 11, 13, 67, 75, 109
Decubitus Ulcer 285
Dehydroepiandrosterone 191
Depot Medroxyprogesterone Acetate 12, 21, 111, 237, 243, 251, 252, 335, 339, 342, 350, 406
Dermoid 379, 382, 383, 384, 385, 387, 388, 396, 397, 453
Detrusor 300, 301, 310, 312, 314
DHEAs 39, 45, 46, 47, 48, 56, 60, 179, 180, 186, 187, 188, 189, 260
Dihydrotestosterone 179, 186
Dilatation 84, 88, 305, 314, 367, 421
Diploid 117, 120, 192, 193, 428
Dopamine 201, 208, 210, 217
Doppler 152, 265, 382, 383, 390, 391, 392, 457, 462, 466
Dysgerminoma 395, 455, 467
Dysmenorrhoea 6, 7, 169, 344, 345
Dyspareunia 8, 144, 152, 159, 164, 165, 166, 167, 168, 169, 170, 173, 177, 195, 200, 255, 282, 284, 286, 296, 345, 347, 400, 409, 448, 449, 456
Dysplasia 59, 64, 163, 356, 407

E

Emergency Contraception 242
Endometriosis 12, 23, 107, 109, 158, 159, 162, 164, 166, 167, 169, 170, 171, 172, 173, 174, 175, 176, 177, 195, 196, 201, 202, 203, 220, 221, 227, 240, 243, 247, 250, 345, 352, 383, 393
Endometrium 5, 6, 10, 11, 13, 14, 17, 19, 20, 21, 23, 24, 25, 26, 45, 47, 53, 67, 72, 73, 94, 151, 154, 156, 172, 193, 198, 200, 203, 215, 219, 224, 237, 242, 244, 249, 258, 265, 266, 267, 268, 271, 329, 345, 347, 420, 435, 436, 437
Endometroid 440
Endopelvic Fascia 275, 292
Enterocoele 276, 278, 284, 299
Ethinyl Oestradiol 64, 232
External OS 8, 83, 93, 107, 109, 154

F

Fallopian Tube 96, 97, 112, 113, 156, 192, 193, 211, 331, 340, 341, 392, 454, 463
Fecundity 218, 331
Ferriman-Gallwey Score 180
Fibroid 20, 22, 23, 28, 29, 100, 315, 329, 330, 336, 344, 381, 464, 465
Fibroma 379, 396
Fitz-Hugh-Curtis Syndrome 138, 152, 153, 167

Flutamide 181
Folinic Acid 102, 103, 112, 124
Follicle 5, 6, 11, 30, 184, 197, 206, 214, 364, 377, 378
Follicle Stimulating Hormone (FSH) 10, 14, 15, 29, 30, 33, 37, 38, 39, 40, 41, 43, 44, 45, 47, 48, 53, 55, 60, 65, 68, 89, 183, 189, 196, 197, 199, 200, 201, 206, 211, 212, 216, 217, 223, 224, 226, 228, 237, 238, 253, 255, 256, 260, 271

G

Gestational Trophoblastic Disease (GTD) 68, 80, 117, 118, 119, 120, 122, 124, 126, 127, 130, 241
Glycine 26
GnRH Agonist 60, 62, 160, 162, 335, 337
GnRH Deficiency 54, 55, 56, 57, 211
Gonadal Dysgenesis 31, 38, 40, 41, 55, 64
Gonadotropin 10, 31, 43, 49, 60, 68, 194, 232, 246, 377
Gonadotropin-Releasing Hormone (GnRH) 9, 10, 17, 20, 25, 29, 35, 42, 43, 46, 53, 54, 55, 56, 57, 58, 59, 60, 62, 63, 64, 160, 162, 171, 172, 179, 184, 199, 201, 211, 215, 219, 227, 230, 232, 249, 255, 335, 337, 338, 339, 340
Gonococcus 152
Grading 278, 407, 417, 420
Granulosa Cell 23, 26, 267

H

Haematocolpos 33, 37, 260
Haematogenous Spread 440, 456, 474
Haematometra 25, 37, 260
Haploid 193
hCG 11, 30, 33, 37, 42, 48, 51, 60, 68, 71, 72, 73, 82, 85, 90, 91, 92, 96, 100, 101, 102, 103, 104, 107, 108, 109, 110, 111, 112, 113, 115, 117, 118, 119, 120, 121, 122, 123, 124, 125, 126, 127, 128, 130, 154, 194, 199, 205, 206, 222, 230, 260, 370, 378, 383, 384, 387, 388, 393, 397, 455, 457, 465, 470
Hereditary Nonpolyposis Colorectal Cancer Syndrome (HNPCC) 419, 437, 470
Hirsutism 37, 181, 182, 183, 186, 188, 189, 245, 247
Hormone Replacement Therapy (HRT) 146, 162, 172, 174, 240, 256, 257, 258, 261, 262, 263, 265, 266, 269, 271, 272, 273, 274, 330, 344, 348, 405, 445, 466
Human Papilloma Virus (HPV) 136, 141, 247, 281, 356, 357, 358, 359, 360, 361, 362, 363, 365, 368, 369, 370, 371, 372, 374, 375, 408, 409, 410, 412, 413,

439, 445, 446, 450, 473, 474, 478, 479
Hyaline Degeneration 436
Hydatidiform Mole 117
Hydrosalpinx 202, 221, 382, 397
Hyperandrogenism 179, 180, 181, 182, 183, 187
Hypergonadotrophic Hypogonadism 222
Hyperinsulinaemia 180, 183, 184, 185, 219
Hyperplasia 17, 20, 23, 24, 37, 38, 39, 49, 51, 59, 63, 118, 168, 179, 182, 189, 208, 224, 240, 247, 258, 259, 264, 265, 266, 267, 268, 270, 271, 272, 273, 274, 330, 345, 348, 379, 380, 381, 397, 409, 422, 429, 430, 436, 459
Hyperprolactinaemia 48, 195, 206, 209, 210, 228
Hypertrichosis 183, 188
Hypogonadotropic Hypogonadism 31, 55, 172, 183, 199
Hypothalamic 10, 29, 30, 31, 37, 46, 48, 49, 50, 53, 55, 56, 58, 199, 230
Hypothyroidism 13, 45, 54, 59, 63, 64, 70, 208
Hysterectomy 9, 20, 21, 93, 105, 106, 122, 130, 149, 160, 172, 173, 176, 266, 268, 273, 278, 280, 285, 286, 289, 291, 292, 294, 296, 299, 315, 319, 335, 337, 339, 344, 351, 352, 353, 372, 373, 375, 391, 417, 418, 422, 424, 425, 429, 430, 431, 432, 444, 445, 446, 448, 450, 452, 454, 458, 460, 463, 469, 470, 482
Hysterosalpingogram 227, 482
Hysteroscopy 7, 8, 47, 86, 197, 227, 265, 266, 268, 334, 349, 374, 421, 482

I

Iliococcygeus 275
Ilioinguinal 399
Imidazole 406
Imiquimod 137, 409
Immunological 70
Imperforate Hymen 29, 37
Implantation 6, 11, 67, 68, 71, 118, 169, 192, 193, 201, 206, 218, 221, 233, 237, 238, 242, 249, 331
Inclusion Cyst 381
Infertility 8, 98, 139, 185, 186, 192, 193, 201, 202, 211, 331, 343, 347, 349, 350
Inflammatory Bowel Disease (IBD) 54, 56, 139, 158, 171
Inhibin 216, 253, 397
Insulin 43, 179, 180, 181, 182, 183, 185, 186, 187, 188, 189, 200, 219
Intermenstrual Bleeding (IMB) 14, 20, 22, 153, 240, 330
Intermittent Self-Catheterisation 314, 320
Internal OS 8, 106, 355

Interstitial 96, 105, 158, 171, 305
Intrauterine Contraceptive Device (IUCD) 2, 20, 21, 24, 26, 50, 97, 98, 110, 114, 126, 144, 146, 147, 153, 162, 172, 239, 240, 241, 242, 243, 246, 249, 250, 252, 265, 266, 267, 268, 274, 330, 335, 338, 346, 347
Intrauterine Insemination 172, 173, 211
Intrinsic Sphincter 301, 306, 308, 309
Invasive Mole (IM) 12, 110, 117, 118, 119, 124, 127, 128, 141, 147, 154, 157, 252
In Vitro Fertilisation (IVF) 94, 104, 106. 111, 124, 197, 202, 204, 206, 214, 216, 220, 221, 227, 268
Irritable Bowel Syndrome (IBS) 158, 160, 161, 162, 170
Ischiocavernosus 297

K

Kallman Syndrome 297
Kegel's Exercises 283, 289
Ketoconazole 406
Koilocytosis 479

L

Laparoscopy 7, 8, 12, 38, 40, 86, 101, 102, 104, 105, 111, 112, 113, 114, 152, 153, 154, 155, 157, 159, 160, 162, 164, 166, 167, 170, 172, 197, 201, 203, 220, 227, 337, 351, 385, 386, 388, 389, 392, 463, 481, 482
Laparotomy 28, 102, 104, 105, 114, 115, 116, 141, 155, 164, 174, 221, 284, 289, 335, 337, 385, 386, 388, 391, 392, 394, 457, 459, 461, 462, 463, 470, 481, 482
Large Loop Excision Of The Transformation Zone (LLETZ) 361, 362, 363, 365, 366, 367, 368, 369, 371, 372, 373, 450
Laser 409, 415, 416, 478
Last Menstrual Period (LMP) 68, 71, 73, 82, 88, 91, 107, 109, 114, 115, 237, 238, 369, 370, 387, 432, 464
Leiomyoma 6, 7, 163, 166, 314, 329, 330, 331, 332, 333, 334, 335, 336, 337, 338, 339, 340, 341, 342, 343, 344, 345, 346, 347, 422, 424, 436
Letrozole 200
Levator Ani 275, 276, 292, 301
Levonorgestrel 7, 26, 99, 114, 162, 172, 236, 237, 239, 240, 242, 246, 250, 251, 252, 268, 274, 330, 335
LH 10, 11, 13, 14, 15, 17, 29, 33, 37, 38, 39, 40, 42, 43, 44, 45, 47, 48, 53, 55, 60, 65, 68, 70, 89, 179, 180, 181, 183, 184, 185, 186, 187, 189, 196, 199, 200, 206, 208, 211, 212, 217, 223, 224, 249,

253, 256, 271

Lichen 40, 146, 400, 401, 402, 403, 409, 411, 414, 415, 416

Ligament 164, 167, 175, 276, 286, 287, 299, 309, 326, 329, 331, 332, 377, 381, 392, 419, 451, 455

Liquid-Based Cytology (LBC) 359, 360, 365, 374

Luteal Phase 9, 194

Luteolysis 10

Luteoma 59, 63

Lymphatic Drainage 355, 456

Lymphogranuloma Venereum 139, 414

Lymphovascular Invasion 419

Lynch Syndrome 419, 421, 433, 434

M

Magnetic Resonance-Guided Focused Ultrasound (MRGFUS) 29, 336, 338, 339, 341, 346

Malignancy 57, 108, 122, 150, 174, 175, 241, 262, 348, 377, 379, 380, 381, 382, 383, 384, 390, 393, 412, 417, 428, 434, 455, 457, 459, 460, 462, 465, 466

Manchester Repair 298

Mayer-Rokitansky-Küster-Hauser Syndrome (MRKH Syndrome) 32, 36, 37

McCall Culdoplasty 298

McCune-Albright Syndrome 59, 60, 63, 64, 65

Mefenamic Acid 7, 226

Meig's Syndrome 379

Menarche 5, 6, 9, 10, 12, 17, 18, 37, 42, 43, 53, 57, 58, 65, 189, 253, 264, 266, 330, 421

Menopausal Hormone Therapy 256. *See Also* Hormone Replacement Therapy

Menopause 5, 6, 28, 43, 47, 175, 188, 195, 201, 224, 253, 254, 255, 256, 257, 258, 260, 261, 262, 263, 264, 266, 271, 273, 274, 280, 302, 336, 352, 399, 418, 421, 431

Menorrhagia 22, 24, 25, 243, 247

Menstruation 6, 8, 10, 11, 12, 15, 22, 29, 42, 57, 158, 170, 171, 172, 194, 253, 256, 260, 383, 395

Mesosalpinx 377, 378

Metaplasia 177, 361, 379, 451

Metformin 89, 181, 183, 184, 185, 187, 190

Methotrexate 102, 103, 104, 108, 110, 111, 112, 113, 114, 124

Midcycle Pain 194

Midluteal Serum Progesterone 196

Mifepristone 242

Minipill 237, 252

Mixed Incontinence 300, 301, 322, 323

Molar Pregnancy 71, 72, 80, 109, 110, 117, 118, 119, 121, 123, 125, 126, 127, 250

Morning-After Pill 242

Mosaic 361, 455

MRI 23, 29, 33, 37, 48, 56, 60, 123, 125, 128, 162, 170, 174, 228, 265, 267, 268, 270, 324, 334, 336, 341, 342, 346, 349, 388, 390, 392, 393, 421, 425, 429, 430, 431, 433, 441, 447, 457, 460, 465, 466, 475

Mucinous Cystadenoma 379, 380, 398

Müllerian Duct 53, 169, 216

Myoma 24, 26, 70, 89, 106, 201, 264, 329, 333, 334, 335, 339, 343

Myomectomy 20, 28, 201, 329, 335, 337, 338, 339, 340, 341, 342

Myometrium 28, 47, 105, 117, 118, 120, 151, 198, 215, 241, 265, 270, 329, 332, 336, 338, 345, 346, 436

N

Nabothian Follicle 364

Neisseria Gonorrhoea 134

Neoadjuvant Chemotherapy 453, 477

New Squamocolumnar Junction 356

Nonsteroidal Anti-Inflammatory Drugs (NSAID) 7, 160

O

Oestradiol 7, 10, 11, 13, 14, 20, 21, 33, 38, 45, 48, 49, 50, 55, 57, 60, 64, 147, 179, 182, 183, 184, 194, 197, 199, 206, 210, 225, 232, 236, 242, 244, 250, 252, 255, 256, 257, 260, 261, 267

Oestriol 14, 252, 273, 274

Oestrogen 14, 19, 49, 53, 88, 142, 149, 150, 191, 234, 236, 248, 252, 256, 257, 258, 259, 261, 262, 267, 273, 308, 381, 418, 423, 429

Oestrone 20, 179, 219, 232, 257

Ointment 473

Oocyte 11, 38, 184, 192, 193, 199, 216, 218, 223, 226, 378, 447

Oophorectomy 9, 40, 141, 160, 163, 172, 173, 260, 268, 351, 352, 353, 377, 385, 394, 421, 422, 424, 425, 429, 430, 455, 458, 459, 460, 462, 463, 465, 466, 470

Osteoporosis 15, 20, 38, 49, 172, 257, 261

Ovarian Cyst 116, 141, 173, 383, 384, 386, 387, 389, 390, 394, 395, 452

Ovarian Drilling 181, 203

Ovarian Failure 37, 45, 47, 48, 183, 194, 214, 229, 341, 469

Ovarian Masses 381, 382, 385, 397, 466

Ovary 10, 11, 63, 98, 105, 116, 141, 158, 168, 169, 170, 173, 176, 184, 193, 200, 201, 214, 215, 216, 232, 253, 260, 352, 377, 378, 381, 383, 390, 391, 392, 394, 396, 398, 456, 457, 459, 460, 462, 463, 465, 469, 470

Overactive Bladder 300

Ovulation 5, 6, 7, 9, 10, 11, 13, 17, 20, 26, 29, 30, 42, 49, 53, 58, 97, 113, 181, 183, 184, 185, 193, 194, 196, 197, 199, 200, 201, 204, 206, 210, 211, 219, 220, 222, 223, 224, 226, 228, 229, 230, 232, 236, 237, 238, 240, 242, 246, 249, 253, 261, 352, 378, 454, 455

Oxybutynin 312, 325

P

Papillary Serous Carcinoma 419, 423, 435

Parametrium 422, 440

Partial Mole (PM) 117, 118, 119, 120, 121, 123, 127, 129, 260, 261

Pearl Index 251

Pelvic Abscess 152, 154, 426, 464

Pelvic Adhesion 173

Pelvic Congestion Syndrome 8

Pelvic Diaphragm 275

Pelvic Floor 219, 275, 276, 280, 291, 292, 293, 320

Pelvic Inflammatory Disease (PID) 12, 26, 97, 98, 100, 107, 109, 136, 151, 152, 153, 154, 156, 157, 158, 159, 162, 165, 167, 168, 195, 233, 241, 247, 251, 387, 481, 482

Pelvic Lymphadenopathy 128

Pelvic Organ Prolapse (POP) 246, 275, 278, 279, 280, 281, 282, 283, 284, 288, 289, 290, 291, 294, 295, 297, 300

Pelvic Pain 32, 37, 82, 83, 102, 112, 115, 151, 152, 153, 158, 160, 162, 163, 164, 169, 170, 173, 177, 220, 221, 232, 294, 334, 394, 456, 460

Perimenopause 253, 254, 267

Perineal Body 277, 285, 289, 292

Perineal Membrane 275, 276, 277

Peritoneal Carcinoma 455

Pessary 165, 266, 283, 289, 290, 291, 294, 295, 299, 406

Pipelle 265, 266, 270, 421

Pituitary 10, 11, 20, 29, 30, 31, 37, 42, 47, 48, 49, 54, 56, 58, 171, 179, 184, 199, 206, 208, 210, 211, 215, 216, 232, 253

Placental Site Trophoblastic Tumour (PSTT) 117, 118, 119, 122, 127, 129

Polycystic Ovarian Syndrome (PCOS) 20, 37, 43, 70, 89, 179, 180, 181, 182, 183, 185, 186, 187, 188, 189, 190, 195, 196, 199, 200, 201, 204, 216, 219, 247, 267, 419

Polyp 6, 23, 70, 163, 266, 267, 333,

334, 349, 350, 364, 422
Pop-Q System 278
Postcoital Bleeding 361
Posterior Vaginal Wall Prolapse 278, 288, 289
Postmenopausal Bleeding 421, 425
Precocious Puberty 42, 58
Progesterone 6, 10, 11, 13, 14, 17, 20, 30, 38, 42, 49, 50, 87, 94, 96, 97, 98, 100, 115, 124, 126, 173, 184, 193, 194, 196, 199, 206, 208, 224, 225, 231, 238, 262, 269, 271, 302, 329, 335, 345, 348, 378
Progesterone Challenge Test 45
Progestin 19, 21, 57, 167, 201, 231, 233, 235, 236, 237, 238, 239, 240, 242, 243, 244, 248, 251, 256, 258, 262
Prolactin 37, 38, 42, 44, 60, 187, 206, 207, 208, 210, 235
Proliferative Phase 13, 203
Prostaglandin 6, 7, 11, 19, 22, 79, 83, 240
Pruritus 400, 401, 403, 404, 405, 411
Pseudomyxoma Peritonei 459
Psoriasis 146, 404, 415
Puberty 42, 43, 53, 54, 55, 56, 57, 58, 59, 60, 61, 62, 63, 64, 65, 253, 356, 397, 399, 402
Pudendal Nerve 291
Punctation 361
Pyosalpinx 152, 154, 383

Q

Q-Tip Test 308

R

Raloxifene 258, 259
Red Degeneration 331, 335, 464
Residual Ovary 352
Resistant 122, 147, 200, 229, 403, 449
Rhabdosphincter 300

S

Sacrocolpopexy 284, 286, 289, 295
Sacrospinous Colpopexy 280, 287, 289, 291, 295, 298
Saline Sonohysterography 18, 270, 334, 342
Second-Look Surgery 453
Secretory Phase 6
Selective Oestrogen Receptor Modulator (SERM) 201, 258, 259, 262, 483
Selective Progesterone Receptor Modulator (SPRM) 335, 338, 339
Semen Analysis 197, 225
Serous 353, 379, 382, 419, 420, 422, 423, 435, 454, 455, 459, 470
Sex Hormone-Binding Globulin (SHBG) 89, 179, 180, 183, 196, 219, 234, 247, 248, 249 184, 187, 191, 219,

234
Simple Cyst 377
Snowstorm 127
Sonohysterography 18, 197, 198, 270, 334, 341, 342, 349
Spinnbarkeit 226
Spironolactone 16, 186
Squamocolumnar Junction 356
Squamous Cell Carcinoma 359, 409, 439
Staging 55, 59, 61, 63, 270, 279, 385, 391, 394, 420, 421, 423, 424, 425, 429, 441, 442, 443, 447, 452, 457, 458, 459, 460, 461, 465, 476
Stress Incontinence 219, 277, 280, 282, 286, 288, 292, 294, 295, 300, 306, 313, 314, 316, 318, 321, 322, 326
Subfertility 170, 192, 227
Syncytiotrophoblasts 68, 103, 120
Syphilis 134, 138, 140, 141, 213, 414

T

Tamoxifen 201, 264, 271, 272, 330, 348, 419, 423, 429, 436, 466
Tanner Stage, Tanner Staging 38, 39, 40, 55, 57, 59, 61, 63
Tension-Free Vaginal Tape 326
Teratoma 59, 379, 395, 398, 453, 455, 459, 468, 469
Testosterone 32, 33, 38, 39, 42, 60, 65, 171, 180, 183, 185, 188, 189, 196, 217, 218, 258, 259
Theca Lutein Cyst 117, 395
Thermal Balloon 24, 25, 28
Thromboprophylaxis Vii, 205, 482
Tibolone 258, 269, 271, 272, 273
Torsion 156, 205, 331, 332, 333, 334, 380, 381, 382, 383, 384, 385, 387, 391, 392, 394, 395, 396, 397, 398, 464
Tranexamic Acid 226, 335
Transformation Zone 356, 358, 361, 362, 366, 367, 450
Trichomonas 134, 374
Triploid 117, 120
Tubo-Ovarian Abscess 153
Tumour 1, 26, 39, 47, 54, 59, 61, 63, 64, 101, 117, 118, 120, 121, 122, 124, 128, 129, 189, 210, 223, 267, 268, 269, 282, 315, 379, 380, 381, 382, 383, 384, 387, 395, 396, 398, 417, 418, 419, 420, 421, 424, 425, 427, 429, 440, 441, 443, 445, 447, 450, 453, 455, 458, 459, 460, 467, 468, 469, 470, 475

U

Urethra 255
Urethrocoele Vi, 278, 282, 288, 299
Urge Incontinence 255, 294, 300, 312, 313, 315, 321, 322, 326
Urodynamic Study 316
Urogenital Diaphragm 302

Uterosacral Ligament 164, 167, 175, 276, 299, 451
Uterus 6, 7, 8, 12, 24, 25, 26, 28, 29, 30, 31, 32, 34, 37, 39, 40, 41, 43, 47, 48, 56, 60, 65, 70, 71, 72, 78, 79, 82, 83, 84, 93, 96, 104, 105, 107, 111, 114, 115, 121, 125, 151, 154, 156, 158, 163, 164, 165, 166, 167, 168, 169, 188, 193, 194, 214, 224, 225, 226, 229, 241, 243, 257, 258, 266, 268, 272, 275, 276, 278, 286, 291, 292, 294, 295, 315, 329, 333, 336, 345, 346, 350, 377, 379, 385, 386, 389, 417, 418, 420, 425, 429, 435, 436, 440, 442, 444, 456, 459, 460

V

Vaginal Discharge 65, 78, 83, 92, 134, 136, 142, 143, 144, 145, 146, 147, 148, 149, 150, 151, 152, 153, 258, 266, 281, 285, 290, 333, 363, 405, 406
Vaginal Intraepithelial Neoplasia (VAIN) 373
Vaginismus 161, 165, 166, 168
Vasomotor Symptoms 200, 335
Vellus Hair 186
Veress Needle 164, 221, 389
Verrucous Carcinoma 474
Vesicovaginal Fistula 65, 320
Vestibule 134, 399
Virilisation 48, 59, 189
Vulva 40, 135, 136, 137, 144, 147, 150, 255, 399, 406, 407, 408, 409, 414, 415, 474, 475, 476, 479
Vulvar Intraepithelial Neoplasia (VIN) 146, 407, 408, 409, 410, 412, 413, 414, 416, 473, 474, 475, 478
Vulvovaginitis 134, 405

W

Whorled Pattern 333

Y

Yuzpe Method 242

Z

Zinc Sulphate 484
Zona Pellucida 11, 192, 193

www.ingramcontent.com/pod-product-compliance
Lightning Source LLC
Chambersburg PA
CBHW080122220326
41598CB00032B/4922